Recent Progress in
Rehabilitation Medicine

Recent Progress in Rehabilitation Medicine

Editor

Masahiro Kohzuki

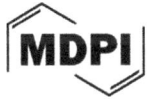

Basel • Beijing • Wuhan • Barcelona • Belgrade • Novi Sad • Cluj • Manchester

Editor
Masahiro Kohzuki
Tohoku University Graduate
School of Medicine
Sendai
Japan

Editorial Office
MDPI
St. Alban-Anlage 66
4052 Basel, Switzerland

This is a reprint of articles from the Special Issue published online in the open access journal *Journal of Clinical Medicine* (ISSN 2077-0383) (available at: https://www.mdpi.com/journal/jcm/special_issues/Rehabilitation_Medicine).

For citation purposes, cite each article independently as indicated on the article page online and as indicated below:

Lastname, A.A.; Lastname, B.B. Article Title. *Journal Name* **Year**, *Volume Number*, Page Range.

ISBN 978-3-7258-0849-6 (Hbk)
ISBN 978-3-7258-0850-2 (PDF)
doi.org/10.3390/books978-3-7258-0850-2

© 2024 by the authors. Articles in this book are Open Access and distributed under the Creative Commons Attribution (CC BY) license. The book as a whole is distributed by MDPI under the terms and conditions of the Creative Commons Attribution-NonCommercial-NoDerivs (CC BY-NC-ND) license.

Contents

Tomasz Marciniak, Weronika Kruk-Majtyka, Patrycja Bobowik and Sławomir Marszałek
The Relationship between Kinesiophobia, Emotional State, Functional State and Chronic Pain in Subjects with/without Temporomandibular Disorders
Reprinted from: *J. Clin. Med.* **2024**, *13*, 848, doi:10.3390/jcm13030848 1

Justyna Mazurek, Błażej Cieślik, Adam Wrzeciono, Robert Gajda and Joanna Szczepańska-Gieracha
Immersive Virtual Reality Therapy Is Supportive for Orthopedic Rehabilitation among the Elderly: A Randomized Controlled Trial
Reprinted from: *J. Clin. Med.* **2023**, *12*, 7681, doi:10.3390/jcm12247681 11

Yuma Hirano, Tomoyuki Fujikura, Kenichi Kono, Naro Ohashi, Tomoya Yamaguchi, Wataru Hanajima, et al.
Decline in Walking Independence and Related Factors in Hospitalization for Dialysis Initiation: A Retrospective Cohort Study
Reprinted from: *J. Clin. Med.* **2022**, *11*, 6589, doi:10.3390/jcm11216589 23

Midori Homma, Misa Miura, Yo Hirayama, Tamao Takahashi, Takahiro Miura, Naoki Yoshida, et al.
Belt Electrode-Skeletal Muscle Electrical Stimulation in Older Hemodialysis Patients with Reduced Physical Activity: A Randomized Controlled Pilot Study
Reprinted from: *J. Clin. Med.* **2022**, *11*, 6170, doi:10.3390/jcm11206170 33

Raffaello Pellegrino, Teresa Paolucci, Fabrizio Brindisino, Paolo Mondardini, Angelo Di Iorio, Antimo Moretti and Giovanni Iolascon
Effectiveness of High-Intensity Laser Therapy Plus Ultrasound-Guided Peritendinous Hyaluronic Acid Compared to Therapeutic Exercise for Patients with Lateral Elbow Tendinopathy
Reprinted from: *J. Clin. Med.* **2022**, *11*, 5492, doi:10.3390/jcm11195492 45

Yuji Iwanami, Kento Ebihara, Keiko Nakao, Naofumi Sato, Midori Miyagi, Yasuhiko Nakamura, et al.
Benefits of Pulmonary Rehabilitation in Patients with Idiopathic Pulmonary Fibrosis Receiving Antifibrotic Drug Treatment
Reprinted from: *J. Clin. Med.* **2022**, *11*, 5336, doi:10.3390/jcm11185336 55

Isabella Schwartz, Ori Safran, Naama Karniel, Michal Abel, Adina Berko, Martin Seyres, et al.
Positive Effect of Manipulated Virtual Kinematic Intervention in Individuals with Traumatic Stiff Shoulder: A Pilot Study
Reprinted from: *J. Clin. Med.* **2022**, *11*, 3919, doi:10.3390/jcm11133919 66

Magdalena Sobiech, Agata Czępińska, Grzegorz Zieliński, Magdalena Zawadka and Piotr Gawda
Does Application of Lymphatic Drainage with Kinesiology Taping Have Any Effect on the Extent of Edema and Range of Motion in Early Postoperative Recovery following Primary Endoprosthetics of the Knee Joint?
Reprinted from: *J. Clin. Med.* **2022**, *11*, 3456, doi:10.3390/jcm11123456 76

Iva Sklempe Kokic, Matko Vuksanic, Tomislav Kokic, Ivan Peric and Ivana Duvnjak
Effects of Electromyographic Biofeedback on Functional Recovery of Patients Two Months after Total Knee Arthroplasty: A Randomized Controlled Trial
Reprinted from: *J. Clin. Med.* **2022**, *11*, 3182, doi:10.3390/jcm11113182 86

Loredana Raciti, Loris Pignolo, Valentina Perini, Massimo Pullia, Bruno Porcari, Desiree Latella, et al.
Improving Upper Extremity Bradykinesia in Parkinson's Disease: A Randomized Clinical Trial on the Use of Gravity-Supporting Exoskeletons
Reprinted from: *J. Clin. Med.* **2022**, *11*, 2543, doi:10.3390/jcm11092543 . . . . **98**

Masahiro Kohzuki
Renal Rehabilitation: Present and Future Perspectives
Reprinted from: *J. Clin. Med.* **2024**, *13*, 552, doi:10.3390/jcm13020552 . . . . **110**

Tomasz Wolny, César Fernández-de-las Peñas, Tomasz Buczek, Magdalena Domin, Arkadiusz Granek and Paweł Linek
The Effects of Physiotherapy in the Treatment of Cubital Tunnel Syndrome: A Systematic Review
Reprinted from: *J. Clin. Med.* **2022**, *11*, 4247, doi:10.3390/jcm11144247 . . . . **122**

Daigo Sakamoto, Toyohiro Hamaguchi, Kai Murata, Atsushi Ishikawa, Yasuhide Nakayama and Masahiro Abo
Study Protocol for a Multicenter, Randomized Controlled Trial to Improve Upper Extremity Hemiparesis in Chronic Stroke Patients by One-to-One Training (NEURO®) with Repetitive Transcranial Magnetic Stimulation
Reprinted from: *J. Clin. Med.* **2022**, *11*, 6835, doi:10.3390/jcm11226835 . . . . **137**

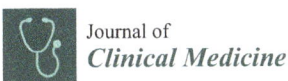 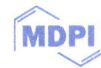

Article

The Relationship between Kinesiophobia, Emotional State, Functional State and Chronic Pain in Subjects with/without Temporomandibular Disorders

Tomasz Marciniak [1,*], Weronika Kruk-Majtyka [1], Patrycja Bobowik [1] and Sławomir Marszałek [2,3]

[1] Faculty of Rehabilitation, Józef Piłsudski Academy of Physical Education in Warsaw, 00-968 Warsaw, Poland; weronika.kruk@awf.edu.pl (W.K.-M.); patrycja.bobowik@awf.edu.pl (P.B.)
[2] Department of Physiotherapy, Poznan University of Medical Sciences, 61-701 Poznan, Poland
[3] Faculty of Physical Education in Gorzow Wielkopolski, Poznan University of Physical Education, 61-871 Poznan, Poland
* Correspondence: tomasz.marciniak@awf.edu.pl

Abstract: Although there is growing evidence that kinesiophobia is correlated with temporomandibular disorders (TMD), its relationship with other characteristic TMD comorbidities, such as depression, anxiety, functional limitations, and pain in the TMD population, has rarely been investigated. This study aims to evaluate the relationship between kinesiophobia, emotional state, functional state and chronic pain in subjects both with and without TMD. A total of 94 subjects participated in the study and were divided into two groups (47 subjects each)—TMD (subjects with temporomandibular disorders) and nTMD (asymptomatic controls)—on the basis of the RDC/TMD protocol. All measurements were taken with self-administered questionnaires: TSK-TMD for kinesiophobia, PHQ-9 and GAD-7 for psychoemotional state, JFLS-20 for jaw functional limitations, and GCPS for chronic pain. The prevalence of kinesiophobia in the TMD group was 38.3% for moderate risk, and 61.7% for high risk. The TMD group showed significantly higher scores in all categories (kinesiophobia, depression, jaw functional limitations and chronic pain), with the exception of anxiety which was right at the cut-off point. Moreover, a significant correlation was found between kinesiophobia (TSK-TMD) and jaw functional limitations (JFLS-20). Results of this study could provide new insight into the relationship between kinesiophobia and TMD, further improving the diagnosis process.

Keywords: kinesiophobia; temporomandibular disorders; TMD; functional limitations

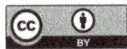

1. Introduction

"Temporomandibular disorders" (TMD) is an umbrella term that refers to one of the main causes of orofacial pain, which consist of a variety of symptoms: myofascial pain or myalgia, intraarticular disorders (disc displacement with or without reduction) and temporomandibular joint pain (arthralgia) [1]. Previous studies showed the prevalence of TMD is between 3–12% in the general population [2–4], and indicated its etiology is multifactorial and includes a wide range of physical and psychoemotional factors, such as emotional stress, depression, anxiety, hormonal changes, occlusion etc. [5,6].

In responding to the emotional influence of TMD in recent years, some authors, in citing its recognition as an important component of chronic pain [7,8], claimed that kinesiophobia could also play a role in a broad spectrum of disorders in TMD.

Kinesiophobia, which is defined as the fear of movement, describes a situation where a patient has an excessive, irrational, and debilitating fear of physical movement and activity, which results from a feeling of vulnerability to painful injury or reinjury [9]. In TMD subjects the fear of movement of the jaw may affect some essential primary activities, such as eating, chewing, emotional expression, or communication [10]. Several studies assessed kinesiophobia and catastrophizing levels in TMD subjects by using standardized tools such as Tampa scale for kinesiophobia for temporomandibular disorders (TSK-TMD) [10–12], with some showing a stronger correlation with painful TMD, compared to nonpainful and control groups. On the other hand, other researchers found this relationship existed, regardless of the existence of pain [10]. It is worth mentioning that the prevalence of kinesiophobia in TMD has only been estimated in one previous study [11]; all other papers investigated the differences between study and control groups, but without showing actual prevalence.

In 2020, von Piekartz et al. [13] published official guidelines related to the international consensus on the most useful assessment tools that physical therapists used to evaluate patients with temporomandibular disorders and, in addition to other tools, recommended PHQ, GAD, JFLS, GCPS, and TSK-TMD questionnaires. Despite the publication of guidelines, no papers have been, to date, been published that investigate the relationship between kinesiophobia, emotional state, functional state and pain, and produce results that can be compared to each other in one global project. While individual studies have tried to address this question in different configurations, their use of different tools produced a limited and selective analysis [10,14–17].

From a clinical perspective, it seems to be important to establish this relationship because it may influence decisions about the therapy modalities that are in the patient's best interest. The presence of kinesiophobia may indicate a need for treatment to be extended beyond just manual therapy.

In taking these different points into consideration, this study sought to (1) evaluate the relationship between kinesiophobia and psychoemotional state, functional state and chronic pain in subjects with temporomandibular disorders and healthy controls; (2) establish the prevalence of kinesiophobia in the studied population.

2. Materials and Methods

2.1. Material

The study involved 94 subjects (aged: 27.14 ± 6.19) aged between 18–45 years-of-age, which were included after providing their (written) consent to participate in the study of temporomandibular joint disorders (orofacial pain, intraarticular disorders, masticatory muscle pain) and associated symptoms. The study excluded those with rheumatoid diseases (e.g., rheumatoid arthritis (RA) and ankylosing spondylitis (AS)), whose jaw had previously been injured (e.g., bone fractures), whose temporomandibular joint ad been injured (e.g., contusions, dislocations), who had undergone facial surgical procedures (e.g., orthognathic surgery, TMJ surgery), or who withheld their written consent and/or did not fall into the study age range.

All participants were divided into two groups based on the presence (TMD group) or absence (nTMD group, i.e., control group) of temporomandibular disorders symptoms, and this division was made on the basis of examination protocol taken from the research diagnostic criteria for temporomandibular disorders (RDC/TMD). After unsuitable candidates were excluded, the TMD group consisted of 47 subjects (10 males, 37 females) aged 27.5 ± 5.6, while the nTMD group consisted of the same number of participants (15 males, 32 females), who were aged 26.8 ± 6.8.

The subjects in the nTMD group did not present any TMD signs nor symptoms, while the prevalence of different groups of symptoms in the TMD group was as follows: muscle pain (Group I) 60% (28 subjects); intraarticular disorders (Group II) 100% (47 subjects); temporomandibular joint pain 27.7% (13 subjects). The concurrence of two or more symptoms, which is very common in TMD patients [18–21], was also observed. The local ethical commission approved the study (signature SKE01-30/2021), after revisions were made to ensure the standards of the Helsinki Declaration, including all participants first providing written consent, were met.

2.2. Methods

After the RDC/TMD examination protocol was completed, all subjects were asked to fill out questionnaires: the Tampa scale for kinesiophobia for temporomandibular disorders (TSK-TMD), patient health questionnaire (PHQ-9), generalized anxiety disorder (GAD-7), jaw functional limitation scale (JFLS-20) and graded chronic pain scale (GCSP). All of questionnaires are standardized and widely used in both clinical and research setups, and show good diagnostic value when applied to the assessment of the TMD population [8,13,16,22]. The whole RDC/TMD examination protocol was performed by a TMD specialist with more than a decade of experience.

TSK-TMD is an 18-item scale that measures levels of kinesiophobia (fear of movement) in subjects with temporomandibular disorder symptoms. Likert scale 1–4 is used to determine the intensity of the situation in each question: 1—strongly disagree, 2—somewhat disagree, 3—somewhat agree, 4—strongly agree. The total score is determined by summing the items: the lowest possible minimum score was 18, and the highest possible maximum was 72. The clinical classification of kinesiophobia was based on TSK-17 questionnaire cut-off points proposed by other researchers, and assessed as low risk (<17 points), moderate risk (17–37 points), and high risk (>37 points) [14,23,24].

Both PHQ-9 and GAD-7 questionnaires seek to assess the psychoemotional state of the subject by establishing the level of depression and anxiety, respectively. PHQ-9 consists of nine questions, which are each scored from 0 to 3 (possible maximum of 27 points in total) and GAD-7 consists of seven questions with the same scoring rules (possible maximum of 21 points). The cut-off point for both clinically significant depression and generalized anxiety disorder is set at 10 points, and the time perspective of both questionnaires is set at the last 14 days [25,26].

The next evaluative instrument used was JFLS-20, which seeks to identify any functional limitations from the last 30 days. Subjects were asked to indicate the severity of limitations of different activities, such as chewing different foods, swallowing, yawning, mouth opening, etc., on a scale from 0 to 10, with 0 meaning "no limitation" and 10 "severe limitation". The global score is calculated via a algorithm proposed by [27].

The graded chronic pain scale (GCSP), which aims to assess pain levels from the last six months, was the last questionnaire to be implemented. In this study, only the results from the characteristic pain intensity (CPI) category will be used for further analysis [28].

2.3. Statistical Analysis

Data was analyzed using STATISTICA 13.0 (StatSoft). The Shapiro-Wilk test assessed the distribution of variables and Levene's test determined homogeneity of variance. Both the T-test and Mann-Whitney U test were used. Effect sizes were assessed by applying Glass's rank-biserial correlation coefficient. Cohen observes the effect size is low if the value of r varies around 0.1, medium if r varies around 0.3, and large if r varies over 0.5 [29]. An ANOVA for factorial designs was conducted, and Spearman's rank correlation test was also performed, with a significance level set at $p \leq 0.05$.

3. Results

The level of kinesiophobia in all subjects from both groups was assessed, showing there was nobody with a low risk of fear of movement. The results of the prevalence of kinesiophobia in subgroups, taken from the TSK-17 cut-off points put forward by Lira et al., Wertli et al. and Dupuis et al. [14,23,24], are presented in Table 1.

Table 1. Kinesiophobia prevalence in the TMD and nTMD groups.

TSK-TMD		TMD Group			nTMD Group		
Level of Kinesiophobia	Points	n = 47			n = 47		
		n	%	Mean ± SD	n	%	Mean ± SD
low risk	<17	-	-	-	-	-	-
moderate risk	17–37	18	38.3	27.72 ± 6.37	44	93.6	21.50 ± 4.11
high risk	>37	29	61.7	44.69 ± 6.27	3	6.4	47.00 ± 6.08

Legend: TMD group—patients with temporomandibular disorders; nTMD group—patients with no signs of temporomandibular disorders; TSK-TMD—Tampa scale for kinesiophobia for temporomandibular disorders.

The analysis showed higher values in the TMD group. Significant differences were observed in TSK-TMD, PHQ-9 and GCPS (CPI), and also in JFLS-20 levels between groups ($p < 0.001$). The detailed results of this analysis are presented in Table 2.

Table 2. Kinesiophobia, emotional state, functional state, and chronic pain differences between the TMD and nTMD groups.

Questionnaire	TMD Group			nTMD Group					
	n = 47			n = 47					
	Mean ± SD	Me	CI 95%	Mean ± SD	Me	CI 95%	Z	p	R
TSK-TMD	38.19 ± 10.41	39.0	35.13–41.25	23.12 ± 7.56	21.0	20.91–25.35	6.03	<0.001	0.723
PHQ-9	7.38 ± 4.64	7.0	6.02–8.75	3.94 ± 3.74	3.0	2.84–5.04	3.78	<0.001	0.453
GAD-7	5.81 ± 4.87	5.0	4.38–7.24	4.15 ± 4.68	3.0	2.77–5.52	1.96	0.050	0.235
JFLS-20	1.08 ± 1.04	0.83	0.78–1.39	0.04 ± 0.15	0.0	−0.01–0.08	6.16	<0.001	0.737
GCPS (CPI)	24.89 ± 21.21	30	18.67–31.12	1.84 ± 7.35	0.0	−0.31–4.00	5.13	<0.001	0.615

Legend: TMD group—patients with temporomandibular disorders; nTMD group—patients with no signs of temporomandibular disorders; TSK-TMD—Tampa scale for kinesiophobia for temporomandibular disorders; PHQ-9—patient health questionnaire; GAD-7—generalized anxiety disorder; JFLS-20—jaw functional limitation scale; GCPS (CPI)—GCPS graded chronic pain scale, CPI—characteristic pain Intensity score; CI—confidence interval; Me—median.

In addition, no interactions between TSK-TMD × TMD × SEX ($F(1, 90) = 0.033$, $p = 0.856$, $\eta = 0.0003$) were found. TSK-TMD levels in females were higher, compared to males, but not at a statistically significant level ($F(1, 90) = 0.053$, $p = 0.818$, $\eta = 0.0006$). The results showed that kinesiophobia levels were significantly different between TMD and nTMD groups ($F(1, 90) = 49.26$, $p < 0.01$, $\eta = 0.354$). The results of the analysis are presented in Figure 1.

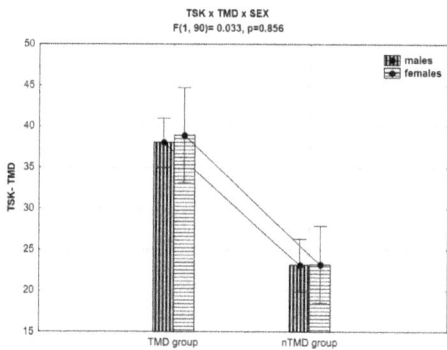

Figure 1. TSK-TMD differences, divided by gender and TMD presence.

Moreover, the TSK-TMD results were correlated with the functional limitations of participants ($p < 0.001$, $r = 0.621$), but not with emotional state nor chronic pain intensity. All results are shown in Table 3.

Table 3. Correlation coefficient values for kinesiophobia (TSK-TMD) levels.

	PHQ-9	GAD-7	JFLS-20	GCPS (CPI)
TSK-TMD	$r = -0.07$; $p = 0.639$	$r = 0.022$; $p = 0.886$	$r = 0.621$; $p < 0.001$	$r = 0.101$; $p = 0.501$

Legend: TSK-TMD—Tampa scale for kinesiophobia for temporomandibular disorders; PHQ-9—patient health questionnaire; GAD-7—generalized anxiety disorder; JFLS-20—jaw functional limitation scale; GCPS (CPI)—GCPS-graded chronic pain scale, CPI—characteristic pain intensity score.

4. Discussion

From a clinical perspective, there is a strong need to screen for kinesiophobia levels in both TMD and nTMD subjects. It seems that the fear of movement is directly correlated with pain intensity, as well as the patient's emotional state. This study therefore aimed to assess the kinesiophobia—psychoemotional state—functional state—pain relationship in subjects with temporomandibular disorders and healthy controls. The second study aim was to assess kinesiophobia prevalance in the studied TMD group.

The results showed that subjects with temporomandibular disorders (TMD group) had significantly higher levels of kinesiophobia ($Z = 6.03$, $p < 0.01$, $R = 0.723$), depression ($Z = 3.78$, $p < 0.01$, $R = 0.453$), chronic pain ($Z = 5.13$, $p < 0.01$, $R = 0.615$), and more severe functional limitations ($Z = 6.16$, $p < 0.01$, $R = 0.737$), compared to the asymptomatic group. Moreover, while TMD patients showed higher levels of anxiety ($Z = 1.96$, $p = 0.05$, $R = 0.235$), the difference with the control group was borderline statistically significant.

The lack of interaction between TSK-TMD × TMD × SEX means that although women show a higher levels of anxiety (compared to men), this difference is not statistically significant. On this basis, it can be assumed that the TSK-TMD questionnaire can be used in both women and men, without fear that one gender has a greater predisposition to kinesiophobia. On the other hand, women experience TMD symptoms more often, and also seek professional medical help more frequently (than men) [18,30,31]: both findings suggest researchers should refrain from claiming definite conclusions, and highlight the need for further research.

4.1. Kinesiophobia and Emotional Status

Although the connection between kinesiophobia and psychoemotional state has been investigated before, only a few studies used TMD-dedicated tools (e.g., TSK-TMD and PHQ questionnaires) [8,10] to assess kinesiophobia and depression levels (i.e., TSK-TMD and PHQ questionnaires) [8,10], finding, in both cases, significant differences between groups (painful TMD, nonpainful TMD, and control group). Other researchers who also assessed emotional status and kinesiophobia in TMD patients by using different measurement tools, such as the hospital anxiety and depression scale (HADS), reached similar conclusions [14]. The results of the current study are consistent with those obtained from previous studies, with the exception of the finding there is no correlation between kinesiophobia and depression levels.

Another aspect of the analysis that should be emphasized is the fear of movement in subjects with joint sounds (clicks due to disk displacement with reduction). Previous studies produced contradictory results on this, but mostly supported this correlation [10,32,33]. Poluha et al., analyzed this extensively, and concluded that subjects with joint sound (regardless of pain existence) showed higher kinesiophobia levels. The authors cited these potential explanations for this phenomenon by using the following arguments put forward by other researchers. First, it seems that the fear of movement is strongly related to mechanical jaw problems, such as sounds or locking [9,34]; second, the pain sensation of the click moment also influences this movement avoidance [35,36]; and finally, the movement-evoked pain conditions are commonly linked to fear of movement [37]. The click sound creates a suspicion the joint is malfunctioning, even in patients without pain [38,39]. Another hypothetical explanation for this could be that joint sounds create a feeling of embarrassment in patients, who therefore avoid movement, as stated by [33]. On the other hand, only Lira et al. displayed no correlation between temporomandibular joint sounds and kinesiophobia in TMD patients [14], but did not identify any possible causes.

The results of the current study are in accordance with the majority of the results available in the literature, as all of the participants experienced joint sounds, and simultaneously showed higher kinesiophobia levels than controls.

The latest systematic review by Dupuis et al. [24] concluded there is a need for further research that compares fear of movement to other similar constructs related to fear/anxiety associated with pain (e.g., pain catastrophizing scale), and claimed this would settle the validity of the TSK-TMD questionnaire. The current study tried to meet this demand by inspecting the kinesiophobia—depression —anxiety —chronic pain relationship, but failed to show a correlation. Moreover, anxiety levels between groups did not even reach the level of significance, and were just above the cut-off point. This could be due to a number of reasons, including the small sample size, the use of different diagnostic tools across individual articles (for example, HADS in the case of depression), the lack of catastrophizing assessment, and the correlation between emotional status and pain presented by others, including [40]. The general consensus holds there is a connection between depression, anxiety and pain perception. However, as the results of the current study did not show significant anxiety level differences between groups, which could potentially influence the emotional status—pain relationship indirectly, resulting in a lack of correlation between kinesiophobia, depression, anxiety and pain in the studied group.

4.2. Kinesiophobia and Functional Limitations (JFLS)

Current results showed a significant correlation between TSK-TMD and the results of JFLS-20, indicating that the functional limitations of TMD subjects increase with the level of kinesiophobia. This is consistent with Kim et al., who suggest that fear of movement may play an important role in mastication impairment [15], and even propose an innovation based on the premise that it would be very useful to compare subcategories from each questionnaire, meaning that jaw function, mastication, and communication for JFLS-20 would be compared with the kinesiophobia (low, moderate and high) risk expressed in TSK-TMD. This is a novelty that future research should consider, and possibly implement.

Some authors conclude that patient-reported outcomes, such as pain perception, pain catastrophizing, and kinesiophobia, are risk factors that seem to have more influence on jaw function than psychological distress, such as depression and anxiety. Current research also supports this by showing a significant correlation between TSK-TMD and JFLS, but not with PHQ or GAD scores. This is another indication that the PCS questionnaire should be used to explore the influence of catastrophizing on functional limitations.

Moreover, the cited study analyzed 145 subjects, more than the current study (94), which could be an influencing factor.

4.3. Kinesiophobia and Chronic Pain (GCPS)

Pain perception is subjective and can be assessed in two ways, first after mechanical induction by using an algometer; and second, with self-administered questionnaires (BPI or GCPS). To date, no studies have investigated the kinesiophobia—pain relationship in the TMD population by applying the Graded Chronic Pain Scale (GCPS). The results of this current study showed no correlation between TSK-TMD and GCPS scores, in contrast to previous studies that demonstrated kinesiophobia is a predictor of pain and disability in TMD patients, and therefore has an important clinical significance in the assessment and treatment of TMD [41]. The current study's lack of significance could be due to the results from the characteristic pain intensity (CPI), rather than the global score of the questionnaire, being used for statistical analysis. Future studies should perhaps use the global score, and may well find it to be more informative.

4.4. Prevalence of Kinesiophobia in TMD

The prevalence of kinesiophobia in both groups (TMD and nTMD) was calculated and presented, and the results showed that nobody in either group presented a low risk of kinesiophobia. Most of the subjects in the TMD group presented a high risk of fear of movement and the majority of the nTMD group presented moderate risk. Scores in the TMD group were, in comparison to the controls, found to be significant in comparison with the controls. One flaw of the kinesiophobia classification, which should be emphasized, resulted in the cut-off points being taken directly from the TSK-17 classification with 17 questions, one less than the TSK-TMD. The risk levels were set at less than 17, 17–37 and more than 37 points for low-, moderate- and high-risk, respectively. The TSK-17 scale was used because there are no TSK-TMD cut-off points in the literature.

This lack is both a limitation of this study and a signpost for future studies, as the creation of subscales (based on cut-off points dedicated to TSK-TMD) that determine levels of kinesiophobia would help to establish a risk assessment that could be used to classify patients, and better address their treatment plans.

To the best of our knowledge, only one paper has, to date, showed prevalence of kinesiophobia in the TMD population [11], in contrast to all the other studies cited in this paper, which merely compare study and control groups. The study group of this one paper only contained 28 subjects, whereas this study had 94, a figure that, while higher, still seems low when generalization of the results to the entire population is considered. Given this, future studies should consider larger study samples.

4.5. Summary

The diagnostics of kinesiophobia in temporomandibular disorder patients seems to be crucial for future treatment selection, including the choice between manual therapy (or physical therapy in general) and other modalities, such as psychotherapy, behavioral therapy or drug administration.

Because the cause of the temporomandibular disorders is multifactorial, the approach to this type of patient should be global and multidisciplinary. In addition to considering the history of the TMJ and undertaking a clinical examination of it, an assessment of the levels of kinesiophobia should also be undertaken, as this seems to be one of the most important elements that affects patient performance. The identification of the risk factor could be a potential indicator that is used for prognostic reasons in assessments of pain chronicity.

There are ongoing scientific projects that aim to lowering kinesiophobia levels by searching for the most effective pain management and functional improvement tools that can be offered on top of conventional TMD treatment. This is important to remember, given that most of the studies cited in this paper only focused on depression and/or anxiety treatment [42].

In conclusion, when kinesiophobia is involved, other specialists should be involved in the multidisciplinary treatment team, as this will ultimately be in the best interests of temporomandibular disorder patients.

4.6. Study Limitations

The findings of this study should be interpreted in light of its limitations, of which the most important are the small sample size and the absence of the PCS questionnaire assessing catastrophizing, which other researchers have shown to be correlated with kinesiophobia, pain and functional limitations. If it was included, the analysis would be even more complete.

A more general limitation is the lack of cut-off points directly dedicated to TSK-TMD in the available literature. Due to this, the authors tried to adapt the scale with cut-off points from TSK-17 despite the strategy being, at the time of writing, unsupported and in need of future validation.

5. Conclusions

This paper's findings displayed significantly higher levels of kinesiophobia, emotional state (except anxiety), functional state, and chronic pain in subjects with temporomandibular disorders, when compared to asymptomatic controls. A correlation between fear of movement and functional limitations of jaw function, mastication, mobility, and communication was also shown.

All TMD and nTMD subjects included in the study showed moderate (38.8% and 93.6, respectively) and high risk (61.7% and 6.4% respectively) of kinesiophobia, and so the prevalence was established at 100%; however, due to various factors, these results cannot be generalized to the whole TMD population.

Further studies should address three of the main weaknesses of this study; first, the study sample should be larger; second, the assessment of catastrophizing levels should complement kinesiophobia characteristics in the TMD population; third, cut-off points dedicated to the TSK-TMD questionnaire should be developed. The creation of subscales that determine levels of kinesiophobia would help the risk assessment to classify patients, and ensure their treatment plans are better addressed.

Author Contributions: Conceptualization, T.M. and W.K.-M.; methodology, T.M. and W.K.-M.; validation, T.M., W.K.-M. and P.B.; formal analysis, T.M. and W.K.-M.; investigation, T.M. and W.K.-M.; resources, T.M.; data curation, P.B.; writing—original draft preparation, T.M., P.B. and W.K.-M.; writing—review and editing, T.M., P.B. and S.M.; visualization, T.M. and W.K.-M.; supervision, T.M. and S.M.; project administration, T.M. and W.K.-M.; funding acquisition, T.M. All authors have read and agreed to the published version of the manuscript.

Funding: The work referred to in this paper was supported by the Ministry of Education and Science in 2022, and was developed by research group no 4 at Józef Piłsudski University of Physical Education in Warsaw, under the project heading: "Physical activity and sports for people with special needs".

Institutional Review Board Statement: The study was conducted in accordance with the Declaration of Helsinki and was approved by the ethical committee of the Józef Piłsudski Academy of Physical Education in Warsaw, Poland (signature SKE 01-30/2021).

Informed Consent Statement: Informed consent was obtained from all study subjects.

Data Availability Statement: Due to privacy restrictions, data is available on request from the corresponding author.

Acknowledgments: We would like to give a special thanks to Katarzyna Kaczmarczyk for her substantive assistance in creating this paper.

Conflicts of Interest: The authors declare no conflicts of interest.

References

1. Schiffman, E.; Ohrbach, R.; Truelove, E.; Look, J.; Anderson, G.; Goulet, J.-P.; List, T.; Svensson, P.; Gonzalez, Y.; Lobbezoo, F.; et al. Diagnostic Criteria for Temporomandibular Disorders (DC/TMD) for Clinical and Research Applications: Recommendations of the International RDC/TMD Consortium Network and Orofacial Pain Special Interest Group. *J. Oral Facial Pain Headache* **2014**, *28*, 6–27. [CrossRef]
2. Conti, P.C.; Miranda, J.E.; Araujo, C.R. Relationship between Systemic Joint Laxity, TMJ Hypertranslation, and Intra-Articular Disorders. *Cranio J. Craniomandib. Pract.* **2000**, *18*, 192–197. [CrossRef]
3. Magnusson, T.; Egermarki, I.; Carlsson, G.E. A Prospective Investigation over Two Decades on Signs and Symptoms of Temporomandibular Disorders and Associated Variables. A Final Summary. *Acta Odontol. Scand.* **2005**, *63*, 99–109. [CrossRef]
4. Zakrzewska, J.M. Temporomandibular Disorders, Headaches and Chronic Pain. *J. Pain Palliat. Care Pharmacother.* **2015**, *29*, 61–63. [CrossRef]
5. Slade, G.D.; Ohrbach, R.; Greenspan, J.D.; Fillingim, R.B.; Bair, E.; Sanders, A.E.; Dubner, R.; Diatchenko, L.; Meloto, C.B.; Smith, S.; et al. Painful Temporomandibular Disorder: Decade of Discovery from OPPERA Studies. *J. Dent. Res.* **2016**, *95*, 1084–1092. [CrossRef]

6. Reiter, S.; Eli, I.; Mahameed, M.; Emodi-Perlman, A.; Friedman-Rubin, P.; Reiter, M.; Winocur, E. Pain Catastrophizing and Pain Persistence in Temporomandibular Disorder Patients. *J. Oral Facial Pain Headache* **2018**, *32*, 309–320. [CrossRef]
7. Vlaeyen, J.W.S.; Kole-Snijders, A.M.J.; Boeren, R.G.B.; van Eek, H. Fear of Movement/(Re)Injury in Chronic Low Back Pain and Its Relation to Behavioral Performance. *Pain* **1995**, *62*, 363–372. [CrossRef] [PubMed]
8. Visscher, C.M.; Baad-Hansen, L.; Durham, J.; Goulet, J.-P.; Michelotti, A.; Roldán Barraza, C.; Häggman-Henrikson, B.; Ekberg, E.; Raphael, K.G. Benefits of Implementing Pain-Related Disability and Psychological Assessment in Dental Practice for Patients with Temporomandibular Pain and Other Oral Health Conditions. *J. Am. Dent. Assoc.* **2018**, *149*, 422–431. [CrossRef] [PubMed]
9. Aguiar, A.S.; Bataglion, C.; Visscher, C.M.; Bevilaqua Grossi, D.; Chaves, T.C. Cross-Cultural Adaptation, Reliability and Construct Validity of the Tampa Scale for Kinesiophobia for Temporomandibular Disorders (TSK/TMD-Br) into Brazilian Portuguese. *J. Oral Rehabil.* **2017**, *44*, 500–510. [CrossRef] [PubMed]
10. Häggman-Henrikson, B.; Jawad, N.; Acuña, X.M.; Visscher, C.M.; Schiffman, E.; List, T. Fear of Movement and Catastrophizing in Participants with Temporomandibular Disorders. *J. Oral Facial Pain Headache* **2022**, *36*, 59–66. [CrossRef]
11. Silva, L.M.C.P.; Rodrigues, B.A.; Lucena, H.Í.d.S.; de Morais, E.P.G.; Rocha, A.C.; de Lucena, L.B.S.; Alves, G.A.d.S.; Benevides, S.D. Prevalence of Kinesiophobia and Catastrophizing in Patients with Temporomandibular Disorders. *Rev. CEFAC* **2022**, *24*, e3322. [CrossRef]
12. He, S.; Wang, J.; Ji, P. Validation of the Tampa Scale for Kinesiophobia for Temporomandibular Disorders (TSK-TMD) in Patients with Painful TMD. *J. Headache Pain* **2016**, *17*, 109. [CrossRef]
13. von Piekartz, H.; Schwiddessen, J.; Reineke, L.; Armijo-Olivio, S.; Bevilaqua-Grossi, D.; Biasotto Gonzalez, D.A.; Carvalho, G.; Chaput, E.; Cox, E.; Fernández-de-las-Peñas, C.; et al. International Consensus on the Most Useful Assessments Used by Physical Therapists to Evaluate Patients with Temporomandibular Disorders: A Delphi Study. *J. Oral Rehabil.* **2020**, *47*, 685–702. [CrossRef] [PubMed]
14. Lira, M.R.; Lemes Da Silva, R.R.; Bataglion, C.; Aguiar, A.D.S.; Greghi, S.M.; Chaves, T.C. Multiple Diagnoses, Increased Kinesiophobia?—Patients with High Kinesiophobia Levels Showed a Greater Number of Temporomandibular Disorder Diagnoses. *Musculoskelet. Sci. Pract.* **2019**, *44*, 102054. [CrossRef] [PubMed]
15. Kim, K.-H.; Park, J.-E.; Kim, M.-E.; Kim, H.-K. Risk Factors of the Masticatory Function in Patients with Temporomandibular Disorders: A Cross-Sectional Cohort Study. *J. Oral Med. Pain* **2019**, *44*, 92–102. [CrossRef]
16. Sousa, C.R.A.; Arsati, Y.B.d.O.L.; Velly, A.M.; da Silva, C.A.L.; Arsati, F. Catastrophizing Is Associated with Pain-Related Disability in Temporomandibular Disorders. *Braz. Oral Res.* **2023**, *37*, e070. [CrossRef]
17. Guzel, H.C.; Tuncer, A. Evaluation of Tongue Strength and Symptoms of Oral Dysphagia in Patients Accompanying Temporomandibular Disorder. *Advances in Rehabilitation* **2021**, *35*, 9–16. [CrossRef]
18. Manfredini, D.; Arveda, N.; Guarda-Nardini, L.; Segù, M.; Collesano, V. Distribution of Diagnoses in a Population of Patients with Temporomandibular Disorders. *Oral Surg. Oral Med. Oral Pathol. Oral Radiol.* **2012**, *114*, e35–e41. [CrossRef] [PubMed]
19. Visscher, C.M.; Lobbezoo, F. The Evolution of Thinking about Temporomandibular Pain. *J. Am. Dent. Assoc.* **2015**, *146*, 925–926. [CrossRef]
20. Loster, J.E.; Osiewicz, M.A.; Groch, M.; Ryniewicz, W.; Wieczorek, A. The Prevalence of TMD in Polish Young Adults. *J. Prosthodont. Off. J. Am. Coll. Prosthodont.* **2017**, *26*, 284–288. [CrossRef]
21. Ayouni, I.; Chebbi, R.; Hela, Z.; Dhidah, M. Comorbidity between Fibromyalgia and Temporomandibular Disorders: A Systematic Review. *Oral Surg. Oral Med. Oral Pathol. Oral Radiol.* **2019**, *128*, 33–42. [CrossRef]
22. Keller, S.; Bocell, F.D.; Mangrum, R.; McLorg, A.; Logan, D.; Chen, A.L.; Steen, A.I.; Woods, P.; Weinberg, J.; Royce, L.; et al. Patient-Reported Outcome Measures for Individuals with Temporomandibular Joint Disorders: A Systematic Review and Evaluation. *Oral Surg. Oral Med. Oral Pathol. Oral Radiol.* **2023**, *135*, 65–78. [CrossRef]
23. Wertli, M.M.; Rasmussen-Barr, E.; Held, U.; Weiser, S.; Bachmann, L.M.; Brunner, F. Fear-Avoidance Beliefs—A Moderator of Treatment Efficacy in Patients with Low Back Pain: A Systematic Review. *Spine J.* **2014**, *14*, 2658–2678. [CrossRef]
24. Dupuis, F.; Cherif, A.; Batcho, C.; Massé-Alarie, H.; Roy, J.-S. The Tampa Scale of Kinesiophobia: A Systematic Review of Its Psychometric Properties in People with Musculoskeletal Pain. *Clin. J. Pain* **2023**, *39*, 236–247. [CrossRef]
25. Kroenke, K.; Spitzer, R.L.; Williams, J.B. The PHQ-9: Validity of a Brief Depression Severity Measure. *J. Gen. Intern. Med.* **2001**, *16*, 606–613. [CrossRef]
26. Spitzer, R.L.; Kroenke, K.; Williams, J.B.W.; Löwe, B. A Brief Measure for Assessing Generalized Anxiety Disorder: The GAD-7. *Arch. Intern. Med.* **2006**, *166*, 1092–1097. [CrossRef] [PubMed]
27. Ohrbach, R.; Larsson, P.; List, T. The Jaw Functional Limitation Scale: Development, Reliability, and Validity of 8-Item and 20-Item Versions. *J. Orofac. Pain* **2008**, *22*, 219–230.
28. Von Korff, M. Assessment of Chronic Pain in Epidemiological and Health Services Research: Empirical Bases and New Directions. In *Handbook of Pain Assessment*; Turk, D., Melzack, R., Eds.; The Guilford Press: New York, NY, USA, 2011; pp. 455–473.
29. Cohen, J. A Power Primer. *Psychol. Bull.* **1992**, *112*, 155–159. [CrossRef] [PubMed]
30. Liu, F.; Steinkeler, A. Epidemiology, Diagnosis, and Treatment of Temporomandibular Disorders. *Dent. Clin. N. Am.* **2013**, *57*, 465–479. [CrossRef]
31. von Piekartz, H.; Rösner, C.; Batz, A.; Hall, T.; Ballenberger, N. Bruxism, Temporomandibular Dysfunction and Cervical Impairments in Females—Results from an Observational Study. *Musculoskelet. Sci. Pract.* **2020**, *45*, 102073. [CrossRef] [PubMed]

32. Poluha, R.L.; De La Torre Canales, G.; Bonjardim, L.R.; Conti, P.C.R. Somatosensory and Psychosocial Profile of Patients with Painful Temporomandibular Joint Clicking. *J. Oral Rehabil.* **2020**, *47*, 1346–1357. [CrossRef]
33. Visscher, C.M.; Ohrbach, R.; van Wijk, A.J.; Wilkosz, M.; Naeije, M. The Tampa Scale for Kinesiophobia for Temporomandibular Disorders (TSK-TMD). *Pain* **2010**, *150*, 492–500. [CrossRef] [PubMed]
34. Vlaeyen, J.W.S.; Linton, S.J. Fear-Avoidance and Its Consequences in Chronic Musculoskeletal Pain: A State of the Art. *Pain* **2000**, *85*, 317–332. [CrossRef]
35. Schwartz, H.C.; Kendrick, R.W. Internal Derangements of the Temporomandibular Joint: Description of Clinical Syndromes. *Oral Surg. Oral Med. Oral Pathol.* **1984**, *58*, 24–29. [CrossRef]
36. Gage, J.P. Mechanisms of Disc Displacement in the Temporomandibular Joint. *Aust. Dent. J.* **1989**, *34*, 427–436. [CrossRef]
37. Corbett, D.B.; Simon, C.B.; Manini, T.M.; George, S.Z.; Riley, J.L.; Fillingim, R.B. Movement-Evoked Pain: Transforming the Way We Understand and Measure Pain. *Pain* **2019**, *160*, 757–761. [CrossRef]
38. Marpaung, C.M.; Kalaykova, S.I.; Lobbezoo, F.; Naeije, M. Validity of Functional Diagnostic Examination for Temporomandibular Joint Disc Displacement with Reduction. *J. Oral Rehabil.* **2014**, *41*, 243–249. [CrossRef] [PubMed]
39. Poluha, R.L.; Canales, G.D.l.T.; Costa, Y.M.; Grossmann, E.; Bonjardim, L.R.; Conti, P.C.R. Temporomandibular Joint Disc Displacement with Reduction: A Review of Mechanisms and Clinical Presentation. *J. Appl. Oral Sci. Rev. FOB* **2019**, *27*, e20180433. [CrossRef] [PubMed]
40. De la Torre Canales, G.; Bonjardim, L.; Poluha, R.; Soares, F.; Guarda-Nardini, L.; Conti, P.; Manfredini, D. Correlation Between Physical and Psychosocial Findings in a Population of Temporomandibular Disorder Patients. *Int. J. Prosthodont.* **2020**, *33*, 155–159. [CrossRef]
41. Gil-Martínez, A.; Grande-Alonso, M.; López-de-Uralde-Villanueva, I.; López-López, A.; Fernández-Carnero, J.; La Touche, R. Chronic Temporomandibular Disorders: Disability, Pain Intensity and Fear of Movement. *J. Headache Pain* **2016**, *17*, 103. [CrossRef]
42. Zhang, Q.; Zhang, J.; Ran, W.; Yu, S.; Jin, Y. Effectiveness of Cognitive Behavioral Therapy on Kinesiophobia and Oral Health-Related Quality of Life in Patients with Temporomandibular Disorders, Study Protocol for a Randomized Controlled Trial. *Medicine* **2020**, *99*, e23295. [CrossRef] [PubMed]

Disclaimer/Publisher's Note: The statements, opinions and data contained in all publications are solely those of the individual author(s) and contributor(s) and not of MDPI and/or the editor(s). MDPI and/or the editor(s) disclaim responsibility for any injury to people or property resulting from any ideas, methods, instructions or products referred to in the content.

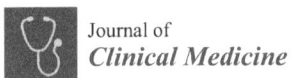
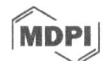

Article

Immersive Virtual Reality Therapy Is Supportive for Orthopedic Rehabilitation among the Elderly: A Randomized Controlled Trial

Justyna Mazurek [1], Błażej Cieślik [2,*], Adam Wrzeciono [3], Robert Gajda [4,5] and Joanna Szczepańska-Gieracha [3]

1. University Rehabilitation Centre, Wroclaw Medical University, 50-556 Wroclaw, Poland
2. Healthcare Innovation Technology Lab, IRCCS San Camillo Hospital, 30126 Venice, Italy
3. Faculty of Physiotherapy, Wroclaw University of Health and Sport Sciences, 51-612 Wroclaw, Poland
4. Department of Kinesiology and Health Prevention, Jan Dlugosz University in Częstochowa, 42-200 Częstochowa, Poland
5. Center for Sports Cardiology, Gajda-Med Medical Center in Pułtusk, 06-100 Pułtusk, Poland
* Correspondence: blazej.cieslik@hsancamillo.it

Abstract: *Objective:* This research aimed to determine the efficacy of VR therapy in mitigating symptoms of depression, anxiety, and stress among older adults following arthroplasty surgery and to comprehend the influence of psychological improvement on changes in functional outcomes. *Methods:* Utilizing a parallel-group randomized controlled trial design, the study involved 68 osteoarthritis patients who had recently undergone either total hip or knee arthroplasty. Subjects were split into two groups. The experimental group underwent eight VR therapy sessions during their rehabilitation, while the control group was given standard care. Assessments encompassed both psychological and functional outcomes, with tools like the Hospital Anxiety and Depression Scale, Perceived Stress Scale, and the Barthel Index, among others. The experimental group showcased notable enhancements in both psychological and functional areas compared to the control group. *Results:* A significant (p value of < 0.001) relationship was found between psychological progress and functional recovery, indicating that psychological factors can serve as predictors for functional outcomes. *Conclusions:* The findings emphasize the promising role of VR therapy as a beneficial addition to the rehabilitation process for older adults' post-hip and knee arthroplasty. The integration of psychological interventions in standard rehabilitation practices appears valuable, but further studies are needed to ascertain the long-term advantages of such an approach.

Keywords: elderly; rehabilitation; physical activity; mood disorders; virtual reality exposure therapy

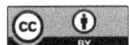

1. Introduction

Osteoarthritis (OA) is currently the most prevalent degenerative disease of the musculoskeletal system. It affects 53% of individuals aged 65+ globally, with a higher prevalence among women [1]. OA of the knee and hip is the third most common musculoskeletal disorder and is ranked as the 11th leading cause of disability worldwide [2]. OA gradually diminishes the patient's ability to be self-reliant, move freely, and engage in social life, thus reducing the overall quality of life [3]. Individuals affected by OA are almost three times more likely to experience very severe pain, and twice as likely to suffer from high levels of psychological distress when compared to those without OA [4]. Many individuals with osteoarthritis experience depression, with a rate of occurrence at 20% [5]. Specifically, patients with both OA and depression have 38.8% higher direct medical costs than those who only have OA [6]. OA can also greatly affect a person's health, resulting in chronic pain and functional limitations leading to decreased physical and mental well-being [7,8].

Similar biological pathways and neurotransmitters are responsible for both chronic pain and psychological impairment like depression and anxiety. Chronic pain is frequently the catalyst that prompts individuals with osteoarthritis to seek medical attention [9]. Chronic pain, depressed mood, stress, and anxiety often occur together, with depression being a frequent comorbidity of various chronic diseases, including OA [10,11]. When a patient has both conditions simultaneously, the effectiveness of standard treatment for each condition alone is decreased (e.g., individuals who have depression and anxiety report more severe pain, greater physical impairment, increased postoperative opioid use, and a lower rate of return to work than those without these mental health conditions) [12]. The considerable number of people affected by osteoarthritis in society results in a significant need for specialized treatment, which frequently surpasses the number of available appointments. As a result, the use of a waitlist is necessary. The public hospitals in Europe are facing long delays, which have been aggravated by the SARS-CoV-2 pandemic, resulting in extensive waiting time for specialist Orthopedic consultations [13]. This postponement in medical care can cause symptoms to worsen and pain to increase. Additionally, it can contribute to a deterioration in mental health (such as depression, stress, anxiety). This is also observed after undergoing a surgical procedure [14].

In the past few decades, joint replacement surgery has become the primary method of Orthopedic surgical treatment of advanced degenerative OA. This is especially true for hip and knee joints. Starting the rehabilitation process immediately after hip and/or knee replacement (total hip replacement—THR, total knee replacement—TKR) is crucial for recovery. Primary interventions for post-operative rehabilitation concentrate on exercises aimed at enhancing joint flexibility and strength, gait reeducation, and retraining functional abilities to optimize independence in tasks such as transferring (from bed to chair, using the toilet, exiting the shower/bath), personal hygiene (bathing and dressing), and broader daily activities [15]. Unfortunately, despite compelling evidence on the link between physical pain and mental well-being, psychological evaluation and intervention are not currently perceived as standard practice in Orthopedic rehabilitation in Europe. Even if all patients had access to the necessary resources to receive suitable treatment, there would still be unaddressed demand due to a shortage of professionally trained mental health clinicians.

Virtual reality (VR) is a technological concept that allows its users to experience the full immersion in a simulated world, providing them with a sense of actual presence through the use of multimodal stimuli [16,17]. The application of VR-based rehabilitation in Orthopedic surgery, especially in THR/TKR, has noticeably and significantly risen [18,19]. Several VR-based protocols have been proposed for rehabilitation following TKR and THR [16,18–20]. However, none of the articles examined the effectiveness of VR-based interventions for symptoms of stress, anxiety, and depression in patients with OA after THR or after TKR. As a result of this research gap, this study was conducted to investigate the impact of VR therapy on the severity of depressive symptoms, anxiety, and stress levels in OA patients who had undergone rehabilitation following THR or TKR. The research hypothesis was as follows: VR therapy has a beneficial effect on the mental and functional state of people undergoing rehabilitation after lower limb arthroplasty. The primary purpose of this study was to determine how effective VR therapy is in alleviating symptoms of depression and anxiety, as well as in reducing perceived stress level in older adults who have undergone arthroplasty surgery. Furthermore, the objective of the study was to evaluate the impact of psychological improvements on changes in functional outcomes.

2. Materials and Methods

2.1. Study Design and Setting

The study took place at St. Hedwig of Silesia Hospital in Trzebnica (Poland) and was designed as a parallel-group randomized controlled trial. Outcomes were evaluated at two intervals: before and after the intervention, with an outcome assessor who was blinded to the group assignments. Participants were evenly divided into two groups using the block randomization method. The sequence for randomization was generated using computer software, and participants were enrolled via sealed, sequentially numbered envelopes. This allocation process remained confidential until the participants were registered and assigned to their respective groups. An independent researcher oversaw the randomization to ensure that the assessors remained blinded throughout. While both the participants and those delivering the intervention were aware of their group assignments during the trial, there were no deviations from the planned intervention due to its context.

The study's design adhered to the recommendations for phase three (VR3) of clinical trials utilizing VR in healthcare, emphasizing the efficacy of the proposed treatment compared to the control group [21]. The protocol was reviewed and approved by the Bioethics Committee at the Wroclaw Medical University (Wroclaw, Poland) under the reference number 119/KB/2023. The study was registered in the ClinicalTrials.gov database (NCT06002139). Participants provided written informed consent to partake in the research.

2.2. Participants

As illustrated in Figure 1, following an initial eligibility assessment, 68 participants were randomly allocated to one of two treatment groups. The experimental group (VR therapy group) consisted of 34 individuals. The remaining 34 participants constituted the control group (CON group). The inclusion criteria specified participants who were 60 years or older and had recently undergone hip or knee joint arthroplasty surgeries. The exclusion criteria included cognitive impairments hindering the independent completion of research questionnaires, recognized consciousness disorders, a history of bipolar affective disorder or other severe mental conditions, use of psychoactive drugs, ongoing psychiatric or individual psychological treatments, contraindications to virtual reality such as epilepsy, vertigo, or notable vision impairments, a functional status that restricts independent movement (although Orthopedic aids like crutches or walkers were acceptable), and refusal to partake in the study at any study stage.

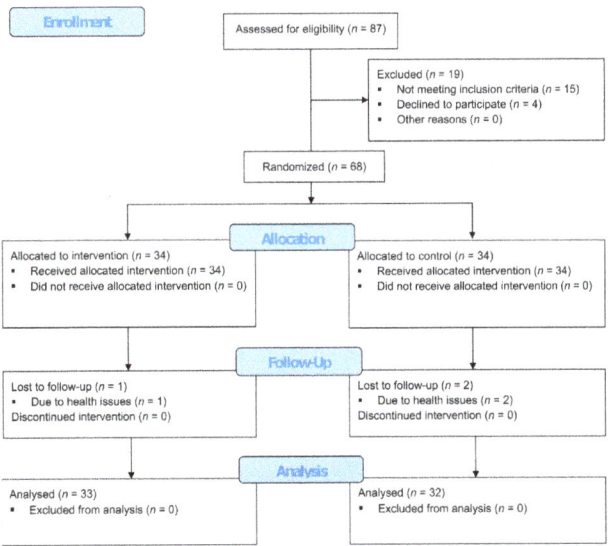

Figure 1. CONSORT study flow diagram.

2.3. Interventions

Both groups underwent a four-week conventional rehabilitation regimen that encompassed two hours of kinesiotherapy (120 min, inclusive of gait training), thirty minutes of ergotherapy, and three individualized physical therapy procedures such as laser therapy, magnetic therapy, and electrotherapy, all tailored to address specific ailments and requirements of each participant.

In addition to their regular treatments, the VR therapy group underwent eight sessions (20 min each, twice weekly) of immersive virtual reality therapy (VR therapy) using the VRTierOne device by Stolgraf®, Stanowice, Poland. This system employed VR HTC VIVE goggles (2017) and two controllers. The VRTierOne goal was to divert patients' attention to a serene virtual environment, allowing relaxation and fostering recognition of their psychological strengths. Sessions began with the patient at a garden door (Figure 2A). As the door opened, the patient entered an evolving garden that became more vibrant each session. Midway, participants colored a mandala using the controllers (Figure 2B). The therapeutic impact of VRTierOne combined Erickson's psychotherapy principles, calming music that grew more uplifting over time, cognitive engagement through mandala coloring, and the mood-enhancing green garden aesthetic rooted in Japanese design (Figure 2C). Therapy included metaphorical communication and posthypnotic therapeutic suggestions [22]. The music was crafted by a therapist–composer duo, and the immersive garden experience aimed to uplift spirits. Further details on the VRTierOne's principles can be found in our prior work [23].

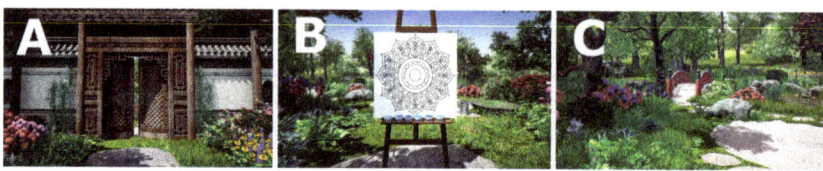

Figure 2. VRTierOne screenshots: (**A**) gate leading to the garden; (**B**) mandala coloring task; (**C**) decorative elements of the garden.

2.4. Outcome Measures

Both primary and secondary outcomes were administered at the beginning and again after a four-week treatment period. The primary outcome measures included the Hospital Anxiety and Depression Scale (HADS) and the Perceived Stress Scale (PSS-10). HADS is a 14-item self-report questionnaire designed to screen for anxiety (using the HADS-A subscale, which comprises seven items) and depression (using the HADS-D subscale, also with seven items) in patients in non-psychiatric settings. Both subscales have a cut-off point of 8/21. The Cronbach's α for the scale ranges from 0.78 to 0.93, and the test-retest correlation stands at r = 0.80, as found by Bjelland et al. in 2002 [24]. The PSS-10 is a ten-item scale assessing the stress an individual perceived over the past month. Its questions are general, making it applicable to various subpopulations [25]. The items evaluate the perceived unpredictability, uncontrollability, and overload in respondents' lives. Scores range from 0 to 40, with higher scores indicating greater perceived stress.

The secondary outcome measures included the Generalized Self-Efficacy Scale (GSES), Barthel Index (BI), Rivermead Mobility Index (RMI), Tinetti's Short Scale, Short Physical Performance Battery (SPPB), the Perception of Stress Questionnaire (PSQ), and the Visual Analogue Scale (VAS) for pain assessment. The GSES is a ten-item psychometric scale assessing optimistic self-beliefs about coping with difficult demands [26]. It measures the confidence one has in addressing a wide variety of stressful or challenging situations. Scores on the GSES range from 10 to 40, with higher scores denoting stronger self-efficacy. The BI, an ordinal scale, evaluates performance in daily living activities, with each activity having an assigned point value [27]. With ten descriptive variables for daily activities and mobility, a higher BI score indicates a greater likelihood of post-hospitalization independent living. The RMI, derived from the Rivermead Motor Assessment Gross Function subscale, quantifies mobility impairment [28]. It comprises 14 items spanning from simple tasks like turning in bed to more demanding ones like running. Each item scores as either 'unable' (0) or 'able' (1), with a perfect score of 14 suggesting full mobility. Tinetti's Short Scale, a condensed version of the Performance-Oriented Mobility Assessment (POMA), gauges a patient's gait and balance. It rates patients based on tasks like moving from sitting to standing and maintaining an upright position for a set time, scored on a 3-point Likert scale. The SPPB combines results from tests on gait speed, chair stands, and balance. It yields a composite score between 0 (worst) and 12 (best), reflecting the overall physical functionality in elderly subjects [29]. Lastly, the PSQ by Plopa and Makarowski is a 27-item scale, with scores from 1 to 5 per item [30]. It assesses stress in areas such as emotional tension, external stress, and internal stress. Overall stress perception scores range from 21 to 105, with a score above 60 indicating elevated stress perception.

2.5. Data Analysis

The required sample size for this study was determined using the G*Power 3.1.9.4 software (Heinrich Heine University Düsseldorf, Germany) [31]. Based on the results of the primary outcome (the depression subscale of HADS) from our previous research on the elderly population, we anticipated an effect size of 0.25, equivalent to a partial eta squared of 0.06 [23]. Setting the significance level (α) at 0.05 and the statistical power $(1-\beta)$ at 0.95, a total of 54 participants was deemed necessary to achieve statistical significance. Taking into account an anticipated 25% dropout rate, we enrolled a sum of 68 participants.

Data were analyzed using JASP version 0.16.3 (University of Amsterdam, The Netherlands). Categorical variables were presented as frequency counts and percentages, while continuous variables were summarized using mean and standard deviation (SD). The Shapiro–Wilk test confirmed the normal distribution of the data. At the outset, baseline demographic variables were cross-compared between groups via unpaired t-tests (for continuous data) and χ^2 tests (for categorical data). Intervention effects between groups (pre- vs. post-intervention) were examined using an analysis of variance (ANOVA), complemented by paired and unpaired *t* tests. The influence of psychological enhancement on functional progress was investigated through Spearman correlation and stepwise linear regression. A significance threshold was set at $\alpha < 0.05$.

3. Results

3.1. Participant Characteristics

Out of 87 potential participants, 68 met the inclusion criteria and were randomized for the study. Three participants dropped out: two from the VR therapy group and one from the control group, all due to health complications requiring re-hospitalization (Figure 1). Table 1 shows that there were no statistically significant differences between the VR therapy and control groups at baseline.

Table 1. Participants baseline characteristics.

Variable	Overall	VR Therapy	Control	*p* Value
N	68	34	34	-
n (%) of women	42 (61.76)	21 (61.76)	21 (61.76)	1.00 [b]
Age, years	69.59 (6.16)	69.71 (6.82)	69.47 (5.52)	0.88 [a]
Body mass, kg	80.25 (16.08)	79.26 (16.60)	81.24 (15.72)	0.62 [a]
Body height, cm	167.69 (10.02)	166.76 (8.07)	168.62 (11.79)	0.45 [a]
Body mass index, kg/m^2	28.54 (5.12)	28.46 (5.25)	28.62 (5.05)	0.89 [a]
Normal (BMI 18.5–24.9), n (%)	13 (19.12)	6 (17.65)	7 (20.59)	0.76 [b]
Overweight (BMI 25–29.9), n (%)	33 (48.53)	18 (52.94)	15 (44.12)	0.47 [b]
Obese (BMI > 30), n (%)	22 (32.35)	10 (29.41)	12 (35.29)	0.60 [b]
Arthroplasty area, n (%)				
Hip	45 (66.18)	22 (64.70)	23 (67.65)	0.80 [b]
Knee	23 (33.83)	12 (35.30)	11 (32.35)	
Marital status, n (%)				
Married	46 (67.65)	21 (61.76)	25 (73.53)	0.30 [b]
Single	1 (1.47)	1 (2.94)	0 (0.00)	-
Widowed	21 (30.88)	12 (35.29)	9 (26.47)	0.43 [b]

Table 1. Cont.

Variable	Overall	VR Therapy	Control	p Value
Education, n (%)				
Primary/vocational	27 (39.71)	13 (38.24)	14 (41.18)	0.80 [b]
Secondary	29 (42.65)	16 (47.06)	13 (38.24)	0.46 [b]
Higher	12 (17.65)	5 (14.71)	7 (20.59)	0.52 [b]

VR: virtual reality; BMI: body mass index; [a] t-test; [b] Chi-square test.

3.2. Effectiveness of the Interventions

Table 2 presents the time × group interaction based on ANOVA, whereas Table 3 illustrates mean values, SD, and the between-group mean difference. The VR therapy group demonstrated significant improvements in their secondary outcomes compared to primary outcomes and compared to the control group. Specifically, for the HADS, the VRT group's scores decreased by 57.8%, while the control group's scores increased by 7.7%. This resulted in a between-group difference of −8.66 ($p < 0.001$). Further analysis of variance revealed a significant group × time interaction for HADS, indicated by an F value of 25.48, effect size ηp^2 of 0.29, and a p value of < 0.001. In the HADS-A assessment, the VRT group's scores decreased by 62.5%, while those in the control group declined by 2.9%.

Table 2. ANOVA results (time × group).

Outcome	Mean Square	F	ηp^2	p Value
Psychological outcomes				
HADS	605.87	25.48	0.29	<0.001
HADS-A	156.29	21.23	0.25	<0.001
HADS-D	146.72	14.79	0.19	<0.001
VAS	53.95	30.88	0.32	<0.001
PSS-10	94.67	17.77	0.22	<0.001
GSES	837.89	47.85	0.43	<0.001
PSQ	4563.31	41.26	0.40	<0.001
ES	345.40	23.88	0.28	<0.001
IS	452.43	30.83	0.33	<0.001
ET	767.11	41.03	0.39	<0.001
Functional outcomes				
Tinetti	92.01	44.79	0.42	<0.001
BI	3520.84	47.48	0.43	<0.001
RMA-GF	35.19	23.74	0.27	<0.001
SPPB	111.54	41.03	0.39	<0.001

HADS: Hospital Anxiety and Depression Scale; HADS-A: anxiety subscale of the HADS; HADS-D: depression subscale of the HADS; VAS: visual analogue scale; PSS-10: Perceived Stress Scale; GSES: General Self-Efficacy Scale; PSQ: Perception of Stress Questionnaire; ES: External Stress; IS: Internal Stress; ET: Emotional Tension; BI: Barthel Index; RMA-GF: Rivermead Motor Assessment Gross-Function; SPPB: Short Physical Performance Battery.

The pronounced difference between the groups was −4.37 ($p < 0.001$). ANOVA for HADS-A supported this with an effect size ηp^2 of 0.25 ($p < 0.001$). For the HADS-D, the VR therapy group's scores decreased by 51.8%, whereas the control group increased 20.1%. This resulted in a significant between-group difference of −4.27 ($p < 0.001$). The group × time interaction for HADS-D was pronounced, with an ηp^2 of 0.19 ($p < 0.001$). Lastly, regarding the PSS-10, the VR group's scores decreased by 11.2%, while those of the control group rose by 2.0%. The between-group difference for PSS-10 was −3.3 ($p < 0.001$), with a group × time interaction marked by an F value of 17.77 and effect size ηp^2 of 0.22 ($p < 0.001$).

A similar pattern emerged for secondary outcomes after treatment. The VR therapy group displayed marked benefits over the control group in both psychological and functional dimensions. In terms of psychological metrics, the VR group exhibited superior improvements: VAS by 2.6 points ($\eta p^2 = 0.32$), GSES by 10.4 points ($\eta p^2 = 0.43$), PSQ by

23.9 points ($\eta p^2 = 0.40$), ES by 6.6 points ($\eta p^2 = 0.28$), IS by 7.7 points ($\eta p^2 = 0.33$), and ET by 9.7 points ($\eta p^2 = 0.39$). In the functional domain, the VR group surpassed the control: Tinetti scores by 3.4 points ($\eta p^2 = 0.42$), BI by 21.2 points ($\eta p^2 = 0.43$), RMA-GF by 2.0 points ($\eta p^2 = 0.27$), and SPPB by 3.8 points ($\eta p^2 = 0.39$). All aforementioned differences were significant with $p < 0.001$.

Table 3. Mean values (SD) of primary and secondary outcomes.

Outcome	VR Therapy ($n = 34$)			Control ($n = 34$)			Between-Group Comparison	
	Baseline	Post-Treatment	p Value	Baseline	Post-Treatment	p Value	Mean Difference	p Value
Psychological outcomes								
HADS	13.15 (5.94)	5.55 (4.64)	<0.001	13.88 (7.68)	14.94 (7.00)	0.02	−8.66	<0.001
HADS-A	7.35 (3.33)	2.76 (2.50)	<0.001	7.56 (3.92)	7.34 (4.04)	0.72	−4.37	<0.001
HADS-D	5.79 (2.59)	2.79 (3.13)	0.004	6.32 (4.35)	7.59 (4.14)	0.06	−4.27	<0.001
VAS	5.27 (1.97)	0.88 (1.02)	<0.001	4.35 (2.07)	2.59 (1.94)	<0.001	−2.63	<0.001
PSS-10	24.94 (3.59)	22.15 (1.77)	<0.001	25.18 (3.77)	25.69 (4.27)	0.14	−3.30	<0.001
GSES	28.59 (6.62)	38.70 (1.29)	<0.001	30.74 (5.71)	30.41 (6.36)	0.88	10.44	<0.001
PSQ	59.32 (18.47)	35.73 (7.71)	<0.001	54.59 (18.64)	54.91 (15.08)	0.94	−23.91	<0.001
ES	18.06 (6.33)	12.73 (3.38)	<0.001	16.47 (6.03)	17.69 (4.97)	0.09	−6.55	<0.001
IS	19.56 (6.65)	11.30 (2.84)	<0.001	18.94 (7.09)	18.38 (6.01)	0.42	−7.70	<0.001
ET	21.71 (7.20)	11.70 (3.85)	<0.001	19.18 (6.52)	18.84 (5.41)	0.69	−9.67	<0.001
Functional outcomes								
Tinetti	3.29 (2.42)	9.64 (0.96)	<0.001	3.59 (2.50)	6.53 (2.27)	<0.001	−3.41	<0.001
BI	54.56 (16.49)	93.94 (6.47)	<0.001	56.18 (17.41)	74.38 (16.84)	<0.001	−21.18	<0.001
RMA-GF	4.56 (2.35)	10.00 (1.00)	<0.001	4.41 (2.55)	7.81 (2.47)	<0.001	−2.04	<0.001
SPPB	2.62 (2.34)	9.12 (2.41)	<0.001	2.88 (2.43)	5.59 (2.98)	<0.001	−3.79	<0.001

HADS: Hospital Anxiety and Depression Scale; HADS-A: anxiety subscale of the HADS; HADS-D: depression subscale of the HADS; VAS: visual analogue scale; PSS-10: Perceived Stress Scale; GSES: General Self-Efficacy Scale; PSQ: Perception of Stress Questionnaire; ES: External Stress; IS: Internal Stress; ET: Emotional Tension; BI: Barthel Index; RMA-GF: Rivermead Motor Assessment Gross-Function; SPPB: Short Physical Performance Battery; SD: standard deviation.

3.3. Correlations and Predictors

Figure 3 depicts the linear correlation heatmap between the change in functional and change in psychological outcomes. All examined parameters showed a significant positive correlation, indicating that higher difference values in one outcome group corresponded to higher values in the other. Notably, significant correlations were observed between psychological parameter differences and SPPB differences (ranging from 0.47 to 0.61), BI (ranging from 0.31 to 0.56), and Tinetti (ranging from 0.27 to 0.61).

Table 4 outlines the psychological predictors of functional improvement based on stepwise regression results. For the change in BI, the change in HADS-A ($B = 1.53$) and the change in PSS-10 ($B = 1.53$) explain 37% of its variance. This model is significant with $F = 18.39$, $p < 0.001$. In the case of the change in Tinetti, the model explains 30% of its variance, primarily driven by changes in GSES ($B = 0.12$) and HADS-A ($B = 0.17$), with $F = 13.25$, $p < 0.001$. For the RMA change, the primary predictors are changes in GSES ($B = 0.09$) and PSS-10 ($B = 0.15$), accounting for 26% of its variance and yielding $F = 10.67$, $p < 0.001$. Finally, for the SPPB change, the key influencers are changes in GSES ($B = 0.11$) and PSS-10 ($B = 0.23$). This model explains 40% of the variance, with $F = 13.46$, $p < 0.001$.

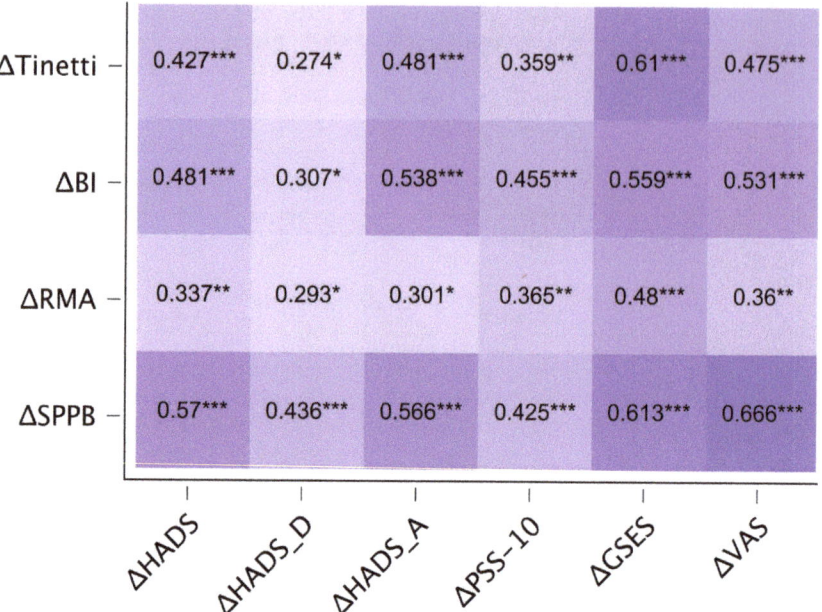

Figure 3. Correlation heatmap. * $p < 0.05$; ** $p < 0.01$; *** $p < 0.001$.

Table 4. Psychological predictors for functional improvement (stepwise regression results).

Variable	B	Beta	t	p Value	F	R^2
ΔBI				<0.001	18.39	0.37
ΔHADS-A	1.53	0.42	4.06			
ΔPSS-10	1.53	0.35	3.38			
ΔTinetti				<0.001	13.25	0.30
ΔGSES	0.12	0.36	2.96			
ΔHADS-A	0.17	0.28	2.33			
ΔRMA-GF				<0.001	10.67	0.26
ΔGSES	0.09	0.34	2.88			
ΔPSS-10	0.15	0.28	2.42			
ΔSPPB				<0.001	13.46	0.40
ΔGSES	0.11	0.29	2.47			
ΔPSS-10	0.23	0.29	2.69			
ΔHADS-A	0.18	0.26	2.32			

HADS-A: anxiety subscale of the HADS; PSS-10: Perceived Stress Scale; GSES: General Self-Efficacy Scale; RMA-GF: Rivermead Motor Assessment Gross-Function; SPPB: Short Physical Performance Battery.

4. Discussion

In recent years, numerous studies have substantiated the efficacy of VR in the context of broadly defined rehabilitation [19]. These studies focused mainly on functional results, i.e., mobility, strength, balance, or range of motion. However, there are no reports on the use of VR to improve the psychological aspects of Orthopedic patients' health, which are important factors affecting the effectiveness of rehabilitation [32,33]. Building upon previous research that has established the efficacy of VR interventions in the treatment of psychiatric disorders, this study aimed to assess the effectiveness of VR therapy in alleviating symptoms of depression and anxiety, as well as in reducing perceived stress levels among older adults recovering from arthroplasty surgery.

Our results showed significant improvements in all examined psychological outcomes in the experimental group, while in the control group, the psychological status did not change and the HADS total score even increased significantly. These findings are consistent with our prior research across diverse rehabilitation domains. Employing the identical procedure within the experimental group, we identified a noteworthy enhancement in the patients' psychological state [17,34]. Furthermore, within the study involving cardiac patients, we also identified a significant increase in the HADS total score, HADS-Anxiety score, and stress level score within the control group following rehabilitation [17]. These findings hold significant implications, highlighting the need to integrate psychological interventions alongside conventional rehabilitation programs.

Among the psychological outcomes assessed, we observed that perceived pain experienced a significant reduction in both groups; notably, the experimental group exhibited a significantly lower level of perceived pain. This study marks the first instance where a noteworthy reduction in pain was achieved within the group utilizing VR therapy. Among stroke patients, no significant reduction in pain was observed [34]. The observed correlation could be attributed to the interplay between pain perception and depression and anxiety. Higher levels of depression and anxiety disorders may lead to heightened pain sensitivity, thereby contributing to the relationship [35]. Pain exerts a considerable influence on the efficacy of rehabilitation programs. Notably, pain can serve as a potent motivational factor, driving patients to actively participate in their rehabilitation. When patients experience relief from or improvements in pain levels, they tend to exhibit greater adherence to prescribed exercises and therapies. Moreover, patients who effectively manage their pain often progress more expeditiously through their rehabilitation programs and are more inclined to express higher satisfaction levels with the quality of care they receive [36,37].

Another significant consideration pertains to the correlation between mental well-being and functional outcomes. Psychological disorders, encompassing conditions such as depression, anxiety, and stress, possess the capacity to exert influence across diverse dimensions of the recovery process. When characterized by heightened severity, these disorders can encumber the efficacy of rehabilitation, extend the recovery time, and reduce the quality of life experienced by patients [32,33,38,39]. Furthermore, numerous studies emphasize the imperative to identify and address mental health issues as an integral component of the rehabilitation process [40–42]. Therefore, the secondary objective of this study was to evaluate how psychological improvements influence changes in functional outcomes.

Our findings revealed significant enhancements in the functional domain within both study groups. Nevertheless, the results of a between-group comparison underline that the VR group exhibited a notably superior performance compared to the control group. Furthermore, the results indicated significant correlations, suggesting that greater differences in psychological outcomes corresponded to higher functional outcomes. In addition, psychological factors have been found to be significant predictors of functional improvements.

Depressive and anxiety disorders have been identified in the literature as potential factors that can impede the efficacy of rehabilitation programs [12]. Nevertheless, it is imperative to highlight the significance of self-efficacy, which was found to be an important determinant of rehabilitation program success [43–45]. Patients who believe in their ability to manage their condition, adhere to treatment plans, and achieve rehabilitation goals are more likely to experience positive outcomes (i.e., improved function, pain relief, and a higher quality of life). Additionally, patients with high self-efficacy may tend to experience less anxiety and depression as they believe they can overcome the challenges posed by their condition. It is noteworthy that our results revealed self-efficacy as a significant predictor of functional domain improvement in patients. This underscores the importance of integrating this often overlooked factor as an important parameter in the patient recovery process assessment [43].

Our study possesses certain limitations that warrant acknowledgment. Notably, the lack of a long-term outcome assessment in the context of recovery from arthroplasty surgery constitutes our primary limitation. This limitation may impact the comprehensiveness of our findings, particularly in assessing the enduring effects of the VR therapy over an extended period. Future research projects may benefit from incorporating follow-up outcome assessments to provide a more thorough understanding of the intervention's efficacy and durability.

5. Conclusions

VR therapy emerges as a compelling therapeutic intervention for elderly patients recovering from arthroplasty surgery, that has the potential to be considered as part of standard treatment. The integration of VR therapy into conventional rehabilitation not only enhances patients' psychological well-being but also fosters improved functional outcomes. The reduction of stress, anxiety, and pain, coupled with the enhancement of self-efficacy, serves as positive prognostic indicators for patients, both during their rehabilitation center stay and upon discharge. These factors are associated with an improved quality of life, increased self-reliance, and sustained physical improvement. Before treatment, patients often find themselves trapped in a vicious cycle where pain and limited mobility worsen their mental health, resulting in decreased physical activity. This, in turn, further deteriorates their functional status, quality of life, and long-term prognosis, potentially leading to permanent disability. The application of our proposed treatment holds the promise of breaking this cycle.

Author Contributions: Conceptualization, J.M. and J.S.-G.; methodology, J.M. and J.S.-G.; software, B.C.; validation, J.M. and B.C.; formal analysis, B.C.; investigation, J.M.; resources, J.M., A.W. and J.S.-G.; data curation, A.W.; visualization, B.C.; writing—original draft preparation, J.M., B.C. and A.W.; writing—review and editing, J.M., R.G. and J.S.-G.; supervision, R.G. and J.S.-G.; project administration, R.G.; funding acquisition, R.G. All authors have read and agreed to the published version of the manuscript.

Funding: This research received no external funding.

Institutional Review Board Statement: The study was conducted in accordance with the Declaration of Helsinki, and approved by the Bioethics Committee at the Wroclaw Medical University (Wroclaw, Poland) under the reference number 119/KB/2023 (27 June 2023).

Informed Consent Statement: Written informed consent was obtained from all subjects involved in the study.

Data Availability Statement: Data are available upon reasonable request to the corresponding author.

Conflicts of Interest: The authors declare no conflict of interest.

References

1. Quicke, J.G.; Conaghan, P.G.; Corp, N.; Peat, G. Osteoarthritis Year in Review 2021: Epidemiology & Therapy. *Osteoarthr. Cartil.* **2022**, *30*, 196–206. [CrossRef]
2. Ackerman, I.N.; Buchbinder, R.; March, L. Global Burden of Disease Study 2019: An Opportunity to Understand the Growing Prevalence and Impact of Hip, Knee, Hand and Other Osteoarthritis in Australia. *Intern. Med. J.* **2023**, *53*, 1875–1882. [CrossRef]
3. World Health Organization Osteoarthritis. Available online: https://www.who.int/news-room/fact-sheets/detail/osteoarthritis (accessed on 26 September 2023).
4. Sambamoorthi, U.; Shah, D.; Zhao, X. Healthcare Burden of Depression in Adults with Arthritis. *Expert. Rev. Pharmacoecon Outcomes Res.* **2017**, *17*, 53–65. [CrossRef]
5. Wang, S.-T.; Ni, G.-X. Depression in Osteoarthritis: Current Understanding. *Neuropsychiatr. Dis. Treat.* **2022**, *18*, 375–389. [CrossRef]
6. Agarwal, P.; Sambamoorthi, U. Healthcare Expenditures Associated with Depression among Individuals with Osteoarthritis: Post-Regression Linear Decomposition Approach. *J. Gen. Intern. Med.* **2015**, *30*, 1803–1811. [CrossRef] [PubMed]
7. Briggs, A.M.; Cross, M.J.; Hoy, D.G.; Sànchez-Riera, L.; Blyth, F.M.; Woolf, A.D.; March, L. Musculoskeletal Health Conditions Represent a Global Threat to Healthy Aging: A Report for the 2015 World Health Organization World Report on Ageing and Health. *Gerontologist* **2016**, *56*, S243–S255. [CrossRef] [PubMed]

8. Shalhoub, M.; Anaya, M.; Deek, S.; Zaben, A.H.; Abdalla, M.A.; Jaber, M.M.; Koni, A.A.; Zyoud, S.H. The Impact of Pain on Quality of Life in Patients with Osteoarthritis: A Cross-Sectional Study from Palestine. *BMC Musculoskelet. Disord.* **2022**, *23*, 248. [CrossRef] [PubMed]
9. Bonanni, R.; Cariati, I.; Tancredi, V.; Iundusi, R.; Gasbarra, E.; Tarantino, U. Chronic Pain in Musculoskeletal Diseases: Do You Know Your Enemy? *J. Clin. Med.* **2022**, *11*, 2609. [CrossRef]
10. Roughan, W.H.; Campos, A.I.; García-Marín, L.M.; Cuéllar-Partida, G.; Lupton, M.K.; Hickie, I.B.; Medland, S.E.; Wray, N.R.; Byrne, E.M.; Ngo, T.T.; et al. Comorbid Chronic Pain and Depression: Shared Risk Factors and Differential Antidepressant Effectiveness. *Front. Psychiatry* **2021**, *12*, 643609. [CrossRef] [PubMed]
11. Zheng, C.J.; Van Drunen, S.; Egorova-Brumley, N. Neural Correlates of Co-Occurring Pain and Depression: An Activation-Likelihood Estimation (ALE) Meta-Analysis and Systematic Review. *Transl. Psychiatry* **2022**, *12*, 196. [CrossRef] [PubMed]
12. Leo, A.J.; Schuelke, M.J.; Hunt, D.M.; Metzler, J.P.; Miller, J.P.; Areán, P.A.; Armbrecht, M.A.; Cheng, A.L. A Digital Mental Health Intervention in an Orthopedic Setting for Patients with Symptoms of Depression and/or Anxiety: Feasibility Prospective Cohort Study. *JMIR Form. Res.* **2022**, *6*, e34889. [CrossRef] [PubMed]
13. Hampton, M.; Riley, E.; Garneti, N.; Anderson, A.; Wembridge, K. The Orthopaedic Waiting List Crisis. *Bone Jt. Open* **2021**, *2*, 530–534. [CrossRef] [PubMed]
14. Patten, R.K.; Asilioglu, A.; Levinger, I.; Tacey, A.; Pascoe, M.; Tran, P.; McKenna, M.J.; Said, C.M.; Coric, N.; De Gori, M.; et al. Prevalence of Diagnosable Depression in Patients Awaiting Orthopaedic Specialist Consultation: A Cross-Sectional Analysis. *BMC Musculoskelet. Disord.* **2023**, *24*, 599. [CrossRef] [PubMed]
15. National Guideline Centre (UK). *Evidence Review for Inpatient Hip and Knee Postoperative Rehabilitation: Joint Replacement (Primary): Hip, Knee and Shoulder: Evidence Review P*; NICE Evidence Reviews Collection; National Institute for Health and Care Excellence (NICE): London, UK, 2020; ISBN 978-1-4731-3722-6.
16. Gazendam, A.; Zhu, M.; Chang, Y.; Phillips, S.; Bhandari, M. Virtual Reality Rehabilitation Following Total Knee Arthroplasty: A Systematic Review and Meta-Analysis of Randomized Controlled Trials. *Knee Surg. Sports Traumatol. Arthrosc.* **2022**, *30*, 2548–2555. [CrossRef] [PubMed]
17. Szczepańska-Gieracha, J.; Jóźwik, S.; Cieślik, B.; Mazurek, J.; Gajda, R. Immersive Virtual Reality Therapy as a Support for Cardiac Rehabilitation: A Pilot Randomized-Controlled Trial. *Cyberpsychol. Behav. Soc. Netw.* **2021**, *24*, 543–549. [CrossRef]
18. Peng, L.; Zeng, Y.; Wu, Y.; Si, H.; Shen, B. Virtual Reality-Based Rehabilitation in Patients Following Total Knee Arthroplasty: A Systematic Review and Meta-Analysis of Randomized Controlled Trials. *Chin. Med. J.* **2021**, *135*, 153–163. [CrossRef]
19. Gumaa, M.; Rehan Youssef, A. Is Virtual Reality Effective in Orthopedic Rehabilitation? A Systematic Review and Meta-Analysis. *Phys. Ther.* **2019**, *99*, 1304–1325. [CrossRef]
20. García-Sánchez, M.; García-Robles, P.; Osuna-Pérez, M.C.; Lomas-Vega, R.; Obrero-Gaitán, E.; Cortés-Pérez, I. Effectiveness of Virtual Reality-Based Early Postoperative Rehabilitation after Total Knee Arthroplasty: A Systematic Review with Meta-Analysis of Randomized Controlled Trials. *Appl. Sci.* **2023**, *13*, 4597. [CrossRef]
21. Birckhead, B.; Khalil, C.; Liu, X.; Conovitz, S.; Rizzo, A.; Danovitch, I.; Bullock, K.; Spiegel, B. Recommendations for Methodology of Virtual Reality Clinical Trials in Health Care by an International Working Group: Iterative Study. *JMIR Ment. Health* **2019**, *6*, e11973. [CrossRef]
22. Matthews, W.J. Ericksonian Approaches to Hypnosis and Therapy: Where Are We Now? *Int. J. Clin. Exp. Hypn.* **2000**, *48*, 418–426, discussion 433–437. [CrossRef]
23. Cieślik, B.; Juszko, K.; Kiper, P.; Szczepańska-Gieracha, J. Immersive Virtual Reality as Support for the Mental Health of Elderly Women: A Randomized Controlled Trial. *Virtual Real.* **2023**, *27*, 2227–2235. [CrossRef] [PubMed]
24. Bjelland, I.; Dahl, A.A.; Haug, T.T.; Neckelmann, D. The Validity of the Hospital Anxiety and Depression Scale. An Updated Literature Review. *J. Psychosom. Res.* **2002**, *52*, 69–77. [CrossRef] [PubMed]
25. Cohen, S. Perceived Stress in a Probability Sample of the United States. In *The Social Psychology of Health*; The Claremont Symposium on Applied Social Psychology; Sage Publications, Inc.: Thousand Oaks, CA, USA, 1988; pp. 31–67. ISBN 978-0-8039-3162-6.
26. Luszczynska, A.; Scholz, U.; Schwarzer, R. The General Self-Efficacy Scale: Multicultural Validation Studies. *J. Psychol.* **2005**, *139*, 439–457. [CrossRef] [PubMed]
27. Collin, C.; Wade, D.T.; Davies, S.; Horne, V. The Barthel ADL Index: A Reliability Study. *Int. Disabil. Stud.* **1988**, *10*, 61–63. [CrossRef] [PubMed]
28. Collen, F.M.; Wade, D.T.; Robb, G.F.; Bradshaw, C.M. The Rivermead Mobility Index: A Further Development of the Rivermead Motor Assessment. *Int. Disabil. Stud.* **1991**, *13*, 50–54. [CrossRef] [PubMed]
29. Lauretani, F.; Ticinesi, A.; Gionti, L.; Prati, B.; Nouvenne, A.; Tana, C.; Meschi, T.; Maggio, M. Short-Physical Performance Battery (SPPB) Score Is Associated with Falls in Older Outpatients. *Aging Clin. Exp. Res.* **2019**, *31*, 1435–1442. [CrossRef]
30. Plopa, M.; Makarowski, R. *The Perception of Stress Questionnaire. Manual*; Vizja Press & IT: Warsaw, Poland, 2010; ISBN 978-83-61086-79-6.
31. Faul, F.; Erdfelder, E.; Lang, A.-G.; Buchner, A. G*Power 3: A Flexible Statistical Power Analysis Program for the Social, Behavioral, and Biomedical Sciences. *Behav. Res. Methods* **2007**, *39*, 175–191. [CrossRef]

32. Vincent, H.K.; Hagen, J.E.; Zdziarski-Horodyski, L.A.; Patrick, M.; Sadasivan, K.K.; Guenther, R.; Vasilopoulos, T.; Sharififar, S.; Horodyski, M. Patient-Reported Outcomes Measurement Information System Outcome Measures and Mental Health in Orthopaedic Trauma Patients During Early Recovery. *J. Orthop. Trauma.* **2018**, *32*, 467–473. [CrossRef]
33. Flanigan, D.C.; Everhart, J.S.; Glassman, A.H. Psychological Factors Affecting Rehabilitation and Outcomes Following Elective Orthopaedic Surgery. *J. Am. Acad. Orthop. Surg.* **2015**, *23*, 563–570. [CrossRef]
34. Kiper, P.; Przysiężna, E.; Cieślik, B.; Broniec-Siekaniec, K.; Kucińska, A.; Szczygieł, J.; Turek, K.; Gajda, R.; Szczepańska-Gieracha, J. Effects of Immersive Virtual Therapy as a Method Supporting Recovery of Depressive Symptoms in Post-Stroke Rehabilitation: Randomized Controlled Trial. *Clin. Interv. Aging* **2022**, *17*, 1673–1685. [CrossRef]
35. Peters, M.L. Emotional and Cognitive Influences on Pain Experience. *Mod. Trends Pharmacopsychiatry* **2015**, *30*, 138–152. [CrossRef]
36. Lin, I.; Wiles, L.; Waller, R.; Goucke, R.; Nagree, Y.; Gibberd, M.; Straker, L.; Maher, C.G.; O'Sullivan, P.P.B. What Does Best Practice Care for Musculoskeletal Pain Look like? Eleven Consistent Recommendations from High-Quality Clinical Practice Guidelines: Systematic Review. *Br. J. Sports Med.* **2020**, *54*, 79–86. [CrossRef]
37. Moseley, G.L.; Vlaeyen, J.W.S. Beyond Nociception: The Imprecision Hypothesis of Chronic Pain. *Pain* **2015**, *156*, 35–38. [CrossRef]
38. Vincent, H.K.; Horodyski, M.; Vincent, K.R.; Brisbane, S.T.; Sadasivan, K.K. Psychological Distress After Orthopedic Trauma: Prevalence in Patients and Implications for Rehabilitation. *PM&R* **2015**, *7*, 978–989. [CrossRef]
39. Shamim, Q.; Fatima, L.; Albab, H. The Impact of Psychological Factors on Rehabilitation Outcomes in Patients with Chronic Pain. *J. Health Rehabil. Res.* **2023**, *3*, 48–52.
40. Cherkin, D.C.; Sherman, K.J.; Balderson, B.H.; Cook, A.J.; Anderson, M.L.; Hawkes, R.J.; Hansen, K.E.; Turner, J.A. Effect of Mindfulness-Based Stress Reduction vs Cognitive Behavioral Therapy or Usual Care on Back Pain and Functional Limitations in Adults with Chronic Low Back Pain: A Randomized Clinical Trial. *JAMA* **2016**, *315*, 1240–1249. [CrossRef] [PubMed]
41. Gil, J.A.; Goodman, A.D.; Mulcahey, M.K. Psychological Factors Affecting Outcomes after Elective Shoulder Surgery. *J. Am. Acad. Orthop. Surg.* **2018**, *26*, e98–e104. [CrossRef] [PubMed]
42. Sheikhzadeh, A.; Wertli, M.M.; Weiner, S.S.; Rasmussen-Barr, E.; Weiser, S. Do Psychological Factors Affect Outcomes in Musculoskeletal Shoulder Disorders? A Systematic Review. *BMC Musculoskelet. Disord.* **2021**, *22*, 560. [CrossRef] [PubMed]
43. Szczepańska-Gieracha, J.; Mazurek, J. The Role of Self-Efficacy in the Recovery Process of Stroke Survivors. *Psychol. Res. Behav. Manag.* **2020**, *13*, 897–906. [CrossRef]
44. Marconcin, P.; Espanha, M.; Teles, J.; Bento, P.; Campos, P.; André, R.; Yázigi, F. A Randomized Controlled Trial of a Combined Self-Management and Exercise Intervention for Elderly People with Osteoarthritis of the Knee: The PLE2NO Program. *Clin. Rehabil.* **2018**, *32*, 223–232. [CrossRef]
45. Khachian, A.; Seyedoshohadaei, M.; Haghani, H.; Amiri, F. Effect of Self-Management Program on Outcome of Adult Knee Osteoarthritis. *Int. J. Orthop. Trauma. Nurs.* **2020**, *39*, 100797. [CrossRef] [PubMed]

Disclaimer/Publisher's Note: The statements, opinions and data contained in all publications are solely those of the individual author(s) and contributor(s) and not of MDPI and/or the editor(s). MDPI and/or the editor(s) disclaim responsibility for any injury to people or property resulting from any ideas, methods, instructions or products referred to in the content.

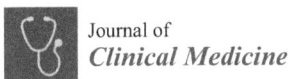

Article

Decline in Walking Independence and Related Factors in Hospitalization for Dialysis Initiation: A Retrospective Cohort Study

Yuma Hirano [1,*], Tomoyuki Fujikura [2], Kenichi Kono [3], Naro Ohashi [2], Tomoya Yamaguchi [1], Wataru Hanajima [1], Hideo Yasuda [2] and Katsuya Yamauchi [1]

1. Department of Rehabilitation Medicine, Hamamatsu University Hospital, 1-20-1 Handayama, Higashi-ku, Hamamatsu City 431-3192, Japan
2. First Department of Medicine, Hamamatsu University Hospital, 1-20-1 Handayama, Higashi-ku, Hamamatsu City 431-3192, Japan
3. Department of Physical Therapy, International University of Health and Welfare School of Health Science at Narita, 4-3, Kozunomori, Narita City 286-8686, Japan
* Correspondence: yuma.h.pt@gmail.com; Tel.: +81-53-435-2746; Fax: +81-053-435-2747

Citation: Hirano, Y.; Fujikura, T.; Kono, K.; Ohashi, N.; Yamaguchi, T.; Hanajima, W.; Yasuda, H.; Yamauchi, K. Decline in Walking Independence and Related Factors in Hospitalization for Dialysis Initiation: A Retrospective Cohort Study. *J. Clin. Med.* **2022**, *11*, 6589. https://doi.org/10.3390/jcm11216589

Academic Editor: Mashahiro Kohzuki

Received: 8 October 2022
Accepted: 4 November 2022
Published: 7 November 2022

Publisher's Note: MDPI stays neutral with regard to jurisdictional claims in published maps and institutional affiliations.

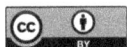

Copyright: © 2022 by the authors. Licensee MDPI, Basel, Switzerland. This article is an open access article distributed under the terms and conditions of the Creative Commons Attribution (CC BY) license (https://creativecommons.org/licenses/by/4.0/).

Abstract: Patients with chronic kidney disease require intervention planning because their physical function declines with worsening disease. Providers can work closely with patients during the induction phase of dialysis. This single-center, retrospective observational study aimed to investigate the rate of decline in walking independence during the induction phase of dialysis and the factors that influence this decline, and to provide information on prevention and treatment during this period. Of the 354 patients who were newly initiated on hemodialysis between April 2018 and January 2022, 285 were included in the analysis. The functional independence measure-walking score was used to sort patients into decreased walking independence (DWI; n = 46) and maintained walking independence (no DWI; n = 239) groups, and patient characteristics were compared. After adjusting for various factors by logistic regression analysis, we observed that age, high Charlson comorbidity index (CCI), C-reactive protein, and emergency dialysis start (EDS) were significant predictors of DWI. Even during the very short period of dialysis induction, as many as 16.1% of patients had DWI, which was associated with older age, higher CCI, higher inflammation, and EDS. Therefore, we recommend the early identification of patients with these characteristics and early rehabilitation.

Keywords: initiation of dialysis; walking independence; rehabilitation

1. Introduction

Physical function plays a role in the life outcomes of patients undergoing dialysis. Reportedly, sarcopenia status, which reflects low muscle mass, low muscle strength, or both, is associated with the survival rate in dialysis patients [1]. This implies that it is important for dialysis patients to maintain a high physical function. Moreover, the physical function of dialysis patients gradually declines as the chronic kidney disease (CKD) stage progresses from the conservative stage [2,3], and continues to decline after the introduction of dialysis. Tamura et al. evaluated the functional status of patients with seven activities of daily living (ADLs) and reported that approximately 60% of patients had a decline in functional status at three months and approximately 75% at six months after dialysis initiation [4]. Goto et al. also evaluated the functional status of 13 ADLs and instrumental ADLs (IADLs) and reported a decline in functional status in approximately 50% of patients six months after dialysis initiation [5]. In other words, the physical function of dialysis patients declined further in increments of months after dialysis introduction.

Rehabilitation from an early stage after the introduction of dialysis may reduce the decline in physical function. However, there are few reports on rehabilitation during this period. Therefore, it is necessary to first identify which patients develop functional decline. This will allow us to identify patients who require intervention at an early stage. Therefore, we focused on the induction phase of dialysis. During this phase, medical staff can work closely with patients for a certain period daily and may be able to provide rehabilitation interventions to prevent the decline in physical function. In addition, analysis of the factors contributing to the decline in physical function during this period will enable intervention from the early stages of dialysis induction. In this study, we focused on the degree of walking independence, which reflects physical function and is greatly related to ADLs, and aimed to clarify the changes in the level of walking independence during the induction phase of dialysis and the factors that influence these changes in walking independence.

2. Materials and Methods

This retrospective observational study was based on a single-center medical record survey. Patients newly initiated on hemodialysis at Hamamatsu University Hospital between April 2018 and January 2022 were included in this study. Exclusion criteria were as follows: patients who withdrew from hemodialysis due to improvement in renal function after hemodialysis induction, patients who did not walk independently before admission, patients who died during hospitalization, and patients who were not transferred to maintenance dialysis for other reasons. All data were extracted from the patients' medical records. In this study, the induction phase of dialysis was defined as the period from just before admission for dialysis induction to the time of discharge. This study was approved by the Ethics Committee of Hamamatsu University School of Medicine (approval number: 22-035). Informed consent was obtained from all study participants.

Sex, age, height, weight, body mass index, medical history, blood data, length of hospital stay, presence of emergency dialysis start (EDS), and rehabilitation were recorded on admission. Blood data included creatinine, C-reactive protein (CRP), albumin, and hemoglobin levels and estimated glomerular filtration rate on admission. EDS was defined as the first dialysis session initiated within 24 h of nephrologist evaluation for life-threatening reasons, in accordance with previous studies [6,7]. Rehabilitation consisted primarily of strength training, aerobic exercise, and training in ADLs. Participants who received at least one rehabilitation session with a physical or occupational therapist during their hospitalization were counted as rehabilitation cases.

The Geriatric Nutritional Risk Index (GNRI) was used to assess nutritional impairment. The GNRI was developed as a screening measure of the risk for morbidity and mortality of disease in hospitalized older adult patients. The GNRI was calculated as $(14.89 + \text{albumin} (g/dL)) + (41.7 \times \text{body weight}/\text{ideal body weight})$ [8], and this nutritional assessment is widely used in maintenance dialysis patients [9–11]. Nutritional impairment was defined as a GNRI less than 92, in accordance with a previous study [12].

Comorbidities were identified and defined using the Charlson comorbidity index (CCI) [13]. This score was developed to calculate predicted mortality from comorbidities on admission. In accordance with previous studies, CCI was divided according to higher or lower than the average [14]. High-CCI participants had a score of 4 or higher. In a previous study of dialysis patients, participants with a CCI of 4 or higher were reported to have a significantly higher mortality rate than those with a CCI of 3 or lower [15].

The gait item (functional independence measure (FIM)-walking score) of the FIM was used as an index to assess walking independence. This rating chart was developed in the U.S. as the Unified Data System's capacity-loss rating method and reflects the patient's "ADLs" that are being done. The FIM-walking score was evaluated on a 7-point scale ranging from independent to full assistance. This has been widely used in previous studies for functional disability assessments [16–18]. To ensure the reliability of the assessment, two physiotherapists (YH and WH) obtained the scores independently. Any discrepancies between them were resolved through discussion and agreement. In this study, the FIM-walking score was used to classify patients as having decreased walking independence (DWI) or maintained walking independence (no DWI). DWI was defined as "a decrease in the FIM-walking score during the hospitalization period" or "an improvement in the FIM-walking score during the hospitalization period but a decrease compared to just before admission".

Statistical Analysis

Descriptive statistics were used for demographic and disease-related data. Inferential statistical analysis with t-test, chi-square test, and Mann–Whitney U test was performed to examine differences in clinical disease information, patient demographics, nutritional status, comorbidities, and blood data between patients with different walking independence statuses. Univariate and multivariate logistic regression analyses were used to determine factors affecting gait independence. Items with correlation coefficients >0.80 were excluded to remove the effects of interrelated factors and multicollinearity between independent variables. Independent variables were analyzed using two models. In Model 1, we entered items of clinical significance from among variables that showed significant differences ($p < 0.001$) between the two groups, referring to previous studies [1,19–21]. In doing so, items that could be intermediate variables for causality (length of hospitalization, FIM-walking score at hospitalization, number of rehabilitations) were excluded. Consequently, age, CCI, CRP, and EDS were entered as independent variables. In Model 2, in addition to the variables in Model 1, sex and nutritional disorders were included as potential confounding variables [3,22]. Statistical significance was set at $p < 0.05$. IBM SPSS version 26 was used for data analysis.

3. Results

3.1. Characteristics of Participants

Of the 354 patients, 285 were included in the analysis, and 69 were excluded. After classification, 46 patients were assigned to the DWI and 239 to the no DWI (Figure 1). The mean age of the participants was 68.4 years (standard deviation (SD) = 14.4); 66.7% were men, and 33.3% were women. Of the participants, 74.0% had hypertension, 41.4% had diabetes, 33.0% had hyperlipidemia, and 43.2% had a history of cardiovascular disease. The median length of hospitalization was 14 days, and 16.1% of the patients had DWI. From admission to discharge, the percentage of FIM-walking score 1 decreased and the percentage of 7 increased (Figure 2). Of the patients, 37.2% underwent EDS. Acute exacerbation of CKD was the reason for EDS in 74.5% of cases, AKI in 17.0%, and other reasons in 8.5%. Other reasons included sepsis and multiorgan failure. In addition, approximately 8% of patients with planned dialysis start and approximately 30% of patients with EDS showed a decrease in walking independence (Figure 3). Only 29.5% of patients were rehabilitated during hospitalization. The mean GNRI was 78.2 (SD = 27.8), and 57.4% of the patients were nutritionally impaired (Table 1).

Table 1. Patients' characteristics (N = 285).

Variable	N, Mean, Median
Sex	
Male [N, (%)]	190 (66.7)
Female [N, (%)]	95 (33.3)
Age (years)	68.4 ± 14.4
Median length of hospitalization (days)	14 (12–28)
DWI [N, (%)]	46 (16.1)
Hypertension [N, (%)]	211 (74.0)
Diabetes mellitus [N, (%)]	118 (41.4)
Hyperlipidemia [N, (%)]	94 (33.0)
Previous history of CVD [N, (%)]	123 (43.2)
Number of rehabilitations [N, (%)]	84 (29.5)
Emergency dialysis start [N, (%)]	106 (37.2)
Creatinine (mg/dL)	7.7 ± 3.0
eGFR (mL/min/1.73 m^2)	7.1 ± 6.3
Geriatric Nutritional Risk Index	78.2 ± 27.8
Malnutrition	159 (57.4)

Data are expressed as percentage in parentheses or as the mean ± SD or median (IQR). *CVD*, cardiovascular disease; *eGFR*, estimated glomerular filtration rate. Nutritional impairment was defined as a GNRI less than 92.

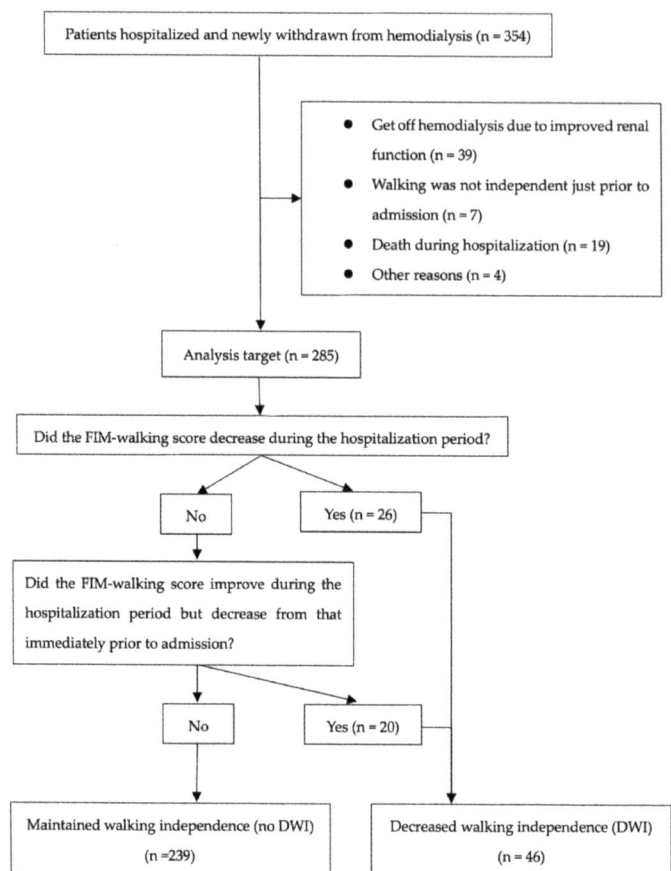

Figure 1. Selection of participants for analysis and assignment to the two groups.

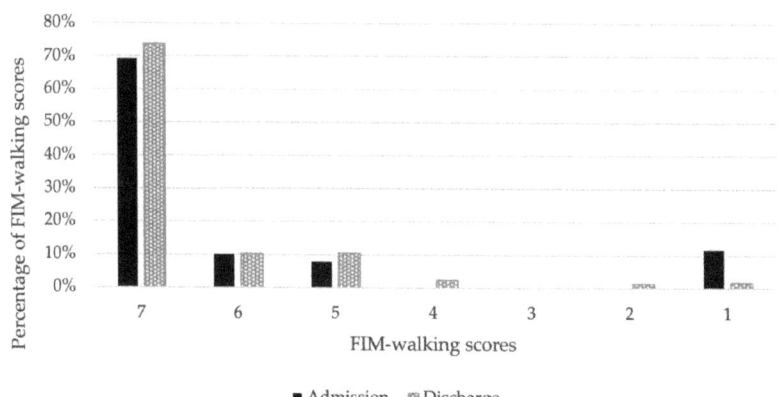

Figure 2. Changes in FIM-walking scores between admission and discharge. On admission, 69% had an FIM-walking score of 7, which increased to 74% at discharge. An FIM-walking score of 1 was present in 12% of patients on admission, but decreased to 2% at discharge.

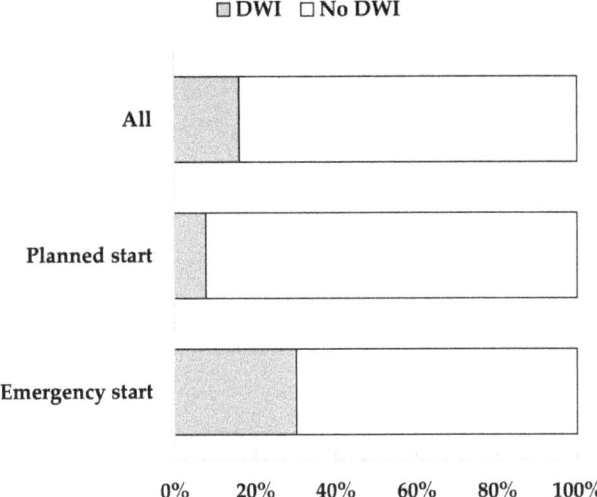

Figure 3. Percentage of decreased walking independence (DWI) in all patients, patients with planned dialysis start, and patients with emergency dialysis start (EDS). The figure shows the percentage of patients with DWI. Walking independence decreased in 16% of all patients, 8% of patients with planned dialysis start, and 30% of patients with EDS.

3.2. Differences between Patients with and without DWI

Patients with DWI were older ($p < 0.001$) and had a longer length of stay ($p < 0.001$). They also had higher rates of rehabilitation ($p < 0.001$), EDS ($p < 0.001$), and nutritional disorders ($p < 0.05$), and a high CCI ($p < 0.001$). Blood tests showed higher CRP levels ($p < 0.001$) (Table 2).

Table 2. Differences between DWI and no DWI patients.

	DWI (N = 46)	No DWI (N = 239)	p-Value
Male [N, (%)]	35 (76.1)	155 (64.9)	0.139
Age (years)	78.5 ± 8.2	66.4 ± 14.6	<0.001 *
Height (cm)	158.0 ± 8.1	159.6 ± 9.4	0.287
Body weight (kg)	56.2 ± 10.0	61.2 ± 15.9	0.127
BMI (kg/m^2)	22.5 ± 3.6	23.9 ± 5.1	0.213
Median length of hospitalization (days)	34 (26–64)	13 (12–22)	<0.001 *
FIM-walking score at hospitalization < 6 [N, (%)]	27 (58.7)	31 (13.0)	<0.001 *
Number of rehabilitations [N, (%)]	33 (71.7)	51 (21.3)	<0.001 *
EDS [N, (%)]	32 (69.6)	74 (31.0)	<0.001 *
Malnutrition [N, (%)]	31 (72.1)	128 (54.7)	0.034 *
High CCI [N, (%)]	37 (80.4)	108 (45.2)	<0.001*
CRP (mg/dL)	0.43 (0.16–0.57)	0.08 (0.03–0.17)	<0.001 *
Alb (g/dL)	3.5 (3.1–3.8)	3.5 (3.2–3.9)	0.145
Hb (g/dL)	9.4 (9.1–10.0)	9.6 (9.0–10.3)	0.645

Data are expressed as percentage in parentheses or as the mean ± SD or median (IQR). *BMI*, body mass index; *EDS*, emergency dialysis start; *CCI*, Charlson comorbidity index; *CRP*, C-reactive protein; *Alb*, albumin; *Hb*, hemoglobin. * Statistically significant.

3.3. Factors Associated with DWI

Univariate logistic regression analysis showed that a reduction in walking independence was significantly associated with age (odds ratio (OR): 1.075, 95% confidence interval (CI): 1.040–1.112), high CCI (OR: 4.987, 95% CI: 2.305–10.788), CRP (OR: 1.296, 95% CI: 1.142–1.471), EDS (OR: 5.097, 95% CI: 2.568–10.113), and malnutrition (OR: 2.139, 95% CI: 1.047–4.370). Multivariate logistic regression analysis showed that age (OR: 1.089, 95% CI: 1.045–1.135), high CCI (OR: 4.540, 95% CI: 1.874–11.001), CRP (OR: 1.163, 95% CI: 1.049–1.291), and EDS (OR: 2.720, 95% CI: 1.217–6.080) remained significant predictors.

Furthermore, after adjusting for factors in Model 2, age (OR: 1.123, 95% CI: 1.067–1.182), high CCI (OR: 4.706, 95% CI: 1.768–12.522), CRP (OR: 1.180, 95% CI: 1.057–1.317), and EDS (OR: 2.957, 95% CI: 1.239–7.059) remained significant predictors (Table 3).

Table 3. Factors related to decreased walking independence.

	Univariate Regression			Multiple Logistic					
				Model 1			Model 2		
	OR	95% CI	p-Value	OR	95% CI	p-Value	OR	95% CI	p-Value
Age	1.075	1.040–1.112	<0.001 *	1.089	1.045–1.135	<0.001 *	1.123	1.067–1.182	<0.001 *
High CCI	4.987	2.305–10.788	<0.001 *	4.540	1.874–11.001	0.001 *	4.706	1.768–12.522	0.002 *
CRP	1.296	1.142–1.471	<0.001 *	1.163	1.049–1.291	0.004 *	1.180	1.057–1.317	0.003 *
EDS	5.097	2.568–10.113	<0.001 *	2.720	1.217–6.080	0.015 *	2.957	1.239–7.059	0.015 *
Sex (male)	0.580	0.280–1.201	0.142				0.839	0.336–2.093	0.706
Malnutrition	2.139	1.047–4.370	0.037 *				1.535	0.645–3.654	0.332

Multivariate logistic regression analysis. CCI, Charlson comorbidity index; CRP, C-reactive protein; EDS, emergency dialysis start; OR, odds ratio; CI, confidence interval. Model 1: Variables with significant differences ($p < 0.001$) that were clearly different between the two groups were selected. However, variables (length of hospitalization, FIM-walking score at hospitalization, number of rehabilitations) that could be "intermediate variables in a causal chain of causes and effects" were excluded. Model 2: Sex and malnutrition were used as adjustment variables. * Statistically significant.

4. Discussion

In this study, we investigated the decline in walking independence during the induction phase of dialysis and identified factors associated with this decline. The analysis showed that 16.1% of the patients had DWI during the induction phase of dialysis, which lasted approximately 14 days. Risk factors for DWI include older age, more severe comorbidities, higher inflammatory levels, and EDS. Interestingly, approximately 8% of patients with a planned dialysis start also had DWI. This is an important finding as it indicates that even patients in stable general conditions are at risk of a short-term decline in walking independence.

Patients with CKD are more likely to have reduced ADLs through loss of muscle mass, and the presence of CKD has been reported to be independently associated with functional impairment, IADL impairment, and basic ADL impairment [23]. The prevalence of sarcopenia in patients with CKD is high (approximately 50%) and is associated with a reduction in physical function [24–26]. In addition, patients with CKD have decreased muscle mass due to increased protein catabolism and nutrient loss due to dialysis, leading to impaired ADLs and IADLs [27]. Similarly, during the induction phase of dialysis, functional status decreases between three and six months after dialysis induction [4,5]. This suggests that the physical function and ADLs of patients with CKD may deteriorate from months to years after the introduction of dialysis.

On the other hand, this study focused on the induction phase of dialysis and, therefore, examined an even shorter period, approximately 14 days. It is clinically important to note that 16.1% of the patients had a decrease in walking independence during this short period. Early rehabilitation after dialysis induction is a potential solution to this problem. In patients with conservative CKD and those undergoing stable dialysis, exercise has been shown to improve muscle strength, exercise tolerance, and quality of life [28,29]. The effectiveness of early rehabilitation has been reported in other areas. Randomized controlled trials of patients with acute stroke have reported that early rehabilitation intervention after stroke onset was associated with a shorter time to independent ambulation and better physical function and ADLs at three and 12 months [30]. Furthermore, early rehabilitation of patients with acute nephrotic syndrome has been reported to improve their motor endurance and SF-36 physical function items without adversely affecting their disease status [31]. However, few studies have examined the effectiveness of rehabilitation during the early post-dialysis period. In this study, only approximately 30% of patients received rehabilitation. Patients immediately before dialysis induction showed a marked decrease in physical activity due to uremia, fluid overload, and renal anemia. Thus, early rehabilitation interventions to correct this decline in physical activity may be beneficial in preventing disuse syndrome and maintaining ADLs.

Our study demonstrated that older age, severity of comorbidities, higher inflammatory levels, and EDS were associated with decreased walking independence.

Generally, ADL independence in older adults decreases with age, which is also true for dialysis patients [5]. In addition to aging, CKD is known to exacerbate frailty and sarcopenia [32], and aging is a very important factor affecting ADLs in chronic inflammatory diseases.

Population aging has led to an increase in the number of patients with comorbidities, with approximately 65% of older people having three or more comorbidities [33]. The CCI is the most commonly used measure to assess comorbidity and is also commonly used in patients with conservative CKD and dialysis patients [34–36]. In dialysis patients, CCI is a strong predictor of mortality, and in older patients with conservative CKD, a higher comorbidity index is associated with functional decline [21,37]. Comorbidities are associated with the severity of depression, anxiety, and fatigue, which reduce the amount of physical activity in patients. This may decrease physical function, which in turn affect the degree of walking independence [38].The presence of comorbidities has received increasing attention worldwide [39] and should also be noted in patients undergoing dialysis induction.

Inflammatory markers such as interleukin-6 and tumor necrosis factor-α increase the factors associated with skeletal muscle destruction in dialysis patients, such as myostatin [40]. They are also associated with low muscle strength in patients on dialysis [1], and inflammation has been implicated in impaired physical function, corroborating previous studies. This inflammation improves with regular exercise [41] and is an important factor that may be targeted for rehabilitation therapy in the future.

Patients with CKD need to be managed so that they can be transferred to dialysis in the best possible condition. However, dialysis is often initiated on an emergency basis [20]. Furthermore, a large epidemiological study in France reported that EDS has an independent impact on mortality [42]. The main causes of EDS are acute systemic diseases, such as cardiovascular disease, sepsis, and autoimmune diseases [43]. Therefore, EDS is an important factor affecting poor prognosis, representing the poor general condition of patients, and in this study, it may have affected the level of walking independence by reflecting the underlying poor general condition of the patients.

It is clinically difficult to provide rehabilitation interventions for more than 40,000 patients undergoing dialysis induction annually in Japan. Therefore, it is necessary for healthcare providers to know in advance which characteristics of patients with CKD need rehabilitation during the induction phase of dialysis and to identify and intervene in patients with a high need for rehabilitation at an early stage. Patients with the characteristics identified in this study (i.e., older age, more comorbidities, higher inflammation, and EDS) are at a high risk of DWI in a short period of time, and it is important to start rehabilitation intervention at an early stage.

The strength of our study is that we focused on a short period during dialysis induction. Similar reports on patients with CKD prior to dialysis conversion and on stable dialysis patients are scattered. However, only few reports describing this period have been published. This study suggests that this period may have an important impact on patients' future ADLs and calls for new interventions, including rehabilitation.

Our study had several limitations. First, some confounders remained unmeasured. Although we attempted to cover the adjustment for confounders related to physical function reported in previous studies, more detailed adjustments need to be considered in future prospective studies. Second, the FIM-walking score assessment was based on medical records, which may be inaccurate for estimating walking independence. To address this issue, two physiotherapists independently conducted the assessment, and we attempted to make it as objective as possible. Third, the GNRI may not accurately reflect the nutritional status of patients. During the induction phase of dialysis, patients may be overweight due to fluid retention, which may lead to an overestimation of the GNRI. However, an accurate nutritional assessment index has not yet been established for the induction phase of dialysis. Therefore, the GNRI, an established index for maintenance dialysis patients, was used in this study. Fourth, 19 of the 69 patients excluded died during hospitalization. The possibility that the exclusion of these 19 cases could be a confounding factor cannot be ruled out. Fifth, our study failed to consider the impact of medical restraints on DWI. Some patients are at risk for dialysis catheter removal due to delirium, insubordination to medical staff, or other reasons. Such patients are subject to medical restraints during hospitalization, which may be one of the risk factors for DWI [44]. However, the hospital has implemented initiatives to eliminate physical restraints, and only six of 285 patients (2.1%) were identified as being physically restrained. Therefore, this study could not clearly examine the impact of physical restraints on DWI.

5. Conclusions

Even during the very short period of dialysis induction, as many as 16.1% of patients had DWI, which was associated with older age, higher CCI, higher inflammation, and EDS. Therefore, we recommend the early identification of patients with these characteristics and early rehabilitation to reduce the decline in physical function and ADLs.

Author Contributions: Study conception and design, participant recruitment, data collection, data interpretation, and drafting of the paper, all authors; literature review and statistical analysis, Y.H., T.F., K.K., T.Y., W.H. and N.O.; supervision, H.Y. and K.Y. All authors have read and agreed to the published version of the manuscript.

Funding: This research received no external funding.

Institutional Review Board Statement: This study was approved by the Ethics Committee of Hamamatsu University School of Medicine (acknowledgment number: 22-035), and all study procedures were performed in accordance with the Declaration of Helsinki.

Informed Consent Statement: Informed consent was obtained from all subjects involved in the study.

Data Availability Statement: The data presented in this study are available on request from the corresponding author. The data are not publicly available because they are the property of the Institute of Hamamatsu University Hospital, Japan.

Acknowledgments: The authors thank the patients at Hamamatsu University Hospital who participated in this study. The authors would also like to thank the staff and nurses for their excellent care of the patients.

Conflicts of Interest: The authors declare no conflict of interest.

References

1. Isoyama, N.; Qureshi, A.R.; Avesani, C.M.; Lindholm, B.; Barany, P.; Heimburger, O.; Cederholm, T.; Stenvinkel, P.; Carrero, J.J. Comparative associations of muscle mass and muscle strength with mortality in dialysis patients. *Clin. J. Am. Soc. Nephrol.* **2014**, *9*, 1720–1728. [CrossRef] [PubMed]
2. Reese, P.P.; Cappola, A.R.; Shults, J.; Townsend, R.R.; Gadegbeku, C.A.; Anderson, C.; Baker, J.F.; Carlow, D.; Sulik, M.J.; Lo, J.C.; et al. Physical performance and frailty in chronic kidney disease. *Am. J. Nephrol.* **2013**, *38*, 307–315. [CrossRef] [PubMed]
3. Hiraki, K.; Yasuda, T.; Hotta, C.; Izawa, K.P.; Morio, Y.; Watanabe, S.; Sakurada, T.; Shibagaki, Y.; Kimura, K. Decreased physical function in pre-dialysis patients with chronic kidney disease. *Clin. Exp. Nephrol.* **2013**, *17*, 225–231. [CrossRef] [PubMed]
4. Kurella Tamura, M.; Covinsky, K.E.; Chertow, G.M.; Yaffe, K.; Landefeld, C.S.; McCulloch, C.E. Functional status of elderly adults before and after initiation of dialysis. *N. Engl. J. Med.* **2009**, *361*, 1539–1547. [CrossRef]
5. Goto, N.A.; van Loon, I.N.; Boereboom, F.T.J.; Emmelot-Vonk, M.H.; Willems, H.C.; Bots, M.L.; Gamadia, L.E.; van Bommel, E.F.H.; Van de Ven, P.J.G.; Douma, C.E.; et al. Association of initiation of maintenance dialysis with functional status and caregiver burden. *Clin. J. Am. Soc. Nephrol.* **2019**, *14*, 1039–1047. [CrossRef]
6. Magalhaes, L.P.; Dos Reis, L.M.; Graciolli, F.G.; Pereira, B.J.; de Oliveira, R.B.; de Souza, A.A.; Moyses, R.M.; Elias, R.M.; Jorgetti, V. Predictive factors of one-year mortality in a cohort of patients undergoing urgent-start hemodialysis. *PLoS ONE* **2017**, *12*, e0167895. [CrossRef]
7. Raffray, M.; Vigneau, C.; Couchoud, C.; Bayat, S. Predialysis care trajectories of patients with ESKD starting dialysis in emergency in France. *Kidney Int. Rep.* **2021**, *6*, 156–167. [CrossRef]

8. Bouillanne, O.; Morineau, G.; Dupont, C.; Coulombel, I.; Vincent, J.P.; Nicolis, I.; Benazeth, S.; Cynober, L.; Aussel, C. Geriatric Nutritional Risk Index: A new index for evaluating at-risk elderly medical patients. *Am. J. Clin. Nutr.* **2005**, *82*, 777–783. [CrossRef]
9. Mahjoub, F.; Mizouri, R.; Ben Amor, N.; Bacha, M.M.; Khedher, A.; Lahmar, I.; Jamoussi, H. Prevalence of malnutrition for elderly hemodialysis patients. *Tunis. Med.* **2019**, *97*, 588–594.
10. Yoshida, M.; Nakashima, A.; Doi, S.; Maeda, K.; Ishiuchi, N.; Naito, T.; Masaki, T. Lower geriatric nutritional risk index (GNRI) is associated with higher risk of fractures in patients undergoing hemodialysis. *Nutrients* **2021**, *13*, 2847. [CrossRef]
11. Kono, K.; Moriyama, Y.; Yabe, H.; Hara, A.; Ishida, T.; Yamada, T.; Nishida, Y. Relationship between malnutrition and possible sarcopenia in the AWGS 2019 consensus affecting mortality in hemodialysis patients: A prospective cohort study. *BMC Nephrol.* **2021**, *22*, 378. [CrossRef] [PubMed]
12. Yamada, K.; Furuya, R.; Takita, T.; Maruyama, Y.; Yamaguchi, Y.; Ohkawa, S.; Kumagai, H. Simplified nutritional screening tools for patients on maintenance hemodialysis. *Am. J. Clin. Nutr.* **2008**, *87*, 106–113. [CrossRef] [PubMed]
13. Charlson, M.E.; Pompei, P.; Ales, K.L.; MacKenzie, C.R. A new method of classifying prognostic comorbidity in longitudinal studies: Development and validation. *J. Chronic Dis.* **1987**, *40*, 373–383. [CrossRef]
14. Visser, W.J.; Egmond, A.; Timman, R.; Severs, D.; Hoorn, E.J. Risk factors for muscle loss in hemodialysis patients with high comorbidity. *Nutrients* **2020**, *12*, 2494. [CrossRef] [PubMed]
15. Lin, Y.T.; Wu, P.H.; Kuo, M.C.; Lin, M.Y.; Lee, T.C.; Chiu, Y.W.; Hwang, S.J.; Chen, H.C. High cost and low survival rate in high comorbidity incident elderly hemodialysis patients. *PLoS ONE* **2013**, *8*, e75318. [CrossRef] [PubMed]
16. Bland, M.D.; Sturmoski, A.; Whitson, M.; Connor, L.T.; Fucetola, R.; Huskey, T.; Corbetta, M.; Lang, C.E. Prediction of discharge walking ability from initial assessment in a stroke inpatient rehabilitation facility population. *Arch. Phys. Med. Rehabil.* **2012**, *93*, 1441–1447. [CrossRef]
17. Ii, T.; Hirano, S.; Tanabe, S.; Saitoh, E.; Yamada, J.; Mukaino, M.; Watanabe, M.; Sonoda, S.; Otaka, Y. Robot-assisted gait training using Welwalk in hemiparetic stroke patients: An effectiveness study with matched control. *J. Stroke Cerebrovasc. Dis.* **2020**, *29*, 105377. [CrossRef]
18. Snowdon, D.A.; Sounthakith, V.; Kolic, J.; Brooks, S.; Scanlon, S.; Taylor, N.F. Many inpatients may not be physically prepared for community ambulation on discharge from a publicly funded rehabilitation centre: A cross-sectional cohort study. *Disabil. Rehabil.* **2021**, *43*, 3672–3679. [CrossRef]
19. Souza, V.A.; Oliveira, D.; Barbosa, S.R.; Correa, J.; Colugnati, F.A.B.; Mansur, H.N.; Fernandes, N.; Bastos, M.G. Sarcopenia in patients with chronic kidney disease not yet on dialysis: Analysis of the prevalence and associated factors. *PLoS ONE* **2017**, *12*, e0176230. [CrossRef]
20. Shimizu, Y.; Nakata, J.; Yanagisawa, N.; Shirotani, Y.; Fukuzaki, H.; Nohara, N.; Suzuki, Y. Emergent initiation of dialysis is related to an increase in both mortality and medical costs. *Sci. Rep.* **2020**, *10*, 19638. [CrossRef]
21. Chang, J.; Hou, W.W.; Wang, Y.F.; Sun, Q.M. Main risk factors related to activities of daily living in non-dialysis patients with chronic kidney disease stage 3–5: A case-control study. *Clin. Interv. Aging* **2020**, *15*, 609–618. [CrossRef] [PubMed]
22. Bakkal, H.; Dizdar, O.S.; Erdem, S.; Kulakoglu, S.; Akcakaya, B.; Katircilar, Y.; Uludag, K. The relationship between hand grip strength and nutritional status determined by malnutrition inflammation score and biochemical parameters in hemodialysis patients. *J. Ren. Nutr.* **2020**, *30*, 548–555. [CrossRef] [PubMed]
23. Smyth, A.; Glynn, L.G.; Murphy, A.W.; Mulqueen, J.; Canavan, M.; Reddan, D.N.; O'Donnell, M. Mild chronic kidney disease and functional impairment in community-dwelling older adults. *Age Ageing* **2013**, *42*, 488–494. [CrossRef]
24. Sabatino, A.; Cuppari, L.; Stenvinkel, P.; Lindholm, B.; Avesani, C.M. Sarcopenia in chronic kidney disease: What have we learned so far? *J. Nephrol.* **2021**, *34*, 1347–1372. [CrossRef]
25. Miyazaki, S.; Iino, N.; Koda, R.; Narita, I.; Kaneko, Y. Brain-derived neurotrophic factor is associated with sarcopenia and frailty in Japanese hemodialysis patients. *Geriatr. Gerontol. Int.* **2021**, *21*, 27–33. [CrossRef] [PubMed]
26. Song, Y.R.; Kim, J.K.; Lee, H.S.; Kim, S.G.; Choi, E.K. Serum levels of protein carbonyl, a marker of oxidative stress, are associated with overhydration, sarcopenia and mortality in hemodialysis patients. *BMC Nephrol.* **2020**, *21*, 281. [CrossRef]
27. Wang, D.X.M.; Yao, J.; Zirek, Y.; Reijnierse, E.M.; Maier, A.B. Muscle mass, strength, and physical performance predicting activities of daily living: A meta-analysis. *J. Cachexia Sarcopenia Muscle* **2020**, *11*, 3–25. [CrossRef]
28. Vanden Wyngaert, K.; Van Craenenbroeck, A.H.; Van Biesen, W.; Dhondt, A.; Tanghe, A.; Van Ginckel, A.; Celie, B.; Calders, P. The effects of aerobic exercise on eGFR, blood pressure and VO2peak in patients with chronic kidney disease stages 3–4: A systematic review and meta-analysis. *PLoS ONE* **2018**, *13*, e0203662. [CrossRef]
29. Villanego, F.; Naranjo, J.; Vigara, L.A.; Cazorla, J.M.; Montero, M.E.; Garcia, T.; Torrado, J.; Mazuecos, A. Impact of physical exercise in patients with chronic kidney disease: Sistematic review and meta-analysis. *Nefrologia* **2020**, *40*, 237–252. [CrossRef]
30. Cumming, T.B.; Thrift, A.G.; Collier, J.M.; Churilov, L.; Dewey, H.M.; Donnan, G.A.; Bernhardt, J. Very early mobilization after stroke fast-tracks return to walking: Further results from the phase II AVERT randomized controlled trial. *Stroke* **2011**, *42*, 153–158. [CrossRef]
31. Iwai, K.; Hatanaka, Y.; Kawaguchi, T.; Araki, S.I. Evaluation of the safety, effectiveness, and health-related QOL impact of early rehabilitation in patients with nephrotic syndrome. *Clin. Exp. Nephrol.* **2019**, *23*, 606–612. [CrossRef] [PubMed]
32. Mori, K. Maintenance of skeletal muscle to counteract sarcopenia in patients with advanced chronic kidney disease and especially those undergoing hemodialysis. *Nutrients* **2021**, *13*, 1538. [CrossRef] [PubMed]

33. Mitsutake, S.; Ishizaki, T.; Teramoto, C.; Shimizu, S.; Ito, H. Patterns of co-occurrence of chronic disease among older adults in Tokyo, Japan. *Prev. Chronic Dis.* **2019**, *16*, E11. [CrossRef] [PubMed]
34. Lin, Y.; Yang, C.; Chu, H.; Wu, J.; Lin, K.; Shi, Y.; Wang, H.; Kong, G.; Zhang, L.; China Kidney Disease Network Working, G. Association between the Charlson Comorbidity Index and the risk of 30-day unplanned readmission in patients receiving maintenance dialysis. *BMC Nephrol.* **2019**, *20*, 363. [CrossRef] [PubMed]
35. Fois, A.; Chatrenet, A.; Cataldo, E.; Lippi, F.; Kaniassi, A.; Vigreux, J.; Froger, L.; Mongilardi, E.; Capizzi, I.; Biolcati, M.; et al. Moderate protein restriction in advanced CKD: A feasible option in an elderly, high-comorbidity population. A stepwise multiple-choice system approach. *Nutrients* **2018**, *11*, 36. [CrossRef]
36. Chae, J.W.; Song, C.S.; Kim, H.; Lee, K.B.; Seo, B.S.; Kim, D.I. Prediction of mortality in patients undergoing maintenance hemodialysis by Charlson Comorbidity Index using ICD-10 database. *Nephron Clin. Pract.* **2011**, *117*, c379–c384. [CrossRef] [PubMed]
37. Di Iorio, B.; Cillo, N.; Cirillo, M.; De Santo, N.G. Charlson Comorbidity Index is a predictor of outcomes in incident hemodialysis patients and correlates with phase angle and hospitalization. *Int. J. Artif. Organs* **2004**, *27*, 330–336. [CrossRef] [PubMed]
38. Wu, Y.H.; Hsu, Y.J.; Tzeng, W.C. Correlation between physical activity and psychological distress in patients receiving hemodialysis with comorbidities: A cross-sectional study. *Int. J. Environ. Res. Public Health* **2022**, *19*, 3972. [CrossRef] [PubMed]
39. Zhou, X.; Zhang, D. Multimorbidity in the elderly: A systematic bibliometric analysis of research output. *Int. J. Environ. Res. Public Health* **2021**, *19*, 353. [CrossRef] [PubMed]
40. Zhang, L.; Rajan, V.; Lin, E.; Hu, Z.; Han, H.Q.; Zhou, X.; Song, Y.; Min, H.; Wang, X.; Du, J.; et al. Pharmacological inhibition of myostatin suppresses systemic inflammation and muscle atrophy in mice with chronic kidney disease. *FASEB J.* **2011**, *25*, 1653–1663. [CrossRef]
41. Sovatzidis, A.; Chatzinikolaou, A.; Fatouros, I.G.; Panagoutsos, S.; Draganidis, D.; Nikolaidou, E.; Avloniti, A.; Michailidis, Y.; Mantzouridis, I.; Batrakoulis, A.; et al. Intradialytic cardiovascular exercise training alters redox status, reduces inflammation and improves physical performance in patients with chronic kidney disease. *Antioxidants* **2020**, *9*, 868. [CrossRef] [PubMed]
42. Michel, A.; Pladys, A.; Bayat, S.; Couchoud, C.; Hannedouche, T.; Vigneau, C. Deleterious effects of dialysis emergency start, insights from the French REIN registry. *BMC Nephrol.* **2018**, *19*, 233. [CrossRef] [PubMed]
43. Arulkumaran, N.; Navaratnarajah, A.; Pillay, C.; Brown, W.; Duncan, N.; McLean, A.; Taube, D.; Brown, E.A. Causes and risk factors for acute dialysis initiation among patients with end-stage kidney disease-a large retrospective observational cohort study. *Clin. Kidney J.* **2019**, *12*, 550–558. [CrossRef] [PubMed]
44. Engberg, J.; Castle, N.G.; McCaffrey, D. Physical restraint initiation in nursing homes and subsequent resident health. *Gerontologist* **2008**, *48*, 442–452. [CrossRef] [PubMed]

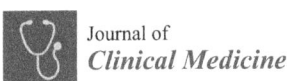

Article

Belt Electrode-Skeletal Muscle Electrical Stimulation in Older Hemodialysis Patients with Reduced Physical Activity: A Randomized Controlled Pilot Study

Midori Homma [1,2], Misa Miura [3], Yo Hirayama [2], Tamao Takahashi [1], Takahiro Miura [1], Naoki Yoshida [1], Satoshi Miyata [4], Masahiro Kohzuki [5] and Satoru Ebihara [1,*]

1. Department of Internal Medicine & Rehabilitation Science, Disability Sciences, Tohoku University Graduate School of Medicine, 1-1 Seiryo-machi, Aoba-ku, Sendai 980-8574, Japan
2. Hirayama Hospital, Hanamigawa 1494-3, Hanamigawa-ku, Chiba 262-0046, Japan
3. Faculty of Health Sciences, Tsukuba University of Technology, Kasuga 4-12-7, Tsukuba 305-8521, Japan
4. Teikyo University Graduate School of Public Health, Kaga 2-11-1, Itabashi-ku, Tokyo 173-8605, Japan
5. Yamagata Prefectural University of Health Sciences, 260 Kamiyanagi, Yamagata 990-2212, Japan
* Correspondence: satoru.ebihara.c4@tohoku.ac.jp; Tel.: +81-22-717-7353

Abstract: Background: Although patients receiving hemodialysis are more likely to develop metabolic disorders and muscle weakness at an earlier stage than healthy individuals, many older dialysis patients have difficulty establishing exercise habits to prevent these problems. Therefore, we evaluated the use of belt electrode-skeletal muscle electrical stimulation (B-SES), which can stimulate a wider area than conventional electrical muscle stimulation (EMS), to examine its application and safety in older hemodialysis patients as a means to improve lower extremity function without voluntary effort. Methods: This study was a randomized controlled trial (RCT) involving 20 older dialysis patients (>65 years old) with reduced physical activity. The control group received 12 weeks of routine care only and the intervention group received 12 weeks of B-SES during hemodialysis in addition to routine care. The primary endpoint was the 6 min walk test (6MWT) distance, while the Short Physical Performance Battery (SPPB), body composition, Functional Independence Measure (FIM), biochemistry test, and blood pressure/pulse measurements were used as secondary endpoints. Results: As a result of the 12-week B-SES intervention, no increase in creatine kinase or C-reactive protein levels was observed after the intervention in either group, and no adverse events attributed to the B-SES intervention were observed in the intervention group. Furthermore, the intervention group showed a significant improvement in the 6MWT and SPPB scores after the intervention. Conclusions: The results of this study suggest that a 12-week B-SES intervention during hemodialysis sessions safely improves 6MWT distance and SPPB scores in older patients with a reduced level of physical activity.

Keywords: electrical muscle stimulation; hemodialysis; older; chronic kidney disease; frailty; 6 min walk test; short physical performance battery

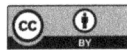

1. Introduction

Hemodialysis patients tend to have increased oxidative stress and inflammatory responses due to uremia and cachexia during the preservation period of chronic kidney disease. Furthermore, as a result of decreased metabolic efficiency and lack of nutrients, hemodialysis patients tend to develop concomitant muscle wasting, cardiovascular disease, joint disease, and arteriosclerosis [1], and more than 70% of older hemodialysis patients are frail [2]. Furthermore, more than 30% of older hemodialysis patients also exhibit sarcopenia, with a prevalence approximately three times higher than that of healthy individuals [3]. Reduced exercise/physical function and a restricted level of physical activity are characteristics of individuals with frailty and sarcopenia and are associated with a decrease in survival rate, an increase in hospitalization rate, and a decrease in the quality of life (QOL) [4,5]. In particular, hemodialysis patients with less than 4000 steps of physical activity on days without hemodialysis sessions have a high mortality risk [6], and they are prone to a reduced tolerance to exercise, muscle strength, and muscle mass, and an increased cardiovascular risk [7,8]. As such, in Japan, where the number of older hemodialysis patients continues to increase, the importance of improving physical functions has been recognized so that older hemodialysis patients can continue to live independently.

In recent years, renal rehabilitation interventions focusing on supervised exercise therapy have been reported to improve muscle strength, exercise tolerance, and inflammation in hemodialysis patients or patients with renal failure [9,10], suggesting the impact of exercise on improved QOL. However, approximately 70% of older hemodialysis patients exhibit frailty, and many patients also have multiple disorders such as locomotor disorders and cardiovascular disorders, making it difficult for many of them to establish exercise habits [11,12]. In the clinical setting, it is often difficult to apply an effective exercise routine through active exercise. Furthermore, since hemodialysis patients receive hemodialysis treatments three times a week for 4 to 5 h per session, it is difficult for them to devote the remaining time to maintaining and improving physical function.

A recent study described the application of electrical muscle stimulation (EMS) using small self-adhesive surface electrode pads in patients with moderate to severe heart failure and respiratory disease and reported improvements in muscle strength, exercise tolerance, and walking ability [13]. Furthermore, improvements in muscle strength and exercise tolerance have also been reported in hemodialysis patients through local functional improvement dependent on surface electrodes [14]. However, in these interventions, the stimulation frequency/time, intervention period, equipment used, electrode pad size, and electrical stimulation intensity have yet to be standardized; thus, supporting evidence is limited [14]. The belt electrode-skeletal muscle electrical stimulation (B-SES) device has a wider electrode attachment area than conventional EMS and is expected to be more effective in improving lower limb muscle strength and the Short Physical Performance Battery (SPPB) score in patients with orthopedic diseases and patients with severe heart failure [15,16].

Furthermore, in recent years, B-SES intervention during hemodialysis sessions has been reported to improve muscle strength, muscle mass, and Timed Up & Go test scores without adverse events in middle-aged patients [17]. However, to date, no B-SES interventions have been conducted in older hemodialysis patients who are more frail and vulnerable to adverse events. Additionally, they are more prone to muscle disuse due to immobility. Therefore, in this study, we hypothesized that B-SES intervention during hemodialysis would improve physical function without adverse events in older hemodialysis patients. Thus, our objective was to investigate the comprehensive impact of B-SES on lower limb function using the 6 min walk test (6MWT) and SPPB as outcome measures.

2. Materials and Methods

2.1. Study Design

This study was a prospective open label randomized controlled trial (RCT). Patients were enrolled at a single center and data analysis was performed in multiple centers. At the start of the study, medical records were screened, and patients were enrolled and divided into an intervention group or a control group. A permuted block design, generated by RAND function in Microsoft Excel, was used to evenly randomize the patients into the two groups. We then collected demographic data from the patients and performed baseline evaluations one week before the intervention. The following variables were evaluated at baseline: physical function (as assessed by the 6MWT and SPPB), post-dialysis weight (dry weight), body composition (skeletal muscle mass of the extremities), activities of daily living (ADL), blood biochemistry, and blood pressure/pulse. Hypertension was diagnosed if, when measured on two different days, both systolic blood pressure (SBP) readings were $\geq$140 mmHg and/or both diastolic blood pressure readings (DBP) were

≥90 mmHg. Dyslipidemia was diagnosed if low-density lipoprotein cholesterol levels were ≥100 mg/dL, high-density lipoprotein cholesterol levels were >40 mg/dL, or triglyceride levels were ≥150 mg/dL. Diabetes mellitus was diagnosed if fasting blood glucose levels were ≥126 mg/dL. We also collected data concerning history of ischemic heart diseases and cerebrovascular diseases from the patients' medical records.

After completion of the 12-week intervention, the same variables were measured again within 1 week (Figure 1). The study period ran from 24 June 2020 to 31 March 2022, and the patient enrollment period was from 24 June 2020 to 31 December 2021.

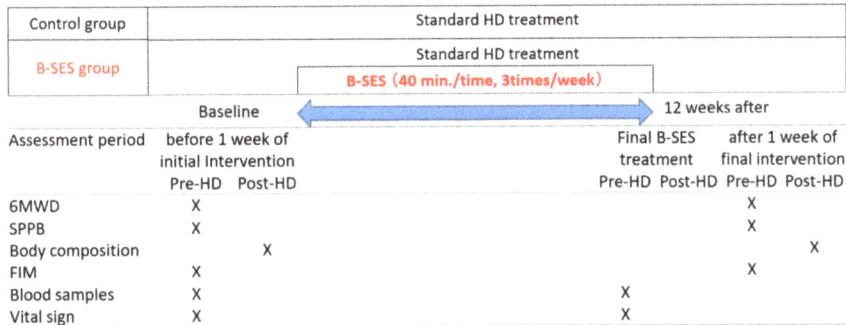

Figure 1. Schematic diagram of study schedule. Most variables were assessed pre-hemodialysis, while body composition was assessed post-hemodialysis. "Vital sign" included assessment of systolic and diastolic blood pressure. 6MWD, 6-Minute Walk Distance; SPPB, Short Physical Performance Battery; and FIM, Functional Independence Measurement.

A note was made in the study notebook of all events that occurred during the intervention. Blood pressure and pulse were measured before the start of each hemodialysis session using the blood pressure monitor of a multipurpose hemodialysis monitoring device (Nikkiso DCS-100NX, Tokyo, Japan).

This study was conducted following approval by the Tohoku University Clinical Research Review Committee (reference number: 2019-6-063) and registration in the Ministry of Health, Labour and Welfare data system (jRCT Protocol No.: jRCTs022200010) and was conducted in accordance with the Declaration of Helsinki. The patients were individually informed of the study rationale using an informed consent form prior to enrollment, and only those who provided their consent were enrolled in the study. The results of this study were reported according to the 2010 CONSORT Guidelines [18].

2.2. Participants

The inclusion criteria for the study were as follows: (1) patients with end-stage kidney disease that had been introduced to hemodialysis, (2) patients who had been receiving hemodialysis for more than 3 months, (3) patients with stable hemodynamics receiving outpatient maintenance hemodialysis, (4) patients aged between 65 and 90 years old at the time of enrollment, (5) patients with daily activity level of less than 4000 steps [6], and (6) patients who were briefed about the study and provided voluntary written consent to participate.

The exclusion criteria were as follows: (1) patients with sensory impairment, (2) patients who had difficulty walking, (3) patients with malignant neoplasms, (4) patients with severe edema, (5) patients with severe skin diseases or wounds on the belt-type electrode attachment site, (6) patients with systolic blood pressure of 180 mmHg or higher or diastolic blood pressure of 110 mmHg or higher, (7) patients participating in other clinical studies, (8) patients requiring acute treatment for acute coronary syndrome, unstable angina, or other conditions, (9) patients with implantable electronic devices (such as pacemakers), (10) patients undergoing temporary pacing or intra-aortic balloon pumping therapy, etc.,

(11) patients with psychiatric disorders or severe dementia, and (12) patients deemed ineligible for the study by the investigator for other reasons.

2.3. Intervention Protocol

B-SES was performed using G-TES (Homer Ion Institute Co., Ltd., Tokyo, Japan), which is an electrical stimulator for general treatment (Figure 2). The stimulation was carried out in "Obsolete mode" (frequency: 20 Hz, on-off: 5 sec–2 sec, pulse width: 250 μs, output waveform: exponentially increasing wave) for 40 min per session, according to the median time reported in a previous study by Schardong et al. [14]. All other stimulation conditions were in accordance with a previous study by Suzuki et al. [17].

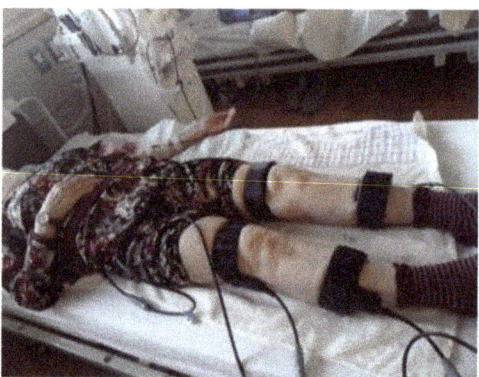

Figure 2. Application of the belt electrode-skeletal muscle electrical stimulation intervention. Patients were placed in the supine position. Five silicon–rubber electrode bands were applied to the patient's waist and bilateral thighs and ankles. Electrical muscle stimulation was administered for 40 min per day.

The intensity of stimulation was the maximum intensity tolerated by the patient. The intervention period was 40 min per day, 3 times a week, for 12 weeks, totaling 36 sessions. Belt-type electrodes were attached to a total of five locations in the trunk, both thighs, and both lower legs of the patients, and electrical stimulation was performed in the first half of the hemodialysis time.

Stimulation intensity was adjusted at two locations, the thigh and lower leg. The median/mean intensity during the first intervention was 1.70/1.79 (minimum 0.8–maximum 2.8) mA at the thigh and 0.95/0.97 (0.4–1.4) mA at the lower leg. At the final intervention, it was 3.15/3.47 (2.1–7.4) mA at the thigh and 1.55/1.74 (1.1–3.9) mA at the lower leg.

Patients in both the control group and the intervention group were instructed to lead the same lifestyle as before the intervention, and no special exercise instructions were given during the intervention period. After the intervention period, all patients underwent voluntary training guidance.

2.4. Outcome Measures

All evaluation variables were measured at the beginning of the study and at the end of the 12-week intervention (Figure 1).

2.4.1. Physical Function Tests

In this study, the 6MWT distance (6MWD), an indicator of exercise intolerance, was the primary endpoint. The 6MWD was assessed using a 15 m one-way corridor and all assessment procedures were performed according to the guidelines of the American Thoracic Society (ATS) [19].

A comprehensive assessment of lower extremity function was performed using the Short Physical Performance Battery (SPPB), according to a previous study [20]. The assessment procedure consisted of (1) tandem stand, (2) 4 m walk test, and (3) 5-Time-Sit-To-Stand (5-STS) tests, and the times and scores were recorded. For all measurement elements, the use of knee braces and walking aids was optional.

2.4.2. Body Compositions

Measurements were taken by a physical therapist after hemodialysis sessions using a body composition analyzer (Tanita Corporation MC-780A-N) [21]. The measurement items were dry weight and skeletal muscle mass in the extremities.

2.4.3. ADL Assessment

ADL were measured by a physiotherapist through an interview survey using the Functional Independence Measure (FIM) [22].

2.4.4. Biochemical Parameters

Blood biochemistry tests were performed during the baseline assessment and on the last day of the intervention. Blood biochemistry tests examined creatine kinase (CK), blood urea nitrogen (BUN), C-reactive protein (CRP), interleukin-6 (IL-6), insulin-like growth factor 1 (IGF-1), total antioxidant capacity (TAC), and irisin levels. In addition, using BUN values before and after hemodialysis, the hemodialysis efficiency (spKt/V) was calculated as spKt/V = −ln (post-dialysis BUN/pre-dialysis BUN − 0.008 * dialysis time) + (4 − 3.5 * post-dialysis BUN/pre-dialysis BUN) * amount of water removed/DW [23].

2.5. Statistical Analysis

All analyses were two-sided with a significance level of 5%. The statistical analysis software was SPSS ver.21 (IBM Corp., Chicago, IL, USA).

Demographic and laboratory data were expressed as mean ± standard deviation or median (interquartile range) for continuous variables, and as number of people (%) for categorical variables. The Shapiro–Wilk test was performed for normality of distribution. For baseline comparisons between the control and intervention groups, continuous variables were analyzed using the unpaired t-test or the Mann–Whitney U test, and categorical variables were analyzed using the chi-square test. For comparison of pre- and post-intervention results between groups, all parameters were analyzed using the paired t-test or Wilcoxon signed rank sum test. For comparisons between the control group and the intervention group after 12 weeks, the unpaired t-test or the Mann–Whitney U test was used. Furthermore, differences in the amount of change between the control and intervention groups were assessed using the unpaired t-test or the Mann–Whitney U test.

The sample size required for the paired analysis of 6MWD was calculated based on a previous EMS study [24], which used a significance level of 5%, a power of 80%, and an effect size of 0.5, resulting in a minimum requirement of 13 participants in each group.

3. Results

A total of 27 older hemodialysis patients were enrolled from 69 candidate participants who met the inclusion criteria and did not violate the exclusion criteria. The 27 patients were randomized into the control group (13 patients) or the intervention group (14 patients) (Figure 3). Seven patients dropped out. Of the four patients who withdrew from the intervention group, two patients were admitted to other hospitals and were unavailable for the endpoint assessment of 6MWD, one patient refused to participate in the endpoint assessment, and one patient had a non-measurable 6MWD due to a thigh injury. Of the three patients who withdrew from the control group, one patient was admitted to another hospital and was unavailable for the 6MWD measurement, and two patients refused to participate in the endpoint assessment.

Therefore, we used a per protocol analysis. A total of 20 patients completed the intervention (control group: 10 patients, intervention group: 10 patients), and their data were analyzed.

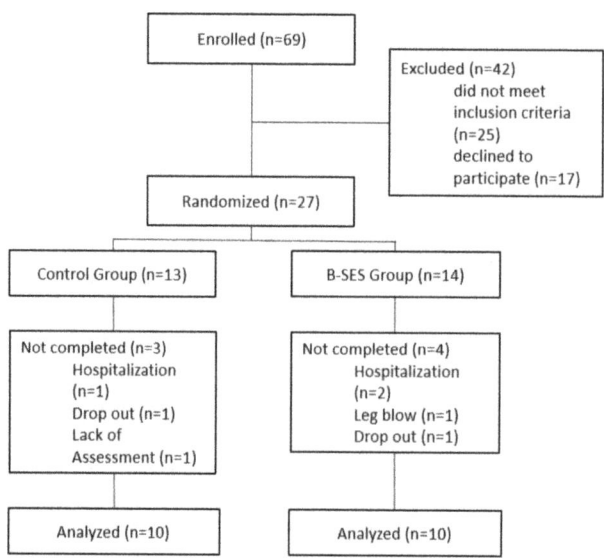

Figure 3. Study flow chart. Among the 69 patients who were screened for eligibility, 42 patients were excluded because of their physical function/medical assessment results or because they declined. Therefore, a total of 20 patients (10 in the control group and 10 in the B-SES group) were included in the final analysis.

Table 1 shows the intergroup comparisons of demographic data at baseline. There were no significant differences between the two groups in terms of age (control group: 78.4 ± 6.2 years old, intervention group: 79.4 ± 6.5 years old), sex ratio (control group: 60.0% male, intervention group: 70.0% male), number of steps (control group: 796.25 (427.50–3276.19) steps/day, intervention group: 1525.38 (735.50–3454.31) steps/day), history of hemodialysis (control group: 34.00 (26.75–50.75) months, intervention group: 28.50 (12.25–79.25) months), or prevalence of diabetes (control group: 40.0%, intervention group: 70.0%).

Table 1. Clinical characteristics.

	Control Group (n = 10)	B-SES Group (n = 10)	p Value
Age (years)	78.40 ± 6.20	79.40 ± 6.50	0.73 [a]
Men, n (%)	6 (60.00)	7 (70.00)	1.00 [c]
Height (cm)	158.11 ± 8.87	154.25 ± 6.49	0.28 [a]
Body composition			
Dry weight (kg)	50.92 ± 12.00	52.35 ± 3.78	0.73 [a]
Skeletomuscular mass (kg)	15.83 ± 3.99	15.05 ± 2.40	0.62 [a]
Physical activity (steps/day)	796.25 [427.50–3276.19]	1525.38 [735.50–3454.31]	0.44 [b]
Duration of hemodialysis (months)	34.00 [26.75–50.75]	28.50 [12.25–79.25]	0.63 [b]
Not completed rate, n (%)	3 (23.08)	4 (28.57)	1.00 [c]
Comorbidity			
Hypertension, n (%)	9 (90)	9 (90)	1.00 [c]
Dyslipidemia, n (%)	1 (10)	4 (40)	0.30 [c]
Diabetes, n (%)	4 (40)	7 (70)	0.37 [c]
History of ischemic heart disease, n (%)	7 (70)	7 (70)	1.00 [c]
History of cerebrovascular disease, n (%)	4 (40)	8 (80)	0.17 [c]
Medication			
Erythropoietin, n (%)	7 (70)	7 (70)	1.00 [c]
L-carnitine, n (%)	9 (90)	8 (80)	1.00 [c]

Values are presented as mean ± standard deviation or median (inter-quartile range (IQR)) unless otherwise indicated; Significance level $p < 0.05$; Baseline, before 1 week of initial intervention; [a] analyzed using the unpaired t-test; [b] analyzed using the Mann–Whitney U test; [c] analyzed using the chi-square test.

Table 2 shows the blood pressure and pulse measurements. There were no significant differences in SBP, DBP, or pulse.

Table 2. Resting vital signs.

	Control Group (n = 10)			B-SES Group (n = 10)			Change from Baseline		
	Baseline	12 Weeks	p Value	Baseline	12 Weeks	p Value	Control Group	B-SES Group	p Value
SBP (mmHg)	153.00 ± 20.36	148.50 ± 21.03	0.21	151.00 ± 23.13	147.70 ± 24.21	0.71	−3.40 ± 10.98	−7.10 ± 15.09	0.54
DBP (mmHg)	74.90 ± 11.57	74.40 ± 10.03	0.76	72.40 ± 16.75	71.00 ± 10.36	0.75	−2.30 ± 11.16	2.90 ± 9.93	0.29
Pulse (bpm)	70.30 ± 13.48	66.40 ± 11.57	0.22	72.50 ± 12.07	75.30 ± 8.15	0.31	1.60 ± 8.34	2.30 ± 7.44	0.85

Values are presented as mean ± standard deviation or median (IQR); Significance level $p < 0.05$; Baseline, before 1 week of initial intervention; SBP, Systolic Blood Pressure; and DBP, Diastolic Blood Pressure.

Table 3 shows the results of 6MWD, the primary endpoint. In the control group, no significant differences were observed between the measurements at baseline and 12 weeks. However, in the intervention group, there was a significant increase in 6MWD from 242.0 ± 94.5 m to 283.0 ± 99.6 m ($p = 0.005$). In addition, there was a significant difference between the amount of change in 6MWD between the two groups, with −18.50 ± 28.29 m in the control group and 41.00 ± 12.65 m in the intervention group ($p < 0.001$).

Table 3 shows the SPPB results. In the control group, there was no significant difference in the total SPPB score at baseline and 12 weeks. However, there was a significant improvement in the intervention group from 8.5 ± 3.3 points to 10.3 ± 2.1 points ($p = 0.008$). There was also a significant difference in the amount of change in SPPB between the two groups ($p = 0.035$). There were no significant differences in dry weight, skeletal muscle mass in the extremities, or FIM (Table 3).

Table 4 shows the results of the blood biochemistry tests. Although there was a significant decrease in albumin levels from baseline to 12 weeks in the control group ($p = 0.027$), this change was not observed in the intervention group and there were no significant differences between the amount of change in albumin levels between the two groups. There were no significant differences in the levels of CK, irisin, IGF-1, TAC, CRP, IL-6, hemoglobin, or in dialysis efficiency.

No locomotor difficulties or cardiovascular events were reported in this study. Four patients in the intervention group withdrew from the study to be hospitalized or withdrew their consent to continue in the study. None of the withdrawals were attributable to effects resulting from the participation in the study.

Table 3. Physical assessments.

	Control Group (n = 10)			B-SES Group (n = 10)			Change from Baseline		
	Baseline	12 Weeks	p Value	Baseline	12 Weeks	p Value	Control Group	B-SES Group	p Value
Physical function test									
6MWD (m)	271.00 ± 90.88	252.50 ± 88.98	0.07	242.00 ± 94.49	283.00 ± 99.62	<0.01	−18.50 ± 28.29	41.00 ± 12.65	<0.001
SPPB Total (score)	8.80 ± 2.53	9.20 ± 2.78	0.10	8.50 ± 3.34	10.30 ± 2.11	0.01	0.40 ± 0.70	1.80 ± 1.81	0.04
SPPB Tandem (score)	2.50 [2.00–4.00]	3.00 [3.00–4.00]	0.18	3.00 [2.75–3.25]	4.00 [3.00–4.00]	0.02	0.00 [0.00–1.00]	1.00 [0.00–1.25]	0.25
SPPB Gait (score)	4.00 [3.00–4.00]	4.00 [3.00–4.00]	0.32	3.00 [2.50–4.00]	3.40 [2.71–4.00]	0.10	0.00 [0.00–0.00]	0.00 [0.00–1.00]	0.17
SPPB 5-STS (score)	2.50 [1.00–3.25]	3.00 [0.75–4.00]	0.48	3.00 [1.00–4.00]	3.50 [2.75–4.00]	0.06	0.00 [−0.25–1.00]	0.00 [0.00–1.00]	0.44
Body composition									
Dry weight (kg)	50.92 ± 12.00	51.49 ± 11.47	0.29	52.35 ± 3.78	52.31 ± 4.18	0.87	0.57 ± 1.59	0.04 ± 0.73	0.29
Skeletomuscular muss (kg)	15.83 ± 3.99	16.05 ± 3.90	0.38	15.05 ± 2.40	15.13 ± 2.53	0.74	0.22 ± 0.76	0.08 ± 0.75	0.68
ADL									
FIM (score)	121.50 [116.75–123.25]	120.50 [117.25–124.00]	0.72	121.00 [118.50–123.00]	121.00 [113.75–123.25]	0.50	0.00 [−3.00–1.50]	0.00 [−2.25–1.00]	0.91

Values are presented as mean ± standard deviation or median (IQR); Significance level $p < 0.05$; Baseline, before 1 week of initial intervention; 6MWD, 6 min walk distance; SPPB, Short Physical Performance Battery; 5-STS, 5-Time-Sit-To-Stand; ADL, activity of daily living; and FIM, functional independence measurement.

Table 4. Biochemical parameters.

	Control Group (n = 10)			B-SES Group (n = 10)			Change from Baseline		
	Baseline	12 Weeks After	p Value	Baseline	12 Weeks After	p Value	Control Group	B-SES Group	p Value
CK (U/L)	81.70 ± 36.99	83.10 ± 50.10	0.93	74.90 ± 28.65	86.80 ± 45.47	0.23	1.40 ± 50.64	11.90 ± 29.32	0.58
Irisin (ng/mL)	6.81 [6.16–7.91]	5.95 [5.68–6.86]	0.14	6.24 [5.78–8.12]	7.00 [5.68–7.82]	0.59	−0.21 [−1.27–1.10]	−0.89 [−2.65–0.29]	0.35
TAC (mM)	2.15 ± 0.49	2.63 ± 0.78	0.13	2.03 ± 0.53	1.82 ± 1.05	0.54	0.49 ± 0.93	−0.21 ± 1.06	0.13
CRP (mg/dL)	0.14 [0.10–0.28]	0.09 [0.05–0.12]	0.19	0.26 [0.06–0.38]	0.13 [0.05–0.51]	0.86	−0.50 [−0.23–0.02]	−0.01 [−0.13–0.23]	0.32
IL-6 (pg/mL)	3.05 ± 1.67	2.58 ± 1.17	0.44	3.87 ± 3.38	3.06 ± 2.15	0.44	−0.48 ± 1.86	−0.81 ± 3.15	0.78
IGF-1 (ng/mL)	84.20 ± 35.56	95.40 ± 41.16	0.27	78.40 ± 18.66	77.70 ± 28.15	0.94	11.20 ± 30.06	−0.70 ± 27.69	0.37
Albumin (mg/dL)	3.58 ± 0.30	3.46 ± 0.33	0.02	3.69 ± 0.26	3.60 ± 0.23	0.24	−0.12 ± 0.14	−0.09 ± 0.22	0.72
Hemoglobin (mg/dL)	9.95 ± 0.96	10.08 ± 0.55	0.53	10.14 ± 1.10	9.92 ± 0.82	0.47	0.13 ± 0.63	−0.22 ± 0.93	0.34
spKt/V	1.46 ± 0.25	1.55 ± 0.26	0.29	1.48 ± 0.28	1.66 ± 0.31	0.05	0.09 ± 0.27	0.18 ± 0.25	0.47

Values are presented as mean ± standard deviation or median (IQR); Significance level $p < 0.05$; Baseline, before 1 week of initial intervention; CK, Creatine Kinase; TAC, Total Antioxidant Capacity; CRP, C-reactive protein; IL-6, interloikin-6; and IGF-1, Insulin-like growth factors-1.

4. Discussion

Many older hemodialysis patients have sarcopenia [3], which has been reported to be associated with decreased physical function, an increased hospitalization rate, and decreased QOL and ADL [10,12]. Therefore, continuous exercise intervention is necessary, but many hemodialysis patients have difficulty establishing exercise habits given the time constraints of hemodialysis treatment, and it is often difficult for older hemodialysis patients with reduced physical function to continue voluntary exercise at an effective load. Therefore, the purpose of this study was to examine the effects of B-SES in older patients on maintenance hemodialysis from the perspective of safety and efficacy in improving physical function.

In this study, to examine the safety of the B-SES intervention in older patients with hemodialysis, we measured CK, CRP, IL-6, blood pressure, and pulse before hemodialysis and verified changes before and after the intervention. To evaluate the effects of electrical stimulation on muscle damage and inflammation, we measured CK, CRP, and IL-6 levels and observed no changes in any parameter before or after the intervention in either group. An increase in CRP and a decrease in albumin have been reported to cause inflammation in the body and contribute to a decrease in muscle mass [25], but in this study, despite the drop in albumin levels in the control group, no changes were observed in albumin levels or skeletal muscle mass of the extremities in the intervention group. No additional inflammatory disease or pneumonia occurred during the intervention, nor did any of the patients change drugs that could affect inflammation, such as antibiotics. Furthermore, neither group showed changes in blood pressure and pulse after the intervention. These observations suggest that B-SES can be implemented for older hemodialysis patients without serious adverse events.

This study is the first to show that a B-SES intervention in older hemodialysis patients with reduced physical activity improved 6MWD, an indirect measure of exercise tolerance, and SPPB scores, an index of comprehensive lower extremity function. A strong correlation between 6MWD and SPPB has been found in previous studies targeting older patients with heart disease and older patients in general [26,27]. Furthermore, SPPB is strongly correlated with lower extremity muscle strength [20], and B-SES interventions have been reported to strengthen lower extremity muscles in previous studies on orthopedic surgery and middle-aged hemodialysis patients [15,17].

Moreover, the improvement in 6MWD and SPPB scores, despite the absence of an increase in muscle mass, may be attributed to their relationship to lower extremity muscle strength. Increases in muscle strength tend to occur earlier than increases in muscle mass, as higher intensity exercise is required to increase muscle mass [28]. Since general EMS passively induces muscle contraction through electrical stimulation via surface electrodes, it has been suggested that even patients who have difficulty moving can achieve exercise effects [14]. Muscle contraction by EMS differs from muscle contraction by general voluntary contraction in that fast-twitch fibers with large fiber diameters (Type II fibers) are mobilized first and muscle contraction is induced only in areas that receive electrical stimulation [29]. In EMS, slow-twitch fibers and fast-twitch fibers capable of continuous contraction (Type II A fibers) have been reported to be predominantly activated by low-frequency stimulation of 20 Hz or less [30]. Increases in muscle strength and muscle mass are often correlated in general resistance training, but there is very little evidence of the effect of EMS on increasing muscle mass [13]. Since the intensity of electrical stimulation was low in this study, the intensity of exercise was weaker than that of resistance training and cannot be regarded as a sufficient load to increase muscle mass. However, we believe that muscle fibers were activated by stimulating the trunk and leg muscles with B-SES, resulting in increased muscle strength. These findings suggest that B-SES improved lower extremity muscle strength as well as 6MWD and SPPB scores.

According to reports in patients with chronic obstructive pulmonary disease (COPD), patients with chronic heart failure, and older patients, the minimal clinically important difference (MCID) of 6MWD ranges from 17 to 54 m [31,32]. In the present study, the change in 6MWD in the intervention group was 41.0 ± 12.0 m, thus falling within this MCID range. Additionally, the change in the total SPPB score in the intervention group was 1.8 ± 1.7 points, exceeding the MCID range of 0.99 to 1.34 points for total SPPB score in older patients [33,34]. These findings show that the B-SES intervention in older hemodialysis patients resulted in clinically significant improvements in both 6MWD and SPPB.

In this study, B-SES intervention for older hemodialysis patients (mean age 78 years) was safe and sustainable. Although there were no changes in muscle mass and blood biochemical parameters, there were improvements in 6MWD and SPPB scores, which may have been as a result of the selective activation of the trunk and leg muscles through electrical stimulation. Dobsak et al. conducted a three-group comparison of EMS vs. exercise training on an ergometer vs. no exercise (control) in middle-aged hemodialysis patients [35]. They found that when comparing the EMS group and the voluntary exercise groups via resistance training and exercise with an ergometer, voluntary exercise had a greater effect on improving physical function. On the basis of the above, B-SES may be useful as a complementary exercise method for older people and patients who have difficulty maintaining voluntary exercise routines.

This study has two limitations, the first being the small sample size. Therefore, we positioned this study as a pilot study. The second is the lack of measurements of muscle strength. In the future, it would be necessary to examine the effects of B-SES on muscle strength by increasing the number of participants and measuring muscle strength.

5. Conclusions

In this study, a 12-week B-SES intervention was performed safely without serious adverse events during hemodialysis sessions in older patients. Furthermore, 6MWD and SPPB scores improved post-intervention, suggesting that B-SES may improve physical function in older people with decreased physical activity.

Author Contributions: Conceptualization, M.M. and S.E.; data curation, M.H., M.M., Y.H., T.T., T.M. and N.Y.; formal analysis, M.H., M.M. and S.M.; funding acquisition, M.K. and S.E.; project administration, M.H., M.M., M.K. and S.E.; supervision, S.E.; writing and editing, M.H., M.M. and S.E.; All authors have read and agreed to the published version of the manuscript.

Funding: Satoru Ebihara is currently receiving grants (19H03984, 19K22821 and 22K19760) from JSPS KAKENHI, and the grant (JP22zf01270019) from AMED. Masahiro Kohzuki is currently receiving the grant (20H04034) from JSPS KAKENHI, the grant from the Specified Clinical Trials Promotion Program for Tohoku University Hospital, and the co-researched fund with Homer ion Laboratory Co., Ltd.

Institutional Review Board Statement: The trial was registered at Japan registry of clinical trials under jRCTs022200010 and was approved by the ethics committee (Tohoku Certified Review Board of Tohoku University, reference number; 2019-6-063, 22 May 2020). It was conducted in accordance with the Declaration of Helsinki and the Clinical Trials Act (Act No. 16 of 14 April 2017).

Informed Consent Statement: Informed consent was obtained from all subjects involved in the study.

Data Availability Statement: The data presented in this study are available on request from the corresponding author.

Conflicts of Interest: Masahiro Kohzuki received partial financial support from Homer ion Laboratory Co., Ltd. However, the company had no control over the interpretation, writing, or publication of the present study. The rest of the authors have no conflicts of interest.

References

1. Kooman, J.P.; Kotanko, P.; Schols, A.M.; Shiels, P.G.; Stenvinkel, P. Chronic kidney disease and premature ageing. *Nat. Rev. Nephrol.* **2014**, *10*, 732–742. [CrossRef] [PubMed]
2. Johansen, K.L.; Chertow, G.M.; Jin, C.; Kutner, N.G. Significance of frailty among dialysis patients. *J. Am. Soc. Nephrol.* **2007**, *18*, 2960–2967. [CrossRef] [PubMed]
3. Kim, J.K.; Choi, S.R.; Choi, M.J.; Kim, S.G.; Lee, Y.K.; Noh, J.W.; Kim, H.J.; Song, Y.R. Prevalence of and factors associated with sarcopenia in elderly patients with end-stage renal disease. *Clin. Nutr.* **2014**, *33*, 64–68. [CrossRef] [PubMed]

4. Painter, P. Physical functioning in end-stage renal disease patients: Update 2005. *Hemodial. Int.* **2005**, *9*, 218–235. [CrossRef] [PubMed]
5. Johansen, K.L.; Chertow, G.M.; Ng, A.V.; Mulligan, K.; Carey, S.; Schoenfeld, P.Y.; Kent-Braun, J.A. Physical activity levels in patients on hemodialysis and healthy sedentary controls. *Kidney Int.* **2000**, *57*, 2564–2570. [CrossRef]
6. Matsuzawa, R.; Roshanravan, B.; Shimoda, T.; Mamorita, N.; Yoneki, K.; Harada, M.; Watanabe, T.; Yoshida, A.; Takeuchi, Y.; Matsunaga, A. Physical Activity Dose for Hemodialysis Patients: Where to Begin? Results from a Prospective Cohort Study. *J. Ren. Nutr.* **2018**, *28*, 45–53. [CrossRef]
7. Hayhurst, W.S.; Ahmed, A. Assessment of physical activity in patients with chronic kidney disease and renal replacement therapy. *Springerplus* **2015**, *4*, 536. [CrossRef]
8. Nelson, M.E.; Rejeski, W.J.; Blair, S.N.; Duncan, P.W.; Judge, J.O.; King, A.C.; Macera, C.A.; Castaneda-Sceppa, C.; American College of Sports, M.; American Heart, A. Physical activity and public health in older adults: Recommendation from the American College of Sports Medicine and the American Heart Association. *Circulation* **2007**, *116*, 1094–1105. [CrossRef]
9. Yamagata, K.; Hoshino, J.; Sugiyama, H.; Hanafusa, N.; Shibagaki, Y.; Komatsu, Y.; Konta, T.; Fujii, N.; Kanda, E.; Sofue, T.; et al. Clinical practice guideline for renal rehabilitation: Systematic reviews and recommendations of exercise therapies in patients with kidney diseases. *Ren. Replace. Ther.* **2019**, *5*, 28. [CrossRef]
10. Sheshadri, A.; Johansen, K.L. Prehabilitation for the Frail Patient Approaching ESRD. *Semin. Nephrol.* **2017**, *37*, 159–172. [CrossRef]
11. Castaneda, C.; Gordon, P.L.; Parker, R.C.; Uhlin, K.L.; Roubenoff, R.; Levey, A.S. Resistance training to reduce the malnutrition-inflammation complex syndrome of chronic kidney disease. *Am. J. Kidney Dis.* **2004**, *43*, 607–616. [CrossRef] [PubMed]
12. Chung, Y.C.; Yeh, M.L.; Liu, Y.M. Effects of intradialytic exercise on the physical function, depression and quality of life for haemodialysis patients: A systematic review and meta-analysis of randomised controlled trials. *J. Clin. Nurs.* **2017**, *26*, 1801–1813. [CrossRef]
13. Jones, S.; Man, W.D.; Gao, W.; Higginson, I.J.; Wilcock, A.; Maddocks, M. Neuromuscular electrical stimulation for muscle weakness in adults with advanced disease. *Cochrane Database Syst. Rev.* **2016**, *10*, CD009419. [CrossRef] [PubMed]
14. Schardong, J.; Stein, C.; Della Mea Plentz, R. Neuromuscular Electrical Stimulation in Chronic Kidney Failure: A Systematic Review and Meta-analysis. *Arch. Phys. Med. Rehabil.* **2020**, *101*, 700–711. [CrossRef] [PubMed]
15. Hasegawa, S.; Kobayashi, M.; Arai, R.; Tamaki, A.; Nakamura, T.; Moritani, T. Effect of early implementation of electrical muscle stimulation to prevent muscle atrophy and weakness in patients after anterior cruciate ligament reconstruction. *J. Electromyogr. Kinesiol.* **2011**, *21*, 622–630. [CrossRef] [PubMed]
16. Tanaka, S.; Kamiya, K.; Matsue, Y.; Yonezawa, R.; Saito, H.; Hamazaki, N.; Matsuzawa, R.; Nozaki, K.; Yamashita, M.; Wakaume, K.; et al. Efficacy and safety of acute phase intensive electrical muscle stimulation in frail older patients with acute heart failure: Results from the ACTIVE-EMS Trial. *J. Cardiovasc. Dev. Dis.* **2022**, *9*, 99. [CrossRef]
17. Suzuki, T.; Ikeda, M.; Minami, M.; Matayoshi, Y.; Nakao, M.; Nakamura, T.; Abo, M. Beneficial Effect of intradialytic electrical muscle stimulation in hemodialysis patients: A randomized controlled trial. *Artif. Organs* **2018**, *42*, 899–910. [CrossRef]
18. Schulz, K.F.; Altman, D.G.; Moher, D. CONSORT 2010 Statement: Updated guidelines for reporting parallel group randomized trials. *Ann. Intern. Med.* **2010**, *152*, 726–732. [CrossRef]
19. ATS Committee on Proficiency Standards for Clinical Pulmonary Function Laboratories. ATS statement: Guidelines for the six-minute walk test. *Am. J. Respir. Crit. Care Med.* **2002**, *166*, 111–117. [CrossRef]
20. Guralnik, J.M.; Ferrucci, L.; Simonsick, E.M.; Salive, M.E.; Wallace, R.B. Lower-extremity function in persons over the age of 70 years as a predictor of subsequent disability. *N. Engl. J. Med.* **1995**, *332*, 556–561. [CrossRef]
21. Kusunoki, H.; Tabara, Y.; Tsuji, S.; Wada, Y.; Tamaki, K.; Nagai, K.; Itoh, M.; Sano, K.; Amano, M.; Maeda, H.; et al. Estimation of Muscle Mass Using Creatinine/Cystatin C Ratio in Japanese Community-Dwelling Older People. *J. Am. Med. Dir. Assoc.* **2022**, *23*, 902.e921–902.e931. [CrossRef] [PubMed]
22. Young, Y.; Fan, M.Y.; Hebel, J.R.; Boult, C. Concurrent validity of administering the functional independence measure (FIM) instrument by interview. *Am. J. Phys. Med. Rehabil.* **2009**, *88*, 766–770. [CrossRef] [PubMed]
23. Daugirdas, J.T. Second generation logarithmic estimates of single-pool variable volume kt/v: An analysis of error. *J. Am. Soc. Nephrol.* **1993**, *4*, 1205–1213. [CrossRef]
24. Iliou, M.C.; Verges-Patois, B.; Pavy, B.; Charles-Nelson, A.; Monpere, C.; Richard, R.; Verdier, J.C. Effects of combined exercise training and electromyostimulation treatments in chronic heart failure: A prospective multicentre study. *Eur. J. Prev. Cardiol.* **2017**, *24*, 1274–1282. [CrossRef] [PubMed]
25. Menon, V.; Wang, X.; Greene, T.; Beck, G.J.; Kusek, J.W.; Marcovina, S.M.; Levey, A.S.; Sarnak, M.J. Relationship between C-reactive protein, albumin, and cardiovascular disease in patients with chronic kidney disease. *Am. J. Kidney Dis.* **2003**, *42*, 44–52. [CrossRef]
26. Kitai, T.; Shimogai, T.; Tang, W.H.W.; Iwata, K.; Xanthopoulos, A.; Otsuka, S.; Nakada, F.; Yokoyama, R.; Kamiya, K.; Saito, H.; et al. Short physical performance battery vs. 6-minute walking test in hospitalized elderly patients with heart failure. *Eur. Heart J. Open* **2021**, *1*, oeab006. [CrossRef]
27. Bean, J.F.; Kiely, D.K.; Leveille, S.G.; Herman, S.; Huynh, C.; Fielding, R.; Frontera, W. The 6-minute walk test in mobility-limited elders: What is being measured? *J. Gerontol. A Biol. Sci. Med. Sci.* **2002**, *57*, M751–M756. [CrossRef]

28. Hikida, R.S.; Staron, R.S.; Hagerman, F.C.; Walsh, S.; Kaiser, E.; Shell, S.; Hervey, S. Effects of high-intensity resistance training on untrained older men. II. Muscle fiber characteristics and nucleo-cytoplasmic relationships. *J. Gerontol. A Biol. Sci. Med. Sci.* **2000**, *55*, B347–B354. [CrossRef]
29. Hamada, T.; Kimura, T.; Moritani, T. Selective fatigue of fast motor units after electrically elicited muscle contractions. *J. Electromyogr. Kinesiol.* **2004**, *14*, 531–538. [CrossRef]
30. Sillen, M.J.; Franssen, F.M.; Gosker, H.R.; Wouters, E.F.; Spruit, M.A. Metabolic and structural changes in lower-limb skeletal muscle following neuromuscular electrical stimulation: A systematic review. *PLoS ONE* **2013**, *8*, e69391. [CrossRef]
31. Shoemaker, M.J.; Curtis, A.B.; Vangsnes, E.; Dickinson, M.G. Clinically meaningful change estimates for the six-minute walk test and daily activity in individuals with chronic heart failure. *Cardiopulm. Phys. Ther. J.* **2013**, *24*, 21–29. [CrossRef] [PubMed]
32. Wise, R.A.; Brown, C.D. Minimal clinically important differences in the six-minute walk test and the incremental shuttle walking test. *COPD* **2005**, *2*, 125–129. [CrossRef]
33. Jacob, M.E.; Travison, T.G.; Ward, R.E.; Latham, N.K.; Leveille, S.G.; Jette, A.M.; Bean, J.F. Neuromuscular attributes associated with lower extremity mobility among community-dwelling older adults. *J. Gerontol. A Biol. Sci. Med. Sci.* **2019**, *74*, 544–549. [CrossRef] [PubMed]
34. Perera, S.; Mody, S.H.; Woodman, R.C.; Studenski, S.A. Meaningful change and responsiveness in common physical performance measures in older adults. *J. Am. Geriatr. Soc.* **2006**, *54*, 743–749. [CrossRef] [PubMed]
35. Dobsak, P.; Homolka, P.; Svojanovsky, J.; Reichertova, A.; Soucek, M.; Novakova, M.; Dusek, L.; Vasku, J.; Eicher, J.C.; Siegelova, J. Intra-dialytic electrostimulation of leg extensors may improve exercise tolerance and quality of life in hemodialyzed patients. *Artif. Organs* **2012**, *36*, 71–78. [CrossRef] [PubMed]

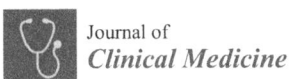

Article

Effectiveness of High-Intensity Laser Therapy Plus Ultrasound-Guided Peritendinous Hyaluronic Acid Compared to Therapeutic Exercise for Patients with Lateral Elbow Tendinopathy

Raffaello Pellegrino [1], Teresa Paolucci [2], Fabrizio Brindisino [3], Paolo Mondardini [4], Angelo Di Iorio [5],*, Antimo Moretti [6] and Giovanni Iolascon [6]

1. Department of Scientific Research, Campus Ludes, Off-Campus Semmelweis University, 6912 Lugano, Switzerland
2. Physical Medicine and Rehabilitation, Department of Oral Medical Science and Biotechnology, "G d'Annunzio" University Chieti-Pescara, 66100 Chieti, Italy
3. Department of Medicine and Health Science "Vincenzo Tiberio", University of Molise c/o Cardarelli Hospital, C/da Tappino, 86100 Campobasso, Italy
4. Department of Sport Science, 40100 Bologna, Italy
5. Department of Innovative Technologies in Medicine & Dentistry, "G. d'Annunzio" University Chieti-Pescara, 66100 Chieti, Italy
6. Department of Medical and Surgical Specialties and Dentistry, University of Campania "Luigi Vanvitelli", 80138 Naples, Italy
* Correspondence: angelo.diiorio@unich.it; Tel.: +39-0871-355-3333

Citation: Pellegrino, R.; Paolucci, T.; Brindisino, F.; Mondardini, P.; Di Iorio, A.; Moretti, A.; Iolascon, G. Effectiveness of High-Intensity Laser Therapy Plus Ultrasound-Guided Peritendinous Hyaluronic Acid Compared to Therapeutic Exercise for Patients with Lateral Elbow Tendinopathy. J. Clin. Med. 2022, 11, 5492. https://doi.org/10.3390/jcm11195492

Academic Editor: Masahiro Kohzuki

Received: 11 August 2022
Accepted: 16 September 2022
Published: 20 September 2022

Publisher's Note: MDPI stays neutral with regard to jurisdictional claims in published maps and institutional affiliations.

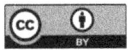

Copyright: © 2022 by the authors. Licensee MDPI, Basel, Switzerland. This article is an open access article distributed under the terms and conditions of the Creative Commons Attribution (CC BY) license (https://creativecommons.org/licenses/by/4.0/).

Abstract: Lateral elbow tendinopathy (LET) is a common painful musculoskeletal disorder. Several treatments have been proposed to provide pain reduction and functional recovery, including laser therapy, hyaluronic acid peritendinous injection (Hy-A), and therapeutic exercise (TE). Our study aims to assess the effectiveness of a combined approach with high-intensity laser therapy (HILT) and Hy-A injections compared to TE on pain, muscle strength, and disability in patients with painful LET. A retrospective longitudinal study was carried out by consulting the medical records of patients with a diagnosis of painful LET formulated by clinical and instrumental findings that received functional evaluations, including the Patient-Rated Tennis Elbow Evaluation (PRTEE) and muscle strength measurement at least four times: T0 ("baseline"), 1-month (T1), 3-month (T2), and 6-month follow-ups (T3). Medical records of 80 patients were analyzed. In the HILT + HyA group, the Peak-strength ($p < 0.001$) and mean strength ($p < 0.001$) significantly increased compared to the TE group between study times. For the PRTEE-total-score as for the subscales, the HILT + HyA group reported statistically significant reductions only for the comparisons of baseline versus T1 and baseline versus T2. No serious adverse events occurred. Our findings suggest that Hy-A associated with HILT might be more effective than TE for people with LET in the short–medium term.

Keywords: hyaluronic acid; high-intensity laser therapy; lateral elbow tendinopathy; Patient-Rated Tennis Elbow Evaluation; muscle strength; disability; ultrasound; rehabilitation

1. Introduction

"Tennis elbow", or lateral elbow tendinopathy (LET), is a noninflammatory condition that affects the tendon insertion or myotendinous junction of wrist muscle extensors [1], causing subacute and chronic symptoms of pain at the lateral epicondyle and disability of the elbow and sometimes of the entire upper limb. LET occurs in between 1% and 3% of the population and typically affects subjects between 30 and 60 years without gender difference [1]. Several determinants were reported to be associated with LET, such as working procedures characterized by the long-term repetitive forearm and hand movement [2], the excessive neuronal activity by nociceptors that derive from the radial nerve leading to axonal sprouting of the free nerve endings and peripheral sensitization, smoking habits, and metabolic factors, such as estrogen decline, hypercholesterolemia, and obesity [1]. LET is a degenerative overuse process of the extensor carpi radialis brevis and of the common extensor tendon [3] characterized by histological micro-rupture, vascular proliferation, and hyaline degeneration without inflammatory cells infiltrating within the tendon tissue [4]. The main clinical manifestation is hyperalgesia during active range of motion of the elbow and at the palpation in the lateral epicondyle area, which is exacerbated by prono-supination of the forearm [5]. Moreover, LET patients complain of painful handgrip with consequent functional limitation, disability in activities of daily living, time lost at work, and poor quality of life [6]. LET is usually considered a self-limiting condition, with the majority of patients recovering in 6–24 months [7], even if some clinical reports noticed symptom recurrence persisting for many years [8]. Several conservative approaches have been proposed to manage LET, including pharmacological therapy, systemic and/or local treatments (corticosteroid injections, botulinum toxin, hyaluronic acid, autologous blood, and platelet-rich plasma) [9], therapeutic exercise (TE), physical modalities, elbow braces, acupuncture, and watchful waiting [8]. Surgery is usually recommended for those patients with persistent pain and disability after a course of conservative therapy [10].

However, no consensus about the best treatment for improving pain and function in people with LET has been reached. Among rehabilitative approaches, manual therapy and TE showed positive effects on people with LET in terms of pain relief and increased tendon strength [11,12]. Among physical modalities commonly used for LET, laser therapy was previously demonstrated to improve grip strength, pain, and functional ability at midterm follow-up (5 to 26 weeks) compared to placebo [8]. The studies on laser treatment in LET have focused mainly on the efficacy of low-level laser therapy (LLLT), and few studies have investigated the efficacy of high-intensity laser therapy (HILT) [8]. However, a meta-analysis highlighted how HILT could be more effective than LLLT in terms of pain control, stiffness, and function in degenerative musculoskeletal conditions [13].

Injection therapy is widely used for the treatment of patients with LET [14]. In particular, peritendinous hyaluronic acid (Hy-A) injection seems to be an effective therapeutic option for pain control and functional improvement in these patients.

We hypothesized that a combined approach with HILT plus peritendinous Hy-A injection could improve pain control and functional recovery, considering the analgesic effect and stimulation of collagen synthesis attributable to HILT [15] and the Hy-A-related enhancement of the activity of the fibroblasts, including their adhesivity, extracellular matrix synthesis, and proliferation [16,17].

Therefore, the main objective of the study is to assess the effectiveness of the combination of HILT and Hy-A peritendinous injection on pain relief, improvement of muscle strength, functional ability, and quality of life, in a mid-long-term period, compared to TE in patients with painful LET.

2. Materials and Methods

2.1. Study Design

A retrospective cohort clinical study was conducted by the Declaration of Helsinki and the STROBE guidelines [18]. The study protocol was planned at the Department of Clinical Research, Ludes Campus, Luganoff Campus of Semmelweis University of Budapest, and written informed consent was obtained from all participants for treatment and data processing. From June 2021 to June 2022, medical records of patients with LET that were treated at the Chiparo Physical Medicine and Rehabilitation Clinic in Lecce, Italy, were consulted and selected by a specialized nurse blinded for the main outcomes of the study.

2.2. Population

We included medical records of patients between 30 and 65 years with elbow pain for at least 2 weeks and the following clinical and instrumental features: (1) no other sources of elbow pain (e.g., cervical radiculopathy); (2) minimal pain at rest (Patient-Rated Tennis Elbow Evaluation, PRTEE, pain subscale < 3); (3) positive wrist extension tests against resistance (Cozen test) [19]; (4) positive palpation test of the epicondyle; (5) ultrasound (US) evaluation showing thickening and heterogeneous echo structure of the common extensor tendon, as well as increased blood flow under Doppler. We did not consider clinical records of patients receiving regular painkillers, previous elbow injections, specific rehabilitation treatments in the previous two months, and those with US-scan-confirmed injury or rupture of any extensor tendon of the carpus or with previous elbow surgery. Additional exclusion criteria were the presence of contraindications to laser therapy and Hy-A injection, such as drug allergy, epilepsy, coagulopathies or anticoagulant therapy, neoplasms, or pregnancy. Patients with fibromyalgia, enthesitis due to seronegative arthritis, and rheumatoid arthritis were also excluded. Finally, patients who had skin infections at the injection site, systemic symptoms (e.g., fever), or were carriers of artificial cardiac pacemakers were also excluded.

2.3. Outcomes

We included medical records of patients who filled the PRTEE questionnaire [20] and who received the measurement of maximum (peak) and mean grip strength by an electronic dynamometer (Activeforce2 Sixtus Prato (PO) Italia) during contraction against the resistance of wrist extensors with the elbow flexed at 90° (Cozen test). Handgrip strength protocol provided 3 maximal contraction trials lasting 5 s each, interspersed with 15 s of rest. The PRTEE is a 15-item questionnaire assessing pain (5 items) and the degree of difficulty in performing various activities (6 specific and 4 usual activities) due to LET over the preceding week [20]. The same functional assessments were performed at different follow-ups: T1 (30 days), T2 (90 days), and T3 (180 days) after the end of treatment.

2.4. Interventions

2.4.1. HILT Plus Hyaluronic Acid (HILT + Hy-A) Group

Our HILT protocol consisted of 10 daily sessions using a LASERIX PRO device (GN med), administered via a fixed tip with a 30 mm spacer. Each HILT session had a total duration of 13 min and was divided into 3 phases. In the first phase lasting 7 min, a frequency of 18 Khz, peak power of 600 W, and 226 Joules of energy was delivered. In the second phase lasting 3 min, a frequency of 14 Khz, peak power of 900 W, and 226 Joules of energy was delivered. In the third phase lasting 3 min, a frequency of 10 Khz, peak power of 1200 W, and 226 Joules of energy was delivered. At the end of the 10 HILT sessions, and on day 7 and day 14 after the last therapeutic session, patients received US-guided (SonoSite M-Turbo ultrasound system with a 6–15 Mhz linear probe) Hy-A injections in the peritendinous area of the elbow epicondyle by the same physiatrist expert in US technique and US-guided injection (Supplementary Figures S1 and S2). The injections were conducted using a pre-filled syringe of 20 mg in 2 mL of linear Hy-A sodium salt with a molecular weight of 500–730 kDa. The needles used were 25G 25 mm. No anesthetic drugs were administered after the injections. During the therapeutic procedure with laser and Hy-A injections, patients were seated, and the affected elbow was positioned at 90° of flexion and in slight pronation. The skin was disinfected with a chlorhexidine wipe. All subjects enrolled in this group were not prescribed any therapeutic exercise and did not receive any other physical or pharmacological therapy.

2.4.2. Therapeutic Exercise Group

Our TE protocol (eccentric exercises series and static stretching exercise) consisted of three/per week clinical supervised sessions for 4 weeks for a total of 12 sessions. Eccentric exercises for LET were performed with the elbow supported on the bed in full extension, forearm in pronation, wrist in maximal extension, and hand hanging over the edge of the bed. In this position, patients were told to flex their wrist slowly until full flexion was achieved and then return to the starting position. Patients were instructed to continue with the exercise even if they experienced mild pain. However, they were instructed to stop the exercise if disabling pain occurred. Each session consisted of three sets of 10 repetitions with at least a 1 min rest interval between each set. When patients were able to perform the eccentric exercises without experiencing any pain or discomfort, the load was increased using free weights or therabands. The starting and final positions of eccentric exercises, the increase in the load, and the degree of mild or disabling pain could not be standardized but were tailored to each patient [11]. The static stretching exercises for LET were performed slowly with the elbow in extension, forearm in pronation, wrist in flexion, and ulnar deviation according to the patient's tolerance to achieve the best stretching position result for the ECRB tendon. This position was held for 30–45 s before and after each set of eccentric exercises [11].

2.4.3. Treatments-Related Adverse Events

We reported adverse events (AEs) in both groups by consulting the clinical records of included patients [21].

2.5. Sample Size

The sample size was calculated for the comparison of the two study groups at a 6-month follow-up for the PRTEE—total score. We assumed as significant minimal change a difference of at least five points in the PRTEE at each follow-up. We also settled for standard deviations of 10. A sample size of N = 36 per study arm (72 overall) provides more than 90% power (alpha = 0.05, two-tailed) applying linear mixed models, with an intraclass-correlation between measures $\rho = 0.50$. To account for 10% attrition during the study period ("dropouts"), we planned to recruit 40 medical records per study group (80 overall) at baseline. Similar values were obtained in the assessment of the sample size according to peak muscle strength [22].

2.6. Statistical Analysis

Data were reported as mean ± standard error (S.E.) for continuous variables and as absolute number and percentage for dichotomous variables; differences between groups were assessed with analysis of variance and chi-square test, respectively. To assess the variation of the PRTEE subscale as the total score, peak, and mean muscle strength, linear mixed models (LMMs) were applied [23]. Intercept and time had a random component. The advantage of this approach is that it increases the precision of the estimate by using all available information concerning performance and, at the same time, allows for handling missing data with more powerful modeling of the analysis.

The LMMs were considered the two treatments: HILT + Hy-A as the reference group, the three times of the study, with baseline as the reference, and lastly, the interaction between time and treatment. Sensitivity analyses were also conducted, excluding from analysis those patients that did not reach a subjective and clinical improvement, applying the same previously described models.

Data were analyzed with SAS software (Rel. 9.4, Cary, NC, USA), and the *p*-value for differences was considered statistically significant for a value less than or equal to 0.05.

3. Results

In this study, the medical records of 80 patients were included (40 for each group). No statistically significant between-group differences were found for main clinical characteristics, for peak and mean strength, and for the PRTEE-total score and PRTEE-subscales (Table 1).

Table 1. Description of the population characteristics according to type of treatment at enrollment. High-intensity laser therapy plus hyaluronic acid (Hilt + Hy-A), therapeutic exercise (TE); Patient-Rated Tennis Elbow Evaluation (PRTEE).

	HILT + Hy-A	TE	*p*-Value
	40	40	
Age (year)	47.3 ± 9.5	50.3 ± 8.1	0.13
Sex female *n* (%)	25 (62.5)	21 (52.5)	0.37
Side pain (right) *n* (%)	19 (47.5)	22 (55.0)	0.50
Weight (kg)	74.1 ± 6.3	74.0 ± 5.5	0.97
Height (m)	1.68 ± 0.1	1.69 ± 0.1	0.75
BMI (kg/m^2)	26.2 ± 2.3	26.1 ± 1.9	0.72
White collar *n* (%)	14 (35.0)	16 (40.0)	0.64
Education			0.78
Junior high school *n* (%)	16 (40.0)	13 (32.5)	
High school *n* (%)	15 (37.5)	17 (42.5)	
University degree *n* (%)	9 (22.5)	10 (25.0)	
Smoke habits (actually) *n* (%)	10 (25.0)	14 (35.0)	0.33
Hypertension *n* (%)	10 (25.0)	9 (22.5)	0.79
Cholesterol mmol/L	184.6 ± 29.7	184.0 ± 28.3	0.94
Hand grip Peak strength (Nw)	91.6 ± 12.2	94.1 ± 7.1	0.28
Hand grip Mean strength (Nw)	77.5 ± 10.0	77.7 ± 7.0	0.96
PRTEE total score	64.2 ± 6.2	63.3 ± 4.7	0.43
PRTEE Pain score	29.6 ± 3.4	29.5 ± 3.2	0.87
PRTEE Specific activities	39.7 ± 4.9	38.6 ± 3.4	0.28
PRTEE Usual activities	29.6 ± 2.8	28.9 ± 2.5	0.27

BMI: Body Mass Index.

Hand-grip peak-strength increased during the study in both groups, and a multiplicative effect was demonstrated for the interaction between treatment and time ($p < 0.001$) (Figure 1).

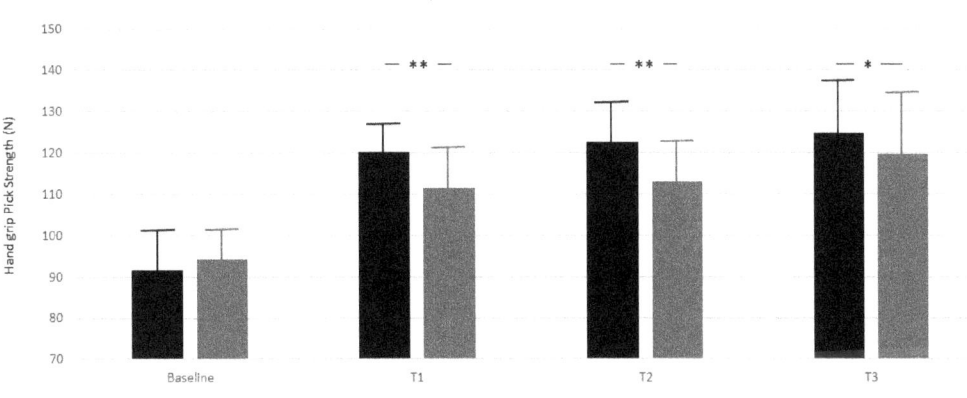

Figure 1. Handgrip peak strength variation according to time and treatment; black box represents high-intensity laser therapy plus hyaluronic acid (HILT + Hy-A) group, whereas grey box represents therapeutic exercise (TE). Results for the linear mixed model analysis (*p*-values for time, treatment, and interaction of time for treatment); Bonferroni adjustment for multiple comparisons were also applied between follow-ups of study compared to baseline; *: $p < 0.05$; **: $p < 0.001$.

In the HILT + Hy-A group, the peak strength significantly increased compared to the TE group in all follow-ups (baseline-T1: 11.21 ± 1.89; $p < 0.001$; baseline-T2: 12.06 ± 2.94;

$p < 0.001$; baseline-T3: 7.57 ± 3.26; $p = 0.02$). Nearly one-quarter ($\rho = 24.5$, Supplementary Table S1, Model A) of the total variation in peak strength was attributable to differences between patients. Moreover, from the unconditional means model, 84% of unexplained residual in the variation of peak strength (Model A: 210.81 ± 18.49 Nw) was associated with linear time (Model B) and 87% with the interaction between time and treatment (Model C). Model goodness increased (AIC decreased between models) with model complexity. Mean strength increased during the study period in both groups, and again a multiplicative effect was demonstrated for the interaction between treatment and time ($p < 0.001$) (Figure 2).

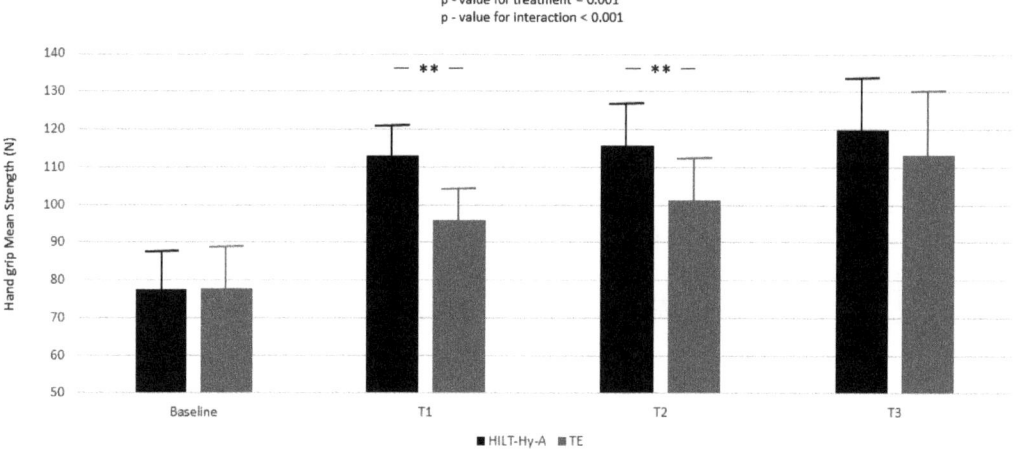

Figure 2. Handgrip mean strength variation according to time and treatment; black box represents high-intensity laser therapy plus hyaluronic acid (HILT+Hy-A) group, whereas grey box represents therapeutic exercise (TE). Results for the linear mixed model analysis (p-values for time, treatment, and interaction for time for treatment). Bonferroni adjustment for multiple comparisons applied between follow-ups of the study compared to baseline; **: $p < 0.001$.

In the HILT + Hy-A group, the mean strength significantly increased compared to the TE group, only between baseline and T1 (17.24 ± 2.20; $p < 0.001$) and between baseline and T2 (14.49 ± 2.81; $p < 0.001$). Almost 15% ($\rho = 14.5$, Supplementary Table S2, Model A) of the total variation in peak strength was attributable to differences between patients. Again, Model B and Model C explained 84 and 89% of the unexplained residuals in the variation of peak strength (335.10 ± 29.21), respectively. Model goodness increased (AIC decreased between models) with model complexity.

Figure 3A–D report the PRTEE total score, the pain subscale score, the specific disability score, and the usual activity score. PRTEE total score and all the subscales decreased during the time points of the study. In the comparison between treatments according to different follow-ups, statistically significant differences were reported only for the comparisons between baseline and T1 and baseline and T2 for the PRTEE-score and all subscales. For the PRTEE score, almost 27% ($\rho = 27.5$, Supplementary Table S3, Model A) of the total variation was attributable to differences between patients. Again, Model B and Model C explained 72 and 76 percent of the unexplained residual in the variation of peak strength (83.93 ± 8.77), respectively. Model goodness increased (AIC decreased between models) with model complexity. After 6 months, 11 patients (13.8%), four in the HILT + HyA group and seven in the TE group (p-value = 0.33), did not improve.

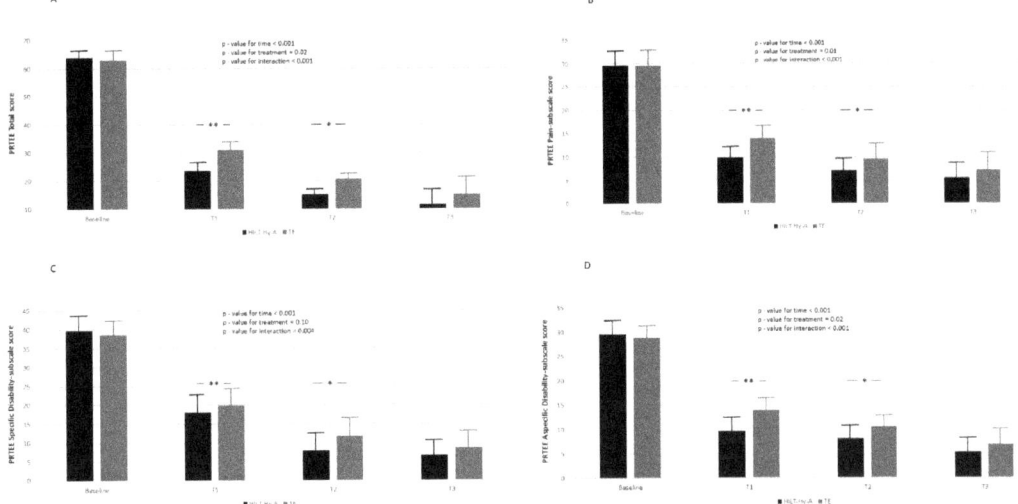

Figure 3. Report the PRTEE total score (**A**), the pain subscale score (**B**), the specific disability score (**C**), and the usual activity score (**D**). according to time and treatment; black box represents high-intensity laser therapy plus hyaluronic acid (HILT + Hy-A) group, whereas grey box represents therapeutic exercise (TE). Results for linear mixed model analysis (p-value for time, treatment, and interaction of time for reatment). Bonferroni adjustment for multiple comparisons applied between follow-ups of the study compared to baseline; *: $p < 0.05$, **: $p < 0.001$.

4. Discussion

To our knowledge, no clinical studies investigated the effectiveness of the combined use of Hy-A and HILT on LET. Our findings suggest that combined peritendinous injections of Hy-A and HILT might be effective for improving pain, muscle strength, and disability in this population at short- and medium-term (1 to 3 month-follow-up) compared to TE.

Tendinopathy can occur because of different insults, such as certain drug treatments (e.g., fluoroquinolones), metabolic disorders (e.g., diabetes mellitus and hypercholesterolemia), and biomechanical factors [24]. In particular, overload and detraining are catabolic stimuli for tendon tissue resulting in increased synthesis of collagenase, proteinase, and pro-inflammatory cytokines [25]. To date, different studies support the use of eccentric exercise to improve pain and muscle strength in patients with LET [26]. Compared with the concentric exercise, the eccentric exercise showed a significant reduction in self-reported pain [26]. Eccentric contraction would appear to stimulate tendon cells, resulting in increased collagen cross-linking [27] and decreased neuro-vascular ingrowth that seem to modulate pain [28]. However, the relationship between exercise type and pain remains unclear in LET, and often, it is debated whether eccentric exercises should be performed with pain [29]. Other therapeutic strategies have been proposed in recent years for the treatment of pain in patients with LET, including injections of different agents, such as platelet-rich plasma (PRP), adipose-derived mesenchymal stromal cells, botulinum toxin, and Hy-A [30]. Hy-A injection seems to inhibit the pro-inflammatory response by local fibroblast [31], reduce pain, improve function, and reduce tendon rubbing in pre-insertion areas during major tendinopathies and post-surgical tendon repair [14]. Among adjunctive interventions for the management of patients with LET, physical modalities are commonly used in clinical practice [24]. In particular, LLLT seems to be useful in different musculoskeletal disorders by reducing edema and inflammation, controlling pain, and promoting tissue healing [32]. However, controversial evidence is available about the benefits of the use of LLLT in patients with LET, where only short-term pain relief was reported [33]. On the other hand, evidence about HILT is scant, with some observational studies suggesting the effectiveness of this intervention in patients with LET on pain control, functional recovery, and quality of life [34]. HILT might have analgesic and regenerative effects attributable to its ability to slow pain transmission, increase the production of morphine-mimetic substances [34], stimulate collagen production, and increase vascular permeability and blood flow within tendons by photochemical and photothermic stimulation [35]. These effects might act synergistically with the analgesic and regenerative effects of Hy-A. For what concerns safety, the combined approach proposed in our study was well tolerated, as demonstrated by the absence of AEs. Moreover, our data suggest that this approach promoted rapid clinical and functional improvement. Lastly, we cannot demonstrate a statistically significant reduction in the therapeutic failure between the two treatments, but this is not the main objective of the study, and probably the study is underpowered against this outcome.

The strengths of our study are the adequate sample size, the long-term follow-up, and no serious adverse effect occurrence in both study groups. Moreover, the character of a real-life study strengthens the results on the efficacy and safety of the combined treatment of Hy-A plus HILT in the treatment of LET. However, our study has some limitations. First, the retrospective design hampered the allocation of patients in the two groups because a randomization procedure was lacking. Moreover, a healthy worker effect could be introduced as further selection bias. In addition, our cohort might not be representative of the general population suffering from LET, such as elderly, overweight-obese people, and workers involved in repetitive and strenuous activities. The choice of a control group treated only with HILT, or alternatively, only with Hy-A, could be more informative to better define the role of each intervention in the control of LET symptomatology.

5. Conclusions

Our findings support the hypothesis that a multimodal approach might provide additional benefits without safety concerns in patients with LET. In particular, our study showed the effectiveness of the combined intervention of HILT and Hy-A injections over TE in subjects affected by LET in the short–medium term. Despite these encouraging findings, randomized controlled trials are required to prove the efficacy of the proposed approach compared to placebo or the efficacy of HILT + Hya + TE over the TE effect.

Supplementary Materials: The following supporting information can be downloaded at: https://www.mdpi.com/article/10.3390/jcm11195492/s1, Table S1: Linear mixed model, variation of handgrip peak strength during the follow-up according to treatment; Table S2: Linear mixed model, variation of handgrip mean-strength during the follow-up according to treatment; Table S3: Linear mixed model, follow-up variation of PRTEE-score according to treatments; Figure S1: Ultra-sound image of the lateral elbow, longitudinal view: (1) humerus, (2) epicondyle, (3) head of radius, (4) extensor tendons, (5) calcific lesion of the tendons; Figure S2: Ultra-sound-guided (6–15 Mhz linear probe) Hyaluronic Acid injections in the peritendinous area of the elbow epicondyle. The injections were done using a pre-filled syringe of 20 mg in 2 mL of linear Hy-A sodium salt with a molecular weight of 500-730 kDa.

Author Contributions: Conceptualization, R.P., A.D.I., A.M. and G.I.; methodology, R.P., T.P., F.B. and P.M.; formal analysis, R.P. and A.D.I.; investigation, F.B. and R.P.; resources, R.P. and A.D.I.; data curation, R.P. and A.D.I.; writing—original draft preparation, R.P., T.P., A.D.I., A.M. and G.I.; writing—review and editing, T.P., F.B., P.M., A.M. and G.I.; supervision, G.I. All authors have read and agreed to the published version of the manuscript.

Funding: This research received no external funding.

Institutional Review Board Statement: Not applicable; this is an observational retrospective study.

Informed Consent Statement: The study was developed following the Good Clinical Practice (GCP) guidelines. It was conducted within the ethical principles outlined in the Declaration of Helsinki and with the procedures defined by the ISO 9001-2015 standards for "Research and experimentation". Written informed consent to provide information included in personal medical records was obtained from all participants.

Data Availability Statement: The datasets used and/or analyzed during the current study are available from the corresponding author upon reasonable request.

Conflicts of Interest: Raffaello Pellegrino, Teresa Paolucci, Fabrizio Brindisino, Paolo Mondardini, Angelo Di Iorio, Antimo Moretti, and Giovanni Iolascon (the authors) certify that there is no conflict of interests with any financial organization regarding the material discussed in this manuscript.

References

1. Cutts, S.; Gangoo, S.; Modi, N.; Pasapula, C. Tennis elbow: A clinical review article. *J. Orthop.* **2019**, *17*, 203–207. [CrossRef]
2. Descatha, A.; Albo, F.; Leclerc, A.; Carton, M.; Godeau, D.; Roquelaure, Y.; Petit, A.; Aublet-Cuvelier, A. Lateral Epicondylitis and Physical Exposure at Work? A Review of Prospective Studies and Meta-Analysis. *Arthritis Care Res.* **2016**, *68*, 1681–1687. [CrossRef] [PubMed]
3. Fahmy, F.S.; ElAttar, M.; Salem, H.F. Hand-Grip Strength and Return to Heavy Manual Work at a Mean 5-Year Follow-up After Arthroscopic Release of Recalcitrant Lateral Epicondylitis. *Orthop. J. Sport. Med* **2022**, *10*, 23259671221078586. [CrossRef] [PubMed]
4. Kheiran, A.; Pandey, A.; Pandey, R. Common tendinopathies around the elbow; what does current evidence say? *J. Clin. Orthop. Trauma* **2021**, *19*, 216–223. [CrossRef] [PubMed]
5. Karabinov, V.; Georgiev, G.P. Lateral epicondylitis: New trends and challenges in treatment. *World J. Orthop.* **2022**, *13*, 354–364. [CrossRef]
6. Stratford, P.W.; Levy, D.R. Assessing valid change over time in patients with lateral epicondylitis at the elbow. *Clin. J. Sport Med.* **1994**, *4*, 88–91. [CrossRef]
7. Ikonen, J.; Lähdeoja, T.; Ardern, C.L.; Buchbinder, R.; Reito, A.; Karjalainen, T. Persistent Tennis Elbow Symptoms Have Little Prognostic Value: A Systematic Review and Meta-analysis. *Clin. Orthop. Relat. Res* **2022**, *480*, 647–660. [CrossRef]
8. Lian, J.; Mohamadi, A.; Chan, J.J.; Hanna, P.; Hemmati, D.; Lechtig, A.; Nazarian, A. Comparative Efficacy and Safety of Nonsurgical Treatment Options for Enthesopathy of the Extensor Carpi Radialis Brevis: A Systematic Review and Meta-analysis of Randomized Placebo-Controlled Trials. *Am. J. Sports Med.* **2019**, *47*, 3019–3029. [CrossRef]
9. de Sire, A.; Lippi, L.; Mezian, K.; Calafiore, D.; Pellegrino, R.; Mascaro, G.; Cisari, C.; Invernizzi, M. Ultrasound-guided platelet-rich-plasma injections for reducing sacroiliac joint pain: A paradigmatic case report and literature review. *J. Back Musculoskelet. Rehabil.* **2022**, *35*, 977–982. [CrossRef]
10. Sanders, T.L.; Maradit Kremers, H.; Bryan, A.J.; Ransom, J.E.; Smith, J.; Morrey, B.F. The epidemiology and health care burden of tennis elbow: A population-based study. *Am. J. Sports Med.* **2015**, *43*, 1066–1071. [CrossRef]
11. Landesa-Piñeiro, L.; Leirós-Rodríguez, R. Physiotherapy treatment of lateral epicondylitis: A systematic review. *J. Back Musculoskelet. Rehabil.* **2022**, *35*, 463–477. [CrossRef] [PubMed]
12. Kachanathu, S.J.; Alenazi, A.M.; Hafez, A.R.; Algarni, A.D.; Alsubiheen, A.M. Comparison of the effects of short-duration wrist joint splinting combined with physical therapy and physical therapy alone on the management of patients with lateral epicondylitis. *Eur. J. Phys. Rehabil. Med.* **2019**, *55*, 488–493. [CrossRef] [PubMed]
13. Ahmad, M.A.; Mohamad, M.S.; Yusof, A. Effects of low-level and high-intensity laser therapy as adjunctive to rehabilitation exercise on pain, stiffness and function in knee osteoarthritis: A systematic review and meta-analysis. *Physiotherapy* **2022**, *114*, 85–95. [CrossRef]
14. Pellegrino, R.; Brindisino, F.; Barassi, G.; Sparvieri, E.; DI Iorio, A.; de Sire, A.; Ruosi, C. Combined ultrasound guided peritendinous hyaluronic acid (500–730 Kda) injection with extracorporeal shock waves therapy vs. extracorporeal shock waves therapy-only in the treatment of shoulder pain due to rotator cuff tendinopathy. A randomized clinical. *J. Sports Med. Phys. Fitness* **2022**, *62*, 1211–1218. [CrossRef]
15. Urdiales-Gálvez, F.; Martín-Sánchez, S.; Maíz-Jiménez, M.; Castellano-Miralla, A.; Lionetti-Leone, L. Concomitant Use of Hyaluronic Acid and Laserin Facial Rejuvenation. *Aesthetic Plast. Surg* **2019**, *43*, 1061. [CrossRef] [PubMed]
16. Oliva, F.; Marsilio, E.; Asparago, G.; Frizziero, A.; Berardi, A.C.; Maffulli, N. The Impact of Hyaluronic Acid on Tendon Physiology and Its Clinical Application in Tendinopathies. *Cells* **2021**, *10*, 3081. [CrossRef]
17. Crimaldi, S.; Liguori, S.; Tamburrino, P.; Moretti, A.; Paoletta, M.; Toro, G.; Iolascon, G. The Role of Hyaluronic Acid in Sport-Related Tendinopathies: A Narrative Review. *Medicina* **2021**, *57*, 1088–2021. [CrossRef]
18. Cuschieri, S. The STROBE guidelines. *Saudi J. Anaesth.* **2019**, *13*, 31–34. [CrossRef]
19. Karanasios, S.; Korakakis, V.; Moutzouri, M.; Drakonaki, E.; Koci, K.; Pantazopoulou, V.; Tsepis, E.; Gioftsos, G. Diagnostic accuracy of examination tests for lateral elbow tendinopathy (LET)—A systematic review. *J. Hand Ther.* **2021**, *in press*. [CrossRef]
20. Cacchio, A.; Necozione, S.; MacDermid, J.C.; Rompe, J.D.; Maffulli, N.; di Orio, F.; Santilli, V.; Paoloni, M. Cross-cultural adaptation and measurement properties of the italian version of the Patient-Rated Tennis Elbow Evaluation (PRTEE) questionnaire. *Phys. Ther.* **2012**, *92*, 1036–1045. [CrossRef]
21. Pahor, M.; Chrischilles, E.A.; Guralnik, J.M.; Brown, S.L.; Wallace, R.B.; Carbonin, P. Drug data coding and analysis in epidemiologic studies. *Eur. J. Epidemiol.* **1994**, *10*, 405–411. [CrossRef]
22. Stroup, W.W. *Generalized Linear Mixed Models Modern Concepts, Methods and Applications*; Taylor & Francis Group: Boca Raton, FL, USA, 2013.

23. Singer, J.D. Using SAS PROC MIXED to Fit Multilevel Models, Hierarchical Models, and Individual Growth Models. *J. Educ. Behav. Stat.* **1998**, *23*, 323–355. [CrossRef]
24. Millar, N.L.; Silbernagel, K.G.; Thorborg, K.; Kirwan, P.D.; Galatz, L.M.; Abrams, G.D.; Murrell, G.A.C.; McInnes, I.B.; Rodeo, S.A. Tendinopathy. *Nat. Rev. Dis. Prim.* **2021**, *7*, 1. [CrossRef] [PubMed]
25. Frizziero, A.; Salamanna, F.; Della Bella, E.; Vittadini, F.; Gasparre, G.; Aldini, N.N.; Masiero, S.; Fini, M. The Role of Detraining in Tendon Mechanobiology. *Front. Aging Neurosci.* **2016**, *8*, 43. [CrossRef] [PubMed]
26. Karanasios, S.; Korakakis, V.; Whiteley, R.; Vasilogeorgis, I.; Woodbridge, S.; Gioftsos, G. Exercise interventions in lateral elbow tendinopathy have better outcomes than passive interventions, but the effects are small: A systematic review and meta-analysis of 2123 subjects in 30 trials. *Br. J. Sports Med.* **2021**, *55*, 477–485. [CrossRef] [PubMed]
27. Chen, Z.; Baker, N.A. Effectiveness of eccentric strengthening in the treatment of lateral elbow tendinopathy: A systematic review with meta-analysis. *J. Hand Ther.* **2021**, *34*, 18–28. [CrossRef]
28. Ryan, C.G.; Gray, H.G.; Newton, M.; Granat, M.H. Pain biology education and exercise classes compared to pain biology education alone for individuals with chronic low back pain: A pilot randomised controlled trial. *Man. Ther.* **2010**, *15*, 382–387. [CrossRef]
29. Yoon, S.Y.; Kim, Y.W.; Shin, I.S.; Kang, S.; Moon, H.I.; Lee, S.C. The Beneficial Effects of Eccentric Exercise in the Management of Lateral Elbow Tendinopathy: A Systematic Review and Meta-Analysis. *J. Clin. Med.* **2021**, *10*, 3968. [CrossRef]
30. Evans, J.P.; Maffulli, N.; Smith, C.; Watts, A.; Valderas, J.; Goodwin, V. Even experts cannot agree on the optimal use of platelet-rich plasma in lateral elbow tendinopathy: An international Delphi study. *J. Orthop. Traumatol.* **2021**, *22*, 47. [CrossRef]
31. Mitsui, Y.; Gotoh, M.; Nakama, K.; Yamada, T.; Higuchi, F.; Nagata, K. Hyaluronic acid inhibits mRNA expression of proinflammatory cytokines and cyclooxygenase-2/prostaglandin E(2) production via CD44 in interleukin-1-stimulated subacromial synovial fibroblasts from patients with rotator cuff disease. *J. Orthop. Res.* **2008**, *26*, 1032–1037. [CrossRef]
32. Cotler, H.B. The Use of Low Level Laser Therapy (LLLT) For Musculoskeletal Pain. *MOJ Orthop. Rheumatol.* **2015**, *2*, 188–194. [CrossRef]
33. Mamais, I.; Papadopoulos, K.; Lamnisos, D.; Stasinopoulos, D. Effectiveness of Low Level Laser Therapy (LLLT) in the treatment of Lateral elbow tendinopathy (LET): An umbrella review. *Laser Ther.* **2018**, *27*, 174–186. [CrossRef] [PubMed]
34. Dundar, U.; Turkmen, U.; Toktas, H.; Ulasli, A.M.; Solak, O. Effectiveness of high-intensity laser therapy and splinting in lateral epicondylitis: A prospective, randomized, controlled study. *Lasers Med. Sci.* **2015**, *30*, 1097–1107. [CrossRef] [PubMed]
35. Akkurt, E.; Kucuksen, S.; Yılmaz, H.; Parlak, S.; Sallı, A.; Karaca, G. Long term effects of high intensity laser therapy in lateral epicondylitis patients. *Lasers Med. Sci.* **2016**, *31*, 249–253. [CrossRef] [PubMed]

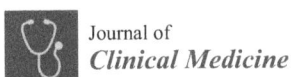

Article

Benefits of Pulmonary Rehabilitation in Patients with Idiopathic Pulmonary Fibrosis Receiving Antifibrotic Drug Treatment

Yuji Iwanami [1], Kento Ebihara [1], Keiko Nakao [1], Naofumi Sato [1], Midori Miyagi [1], Yasuhiko Nakamura [2], Susumu Sakamoto [2], Kazuma Kishi [2], Sakae Homma [3] and Satoru Ebihara [1,4,*]

1. Department of Rehabilitation Medicine, Toho University Omori Medical Center, 6-11-1 Omori-nishi, Ota-ku, Tokyo 143-8541, Japan
2. Department of Respiratory Medicine, Toho University School of Medicine, 6-11-1 Omori-nishi, Ota-ku, Tokyo 143-8541, Japan
3. Department of Advanced and Integrated Interstitial Lung Diseases Research, Toho University School of Medicine, 6-11-1 Omori-nishi, Ota-ku, Tokyo 143-8541, Japan
4. Department of Internal Medicine and Rehabilitation Science, Tohoku University Graduate School of Medicine, 1-1 Seiryo-machi, Aoba-ku, Sendai 980-8574, Japan
* Correspondence: satoru.ebihara.c4@tohoku.ac.jp

Abstract: Background: Although patients with idiopathic pulmonary fibrosis (IPF) often receive treatment with antifibrotic drugs (AFDs) and pulmonary rehabilitation (PR) concurrently, there are no reports on the effect of PR on patients with IPF receiving AFDs. Therefore, we investigated the effect of PR on patients with IPF receiving AFDs. Methods: Eighty-seven eligible patients with IPF (61 male; 72.0 ± 8.1 years; GAP severity stage I/II/III: 26/32/12) were recruited for the study. Patients who completed a 3-month outpatient PR program and those who did not participate were classified into four groups according to use of AFDs: PR group (n = 29), PR+AFD group (n = 11), treatment-free observational group (control group; n = 26), and AFD group (n = 21). There was no significant difference in age, sex, or severity among the groups. Patients were evaluated for physical functions such as 6-min walk distance (6MWD) and muscle strength, dyspnea, and health-related quality of life (HRQOL) at baseline and at 3 months. Results: In the PR group, dyspnea and 6MWD showed significant improvement after the 3-month PR program ($p < 0.05$ and $p < 0.01$, respectively). HRQOL was significantly worse at 3 months ($p < 0.05$) in the AFD group, but not in the other groups. The change in 6MWD from baseline to the 3-month time point was significantly higher in the PR+AFD group than in the AFD groups ($p < 0.01$). Conclusions: It was suggested that AFD treatment reduced exercise tolerance and HRQOL at 3 months; however, the concurrent use of PR may prevent or mitigate these effects.

Keywords: antifibrotic drugs; pulmonary rehabilitation; idiopathic pulmonary fibrosis

Citation: Iwanami, Y.; Ebihara, K.; Nakao, K.; Sato, N.; Miyagi, M.; Nakamura, Y.; Sakamoto, S.; Kishi, K.; Homma, S.; Ebihara, S. Benefits of Pulmonary Rehabilitation in Patients with Idiopathic Pulmonary Fibrosis Receiving Antifibrotic Drug Treatment. *J. Clin. Med.* 2022, *11*, 5336. https://doi.org/10.3390/jcm11185336

Academic Editors: Masahiro Kohzuki and Francisco Dasí

Received: 9 August 2022
Accepted: 8 September 2022
Published: 11 September 2022

Publisher's Note: MDPI stays neutral with regard to jurisdictional claims in published maps and institutional affiliations.

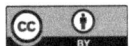

Copyright: © 2022 by the authors. Licensee MDPI, Basel, Switzerland. This article is an open access article distributed under the terms and conditions of the Creative Commons Attribution (CC BY) license (https://creativecommons.org/licenses/by/4.0/).

1. Introduction

Idiopathic pulmonary fibrosis (IPF) is an irreversible, chronic, and progressive disease with a poor prognosis due to severe fibrosis [1,2]. As IPF progresses, it leads to decreased forced vital capacity (FVC), severe hypoxemia, impaired exercise tolerance, and reduced health-related quality of life (HRQOL) [3]. The antifibrotic drugs (AFDs) pirfenidone and nintedanib are recommended for the treatment of IPF [2,4–6].

AFDs suppress the decline in FVC and progression of the disease [4–7]. However, AFDs have not been reported to improve IPF-associated dyspnea, impaired exercise tolerance, and reduced HRQOL. Therefore, other nonpharmacological interventions are important for managing the symptoms experienced by patients with IPF [8]. One of the pillars of nonpharmacological therapy is pulmonary rehabilitation (PR). A Cochrane meta-analysis on patients with interstitial lung disease (ILD) showed that PR improves dyspnea, exercise tolerance, and HRQOL [9]. However, the effect of PR on indicators of lung function, such as predicted forced vital capacity (%FVC) and lung diffusion capacity for carbon monoxide was limited [10].

AFDs and PR are recommended in national and international guidelines [1,8]. Therefore, patients with IPF often receive AFD treatment and PR concurrently, but no study has reported the effect of PR on patients with IPF receiving AFDs. AFDs and PR have different mechanisms of action and may have a synergistic effect. PR is the only treatment that improves exercise tolerance and HRQOL, but its effectiveness is limited in advanced stages of the disease [11]. Therefore, concomitant use of AFDs, which suppress disease progression, may enhance the effect of PR and compensate for its shortcomings.

Side effects have been reported to occur in approximately 60% and 30% of patients receiving nintedanib and pirfenidone, respectively [6,12]. Therefore, there is concern that side effects (e.g., photosensitivity reaction, diarrhea, anorexia, fatigue from liver dysfunction) of AFDs may limit daily life and lead to a decline in HRQOL and 6-min walk distance (6MWD) [13]. Consequently, we investigated the effect of PR on patients with IPF receiving AFDs.

2. Materials and Methods

2.1. Study Design

This study analyzed data from a subgroup of 114 patients with IPF among the participants of the Toho Rehabilitation for Interstitial Pneumonia (TRIP) study enrolled between July 2014 and February 2019 [14]. The TRIP study is an ongoing project at the Toho University Medical Center Omori Hospital (Tokyo, Japan) to assess the long-term effects of PR in patients with interstitial lung disease (ILD) through a two-year follow-up. The study was approved by the Ethics Committee of Toho University Omori Medical Center (approval 27–82 and M21153). The study was registered with the authorized clinical trial registry of International Committee of Medical Journal Editors (UMIN Clinical Trials Registry: UMIN000047241). Written informed consent for participation was obtained from all patients before enrollment in the study. This is a prospective, nonrandomized, controlled observational study in which stable patients with ILD undergo a 3-month outpatient pulmonary rehabilitation program (PRP). Participation in the PRP is elective, and if a patient chooses not to participate, evaluation is performed at baseline and 3 months later.

2.2. Participants

Of the 164 patients who were recruited in the TRIP study between July 2014 and February 2019, 114 patients who were diagnosed with IPF, medically stable, and able to walk independently were included in this study. IPF was diagnosed in accordance with the American Thoracic Society/European Respiratory Society statement via multidisciplinary discussion [1].

Exclusion criteria were as follows: patients with orthopedic or central nervous system disorders that cause gait disturbance, dementia, and other diseases with poor prognosis (e.g., terminal malignant tumors, severe heart failure). Further, patients who had participated in PRP at least once in the past or changed medications within the past 3 months, including AFDs, were excluded.

Patients who completed outpatient PRP (once a week for 3 months) and those who did not participate were classified into four groups according to use of AFDs: PR group (n = 29), PR+AFD group (n = 11), treatment-free observational group (control group, n = 26), and AFD group (n = 21) (Figure 1).

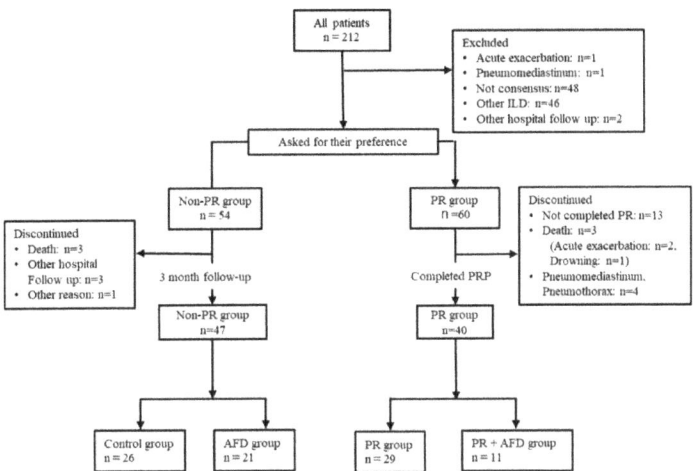

Figure 1. Participant selection flow diagram. Abbreviations: ILD, interstitial lung disease; PR, pulmonary rehabilitation; AFD, antifibrotic drugs.

AFD treatment was appropriately commenced by the treating pulmonologist once IPF was diagnosed. Some patients received AFDs before the start of rehabilitation and some started both simultaneously.

2.3. Pulmonary Rehabilitation Program

Participants underwent a weekly PR session for three months on an outpatient basis, and each session lasted 60 min. PRP consisted of aerobic exercise, upper and lower limb resistance training, breathing exercises (pursed lip breathing, diaphragmatic breathing), trunk-centered stretching, and patient education (disease knowledge, self-management of disease, and how to use oxygen). PRP was individually supervised by a physical therapist.

Aerobic exercise was performed using a treadmill at 60–80% of the patient's maximum walking speed for at least 20–30 min. The maximum walking speed was calculated based on the 6MWD at baseline. Weights were used for resistance training of the upper and lower limbs. Each set consisted of 10–15 repetitions, and the volume was gradually increased to 3–5 sets.

The PR group was also instructed to perform aerobic exercise, including resistance training, limb/trunk stretching, and walking, at least 2–3 days a week as a home exercise program. Patients were also asked to record whether they had a home exercise program. In addition, physical activity (number of steps by the pedometer), degree of dyspnea, and vital signs (blood pressure, pulse and SpO_2 as measured by the patients) were recorded daily to improve self-management ability. The recorded content was confirmed and discussed by the physiotherapist at the outpatient visits.

For patients who did not wish to have outpatient PR (control and AFD groups), we provided guidance, using a pamphlet on how to exercise at home, at the initial evaluation.

2.4. Measurements

Patients were evaluated at baseline and at 3 months. At baseline, medication history, use of oxygen therapy, and respiratory function were evaluated. Vital function tests including FVC, forced expiratory volume in 1 s (FEV_1), FEV_1/FVC, and lung diffusion capacity for carbon monoxide were measured according to guidelines [15,16]. Arterial blood gas analysis was conducted using a spectrophotometer (ABL800 Flex; Radiometer Medical) on arterial blood collected at rest. The severity of IPF was assessed using a multidimensional index and staging system (Sex-Age-Physiology Index Stage) [17].

Dyspnea, HRQOL, 6MWD, quadriceps force (QF), and hand grip strength (HGS) were assessed at baseline and 3 months later. Subjective dyspnea was assessed using the modified Medical Research Council dyspnea scale (mMRC scale) and graded from 0 to 4 [18]. Quadriceps force (QF) was measured using a hand-held dynamometer (a Mobie: Sakai Medical Corp., Tokyo, Japan) to measure isometric knee extension muscle [19]. Patients sat on a training bench and adjusted the position of their gluteal region so that a bench leg was behind the lower extremity on the measurement side. Measurements were performed three times for each leg at intervals of 30 s and the largest value was used to calculate the ratio of knee extension strength to body weight. Hand grip strength (HGS) was measured using a hand dynamometer in the standing, supinated position. HGF was assessed for each hand with the shoulder and wrist in neutral position. Measurements were performed three times for each hand and the largest value was used as HGF.

HRQOL was evaluated using the chronic obstructive pulmonary disease (COPD) Assessment test (CAT) and St. George's Respiratory Questionnaire (SGRQ) scores [20,21]. CAT includes a simple questionnaire consisting of eight questions. Each item is evaluated from 0 to 5, and the higher the score, the worse the health condition. The SGRQ consists of 72 questions, and the higher the score, the lower the HRQOL. Both questionnaires were initially developed for patients with COPD but have been shown to be effective in the evaluation of patients with IPF [22,23].

The 6-min walk test was conducted in accordance with the American Thoracic Society guidelines [24]. Patients on long-term oxygen therapy were tested at the oxygen flow rate during exertion, as directed by their physician. The ratio of the predicted values was calculated using the prediction formula of Enright et al. (%6MWD) [25].

2.5. Statistical Analysis

Baseline values were subtracted from the 3-month values for 6MWD, %6MWD, QF, HGS, mMRC, and SGRQ and CAT scores, and the change from baseline to the 3-month time point (delta [Δ]) was calculated.

The Wilcoxon rank-sum test was used for comparison between values at baseline and at the 3-month time point because the data were not normally distributed based on the estimation using the Shapiro–Wilk test. One-way analysis of variance (one-way ANOVA), multiple comparisons (post hoc Tukey's test), and χ^2 tests were used for between-group comparisons of changes from baseline. Spearman's correlation coefficient was used to assess the relationship between Δ6MWD, ΔmMRC, and ΔSGRQ. Statistical significance was set at $p < 0.5$. All analyses were conducted using SPSS ver.17 (SPSS Inc., Chicago, IL, USA).

3. Results

Sixty participants requested PR and 54 patients were not interested in participating in PR. Of the 60 patients, 40 completed PRP, and we successfully followed-up 47 patients who did not participate in PR.

Table 1 shows the patient characteristics at baseline. There were no significant differences between the four groups with regard to age, body mass index, use of oxygen therapy, severity, and lung function other than FEV_1/FVC.

Table 2 shows the results of the mMRC, 6MWD, HGS, QF, and HRQOL (SGRQ and CAT scores) at baseline and at 3 months. As for mMRC, the PR group showed significant improvement ($p < 0.05$) whereas other groups did not. Similarly to the 6 min walk test, the PR group showed significant improvement in both 6MWD ($p < 0.01$) and %6MWD ($p < 0.01$), whereas other groups did not. In muscle strength, there were no significant changes in any group. As for HRQOL, the CAT score was significantly worse at 3 months compared to that at baseline ($p < 0.05$) in the AFD group, but not in the other groups.

Table 1. Baseline characteristics of each group.

	All (n = 87)	Control (n = 26)	AFD (n = 21)	PR (n = 29)	PR+AFD (n =11)	p Value
Age, year	72.0 ± 8.1	73.0 ± 8.5	70.3 ± 6.6	73.5 ± 8.9	69.0 ± 7.4	0.29 [a]
Sex, male/female	61/26	14/12	18/3	18/11	11/0	<0.05 [b]
BMI, kg/m²	22.9 ± 3.9	24.0 ± 3.6	22.3 ± 4.2	22.5 ± 3.9	22.5 ± 4.1	0.38 [a]
Oxygen use (%)	21 (30)	3 (15)	6 (40)	9 (33)	3 (37.5)	0.34 [b]
Smoking status (current/former/never)	1/44/25	1/13/12	0/14/7	0/19/10	0/9/2	0.47 [b]
Medications						
Azathioprine	0	0	0	0	0	
Cyclophosphamide	0	0	0	0	0	
Cyclosporine	2	1	0	1	0	
Tacrolimus	0	0	0	0	0	
Prednisolone	19	5	6	3	4	
Pirfenidone	15	0	10	0	5	
Nintedanib	17	0	11	0	6	
N-Acetylcysteine	18	4	4	6	2	
Severity						
GAP stage	1.6 ± 0.7	1.4 ± 0.6	1.6 ± 0.7	1.7 ± 0.7	2.0 ± 0.7	0.15 [a]
(I/II/III)	26/32/12	16/8/2	10/8/3	11/13/5	3/5/3	
Pulmonary function						
FVC, % pred	77.1 ± 20.5	84.2 ± 18.2	71.6 ± 15.7	77.9 ± 23.2	68.5 ± 22.1	0.08 [a]
FEV_1, % pred	91.2 ± 22.6	95.7 ± 18.6	85.5 ± 17.3	95.1 ± 28.6	81.5 ± 19.5	0.15 [a]
FEV_1/FVC, %	86.1 ± 13.2	79.9 ± 8.0 [c]	90.5 ± 14.5	87.7 ± 15.7	88.3 ± 9.4	<0.05 [a]
DL_{CO}, % pred	60.1 ± 21.1	69.6 ± 22.4	55.8 ± 22.1	57.8 ± 18.1	53.1 ± 18.9	0.056 [a]
PaO_2, torr	81.9 ± 13.4	86.1 ± 13.2	84.1 ± 14.2	77.2 ± 12.0	79.9 ± 13.8	0.07 [a]
$PaCO_2$, torr	41.7 ± 5.2	41.2 ± 4.1	41.4 ± 3.6	41.7 ± 6.7	43.7 ± 5.6	0.61 [a]
IP marker						
KL-6, U/mL	1040.3 ± 743.5	790.8 ± 428.0	1185.8 ± 921.6	1098.9 ± 759.5	1198.0 ± 859.2	0.22 [a]
SP-A, U/mL	68.3 ± 30.9	67.6 ± 33.7	68.5 ± 36.5	67.5 ± 27.8	71.7 ± 22.7	0.98 [a]
SP-D, U/mL	239.5 ± 163.6	176.7 ± 102.5	258.5 ±108.6	282.4 ± 236.9	239.1 ± 82.6	0.10 [a]

Data are reported as means ± SD or number (n). [a] p values calculated using a one-way analysis of variance with post hoc Tukey test. [b] p values calculated using a χ² test. [c] p < 0.05 vs. AFD. Abbreviations: n.s., not significant; AFD, antifibrotic drug; PR, pulmonary rehabilitation; BMI, body mass index; JRC, the Japanese Respiratory Society IPF disease severity classifications; GAP stage, Sex-Age-Physiology Index Stage; FVC, forced vital capacity; % pred, percent predicted; FEV_1, forced expiratory volume in 1 s; DLCO, lung diffusion capacity for carbon monoxide; IP marker; interstitial pneumonia serum marker, KL-6, Krebs von den Lungen-6; SP-A, surfactant protein-A; SP-D, surfactant protein-D.

Table 2. Comparison of results at baseline and 3 months in each group.

	Control		AFD		PR		PR+AFD	
	Baseline	3 Months	Baseline	3 Months	Baseline	3 Months	Baseline	3 Months
mMRC scale	1.3 ± 1.1	1.2 ± 0.9	1.4 ± 1.0	1.7 ± 1.2	1.5 ± 1.0	1.1 ± 0.8 [a]	1.9 ± 1.1	1.7 ±1.1
6 min walk test								
6MWD (m)	410.5 ± 98.1	413.2 ± 112.3	409.2 ± 115.1	374.7 ± 155.2	365.8 ± 96.9	410.5 ± 107.1 [b]	386.3 ± 91.1	420.4 ±124.4
% 6MWD (%)	86.0 ± 21.6	86.6 ± 24.8	83.1 ± 21.2	76.0 ± 30.4	73.5 ± 20.2	84.1 ± 23.7 [b]	78.5 ± 16.5	84.5 ±19.1
Muscle strength								
QF (Nm/kg)	1.2 ± 0.4	1.2 ± 0.5	1.3 ± 0.3	1.4 ± 0.5	1.3 ± 0.4	1.3 ± 0.3	1.3 ± 0.5	1.3 ±0.6
HGS (kg)	24.0 ± 7.8	24.2 ± 7.8	29.1 ± 7.3	28.5 ± 7.0	26.2 ± 8.3	26.4 ± 8.0	29.4 ± 7.7	30.2 ±7.8
HRQOL								
SGRQ total	32.3 ± 20.1	30.3 ± 16.5	38.3 ± 21.1	42.9 ± 20.4	39.6 ± 18.5	40.0 ± 20.2	52.1 ± 20.2	52.0 ±20.2
CAT	11.8 ± 9.1	11.8 ± 7.5	13.2 ± 9.1	15.9 ± 7.2 [c]	14.0 ±7.4	14.5 ± 7.4	20.1 ± 9.5	21.5 ±10.2

Data are reported as means ± SD. p values were calculated using the Wilcoxon rank-sum test. [a] p < 0.05 vs. PR at baseline; [b] p < 0.01 vs. PR at baseline; [c] p < 0.05 vs. AFD at baseline. Abbreviations: AFD, antifibrotic drugs; PR, pulmonary rehabilitation; mMRC, modified Medical Research Council test; 6MWD, six-minute walk distance; % 6MWD, percent predicted six-minute walk distance; QF, quadriceps force; HGS, hand grip strength; HRQOL, Health-Related Quality of Life; SGRQ, St George Respiratory Questionnaire; CAT, Chronic obstructive pulmonary disease assessment test.

Table 3 shows the changes in mMRC, 6MWD, HGS, QF and HRQoL over the 3-month intervention period. A comparison of the four groups using one-way ANOVA showed that

ΔmMRC was significantly worse in the AFD group than in the PR group ($p < 0.05$) while this was not the case for the other groups. There were no significant differences between groups in other variables (Table 3).

Table 3. Comparison of the change between baseline and 3 months between the groups.

	Control	AFD	PR	PR+AFD
Dyspnea				
ΔmMRC scale	−0.07 ± 0.6	0.3 ± 0.9 [a]	−0.4 ± 0.9	−0.1 ± 0.6
	(−0.3 to 0.2)	(−0.1 to 0.7)	(−0.7 to −0.06)	(−0.5 to 0.2)
Peripheral muscle strength				
ΔQF (Nm/kg)	0.06 ± 0.2	0.1 ± 0.4	−0.01 ± 0.3	−0.04 ± 0.4
	(−0.03 to 0.1)	(−0.08 to 0.3)	(−0.1 to 0.1)	(−0.3 to 0.3)
ΔHGS (kg)	0.2 ± 2.8	−0.5 ± 2.8	0.2 ± 2.1	0.6 ± 1.5
	(−0.9 to 1.3)	(−1.8 to 0.7)	(−0.5 to 1.0)	(−0.2 to 1.8)
HRQOL				
ΔSGRQ total	−1.9 ± 13.7	4.5 ± 9.6	0.4 ± 14.9	−0.04 ± 12.5
	(−7.5 to 3.6)	(0.7 to 8.9)	(−5.2 to 6.0)	(−8.4 to 8.4)
ΔCAT	−0.03 ± 6.2	2.6 ± 5.6	0.5 ± 6.6	1.3 ± 7.6
	(−2.5 to 2.4)	(0.04 to 5.1)	(−2.0 to 3.0)	(−3.7 to 6.5)

Data are reported as means ± SD. (95% confidence interval). p values were calculated using a one-way analysis of variance post hoc Tukey's test. [a] $p < 0.05$ vs. PR. Abbreviations: AFD, antifibrotic drugs; PR, pulmonary rehabilitation; Δ, delta; mMRC, modified Medical Research Council; QF, quadriceps force; HGS, hand grip strength; HRQOL, Health-Related Quality of Life; SGRQ, St George Respiratory Questionnaire; CAT, COPD assessment test.

The changes in 6MWD and %6MWD are shown in Figure 2A,B, respectively. Δ6MWD was significantly higher in the PR group than in the control and AFD groups ($p < 0.05$ and $p < 0.001$, respectively). In addition, the values in the PR+AFD group were significantly higher than those in the AFD group ($p < 0.01$). Similarly, Δ%6MWD was significantly higher in the PR group than in the control and AFD groups ($p < 0.05$ and $p < 0.001$ respectively). Moreover, the values in the PR+AFD group were significantly higher values than those in the AFD group ($p < 0.05$).

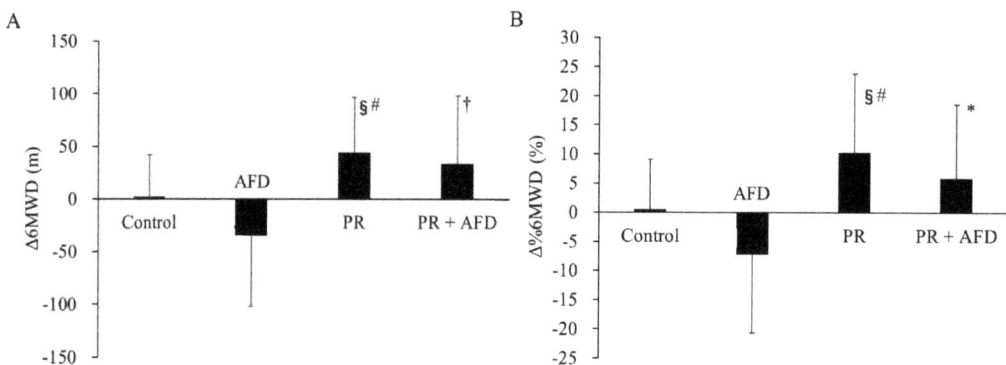

Figure 2. Comparison of the (**A**) change in six-minute walk distance (Δ6MWD) and (**B**) change in the percentage of predicted six-minute walk distance (Δ%6MWD) at 3 months between groups. Abbreviations: PR, pulmonary rehabilitation; AFD, antifibrotic drugs; 6MWD, six-minute walk distance; %6MWD, percent predicted six-minute walk distance. Vertical columns indicate means ± SD. p values were calculated using a one-way analysis of variance with post hoc Tukey's test. §: $p < 0.05$ vs. control, #: $p < 0.001$ vs. AFD, †: $p < 0.01$ vs. AFD, *: $p < 0.05$ vs. AFD.

Further, we investigated the association between Δ6MWD and ΔmMRC and ΔSGRQ in all patients. A significant negative correlation was found between ΔmMRC and Δ6MWD/Δ%6MWD ($r = -0.337$, $p < 0.05$ and $r = -0.331$, $p < 0.05$, respectively, Figure 3A,B). In addition, Δ6MWD and Δ%6MWD showed a significant negative correlation with ΔSGRQ ($r = -0.277$, $p < 0.05$ and $r = -0.301$, $p < 0.05$, respectively; Figure 3C,D).

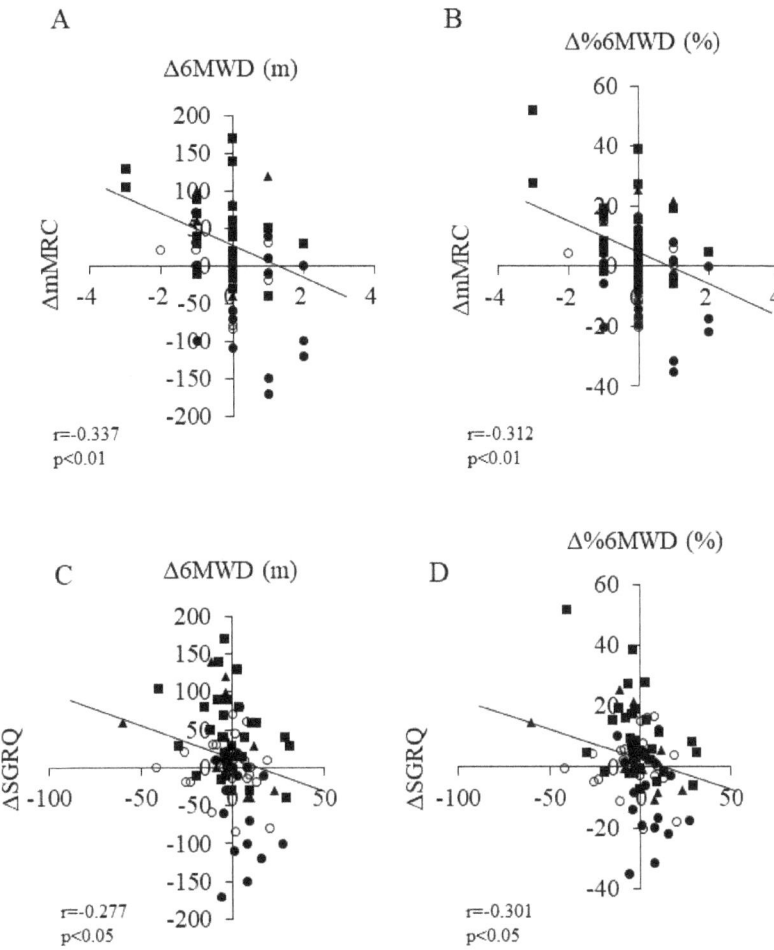

Figure 3. Relationship between (**A**) Δ6MWD and ΔmMRC scale scores, (**B**) Δ%6MWD and ΔmMRC scale scores, (**C**) Δ6MWD and ΔSGRQ scores, and (**D**) Δ%6MWD and ΔSGRQ scores in all patients. ○: control group, ■: PR group, ●: AFD group, ▲: PR+AFD group. Abbreviations: AFD, antifibrotic drugs; PR, pulmonary rehabilitation; Δ, delta; 6MWD, six-minute walk distance; mMRC, modified Medical Research Council; SGRQ, St George Respiratory Questionnaire.

Table 4 shows the AFD administration period at baseline in the PR+AFD and AFD groups, frequency of side effects, and their breakdown. There were no significant differences in the duration of AFD administration, incidence of overall side effects, or incidence of each side effect between the PR+AFD and AFD groups.

Table 4. Treatment adverse events in the AFD and PR+AFD groups.

	AFD	PR+AFD	p Value
Duration of AFD treatment at baseline, (days)	6.9 ±13.4	6.2 ±15.2	0.85 [a]
Number of patients with adverse events, n (%)			0.37 [b]
(−)	12 (57.1)	4 (36.3)	
(+)	9 (42.8)	7 (63.6)	
Adverse events			
Nausea, n (%)	0	1 (9.0)	0.16 [b]
Diarrhea, n (%)	5 (23.8)	3 (27.2)	0.37 [b]
Liver dysfunction, n (%)	3 (14.2)	1 (9.0)	0.67 [b]
Decreased appetite, n (%)	2 (9.5)	3 (27.2)	0.18 [b]
Fatigue, n (%)	0	1 (9.0)	0.16 [b]
Dizziness, n (%)	0	1 (9.0)	0.16 [b]
Photosensitivity reaction, n (%)	1 (4.7)	0	0.46 [b]
Thrombocytopenia, n (%)	0	1 (9.0)	0.16 [b]

Data are reported as means ± SD or number (%). [a] p values calculated using Mann–Whitney U test. [b] p values calculated using χ^2 test. Abbreviations: n.s., not significant; AFD, antifibrotic drugs; PR, pulmonary rehabilitation.

4. Discussion

To the best of our knowledge, this is the first study to examine the effects of PR on patients with IPF receiving AFDs. In the AFD group, a decrease in 6MWD was observed, and a significant improvement in Δ6MWD was observed in the PR+AFD group compared to the AFD group, suggesting a beneficial effect of PR on patients receiving AFDs.

In recent systemic reviews, PR was shown to improve exercise tolerance (6MWD and peak volume of oxygen consumed), reduce dyspnea, and improve HRQOL in patients with IPF [9,10]. In our study, the PR group showed a significant increase in 6MWD compared to the control group, which is consistent with the findings in previous studies [9]. It is also consistent with previous findings that the extended distance was about 40 m [9]. In contrast, previous studies on AFDs reported that pirfenidone suppressed the decline in FVC, 6MWD, and dyspnea scores after 52 weeks of intervention [4,12,26]. In addition, nintedanib has been shown to significantly suppress the decrease in FVC compared to placebo after 52 weeks of intervention and, in subgroup analyses, it suppressed deterioration in SGRQ scores in patients with severe IPF [6,13]. However, no study has reported the effects of AFDs after administration for only 3 months [4,13]. Therefore, in this study, we investigated the effect of PR with concurrent AFD administration and AFD monotherapy on 6MWD and HRQOL at 3 months.

An important consideration in AFD administration is side effects. The most common side effects are gastrointestinal symptoms, such as nausea, diarrhea, loss of appetite, and liver damage. These symptoms are likely to impair activities of daily living and HRQOL in patients with IPF [13]. In addition, pirfenidone has been reported to cause photosensitivity and rashes, which may limit outdoor activities of daily life and affect exercise tolerance and quality of life [6].

In this study, side effects similar to those in a previous study were observed in the AFD and PR+AFD groups (approximately 40% and 60% of participants, respectively), but no patient required discontinuation of medication due to side effects. However, in the AFD group, an average decrease of approximately 35 m in 6MWD was observed at 3 months from baseline. Since the minimum clinically significant difference in 6MWD in patients with IPF is 28 m, this change is clinically relevant, despite not being significant [27]. This suggests that AFD use affected 6MWD. In contrast, Δ6MWD in the PR+AFD group was significantly higher than that in the AFD group. This suggests that PR can prevent the decrease in 6MWD caused by AFDs in patients with IPF.

In this study, mMRC scale scores, which are an index of shortness of breath, showed a significant improvement after PR in the PR group. In addition, a significant difference was found in ΔmMRC values between the AFD and PR groups. Thus, the findings suggest that PR improves dyspnea.

Regarding the effect of AFDs on dyspnea, Kreuter et al. used the University of California San Diego shortness of breath questionnaire (UCSD-SOBQ) and reported that AFDs suppressed deterioration in the UCSD-SOBQ score compared to that with a placebo. However, this effect was not sufficient to improve dyspnea [13,28]. Therefore, it was suggested that PR is important for improving dyspnea. In the present study, ΔmMRC was found to have a significant negative correlation with Δ6MWD and Δ% 6MWD (Figure 3A,B). Thus, improvement in dyspnea contributes to improvement in the 6MWD.

In contrast, no significant improvement in dyspnea was observed in the PR+AFD group. This may be due to the small sample size of the PR+AFD group.

HRQOL is an important outcome of the effect of PR on IPF. In this study, SGRQ and CAT scores showed no significant difference in HRQOL between the groups. A previous study showed that compared to a placebo, AFDs significantly suppressed the deterioration of HRQOL assessed using SGRQ scores [13]. However, no significant change observed in the present study may be attributed to the short study period of 3 months (12 weeks) compared to the 52-week intervention in the previous study. Quality of life is influenced by a variety of factors such as exercise performance, daily symptoms and emotional factors, which can lead to variability in data [29]. In this study there was wide variability of change in SGRQ scores, which may have prevented detection of significant differences. In contrast, significant deterioration in CAT scores was observed only in the AFD group. It is possible that AFD can worsen quality of life at 3 months, as this is when side effects are likely to occur.

We also investigated the relationship between ΔSGRQ, Δ6MWD, and Δ% 6MWD in patients with IPF and found a significant negative correlation (Figure 3 C,D). In a previous cross-sectional study on the relationship between 6MWD and HRQOL, Verma et al. showed a significant correlation between SGRQ and 6MWD in 82 patients with IPF [30]; however, our study was longitudinal. Regarding the amount of change observed over three months, the fact that improvement in 6MWD contributed to the improvement of the SGRQ score was a new finding.

In a subanalysis of a larger multicenter study, patients with IPF under AFD treatment showed a trend for higher improvement in exercise capacity as compared to those not treated, suggesting a synergistic effect of AFD and PR. In contrast, our result showed PR tended to counteract the adverse effects of AFD on 6WMD [31]. This might be due to racial differences and differences in the frequency and duration of PR. Further study is warranted to clarify these points.

This study had some limitations. First, the sample was small, thus making the power of our inferences low. Using the mean and standard deviation data provided in our previous TRIP study report [14], the calculated sample sizes with power of 80% to detect significant change were 22 and 15 in each group for 6MWD and %6MWD, respectively. However, since IPF is a rare disease, this obstacle is difficult to overcome, and the sample size used here is not drastically different from that in previous studies. Second, the possibility of bias cannot be ruled out because this study was not randomized, and it was a single-center study.

Third, the large number of dropouts may have affected the results. In this study, the participants were older than those in previous studies. Thus, many patients had difficulty in reaching the hospital. In addition, since IPF is a progressive disease, there were cases of death due to acute worsening of patient condition.

Fourth, nintedanib and pirfenidone were not examined separately. Each has a different mechanism of action and side effects [4,5]; therefore, it is necessary to investigate these AFDs separately in the future. Fifth, we found no difference in the onset of side effects between the AFD group and the PR+AFD group (Table 4). Therefore, it could not be proven that PR suppresses side effects.

Lastly, the length of follow-up was just 3 months in this study. Both AFD and PR are treatments that should be continued as long as possible unless there is a reason to stop. Currently, a randomized controlled study to evaluate the 12-month effects of pulmonary rehabilitation in IPF treated with nintedanib is ongoing [32]. That study may reveal the contribution of concomitant use of nintedanib to the maintenance of long-term effects of pulmonary rehabilitation.

5. Conclusions

This study examined the effects of PR with concurrent AFD treatment in patients with IPF. It was suggested that while AFDs reduced exercise tolerance and HRQOL at 3 months, the concurrent use of PR may prevent or mitigate these effects.

Author Contributions: Conceptualization, Y.I., S.H. and S.E.; validation, Y.I. and S.E.; formal analysis, Y.I.; investigation, Y.I, K.E., K.N. and N.S.; data curation, Y.I., K.E., K.N. and N.S.; writing—original draft preparation, Y.I.; writing—review and editing, M.M., Y.N., S.S., K.K., S.H. and S.E.; visualization, Y.I.; supervision, S.E.; project administration, Y.I. and S.E.; funding acquisition, Y.I. and S.E. All authors have read and agreed to the published version of the manuscript.

Funding: Yuji Iwanami is currently receiving a grant (21H04317) from JSPS KAKENHI, and Satoru Ebihara is currently receiving grants (19H03984, 19K22821 and 22K19760) from JSPS KAKENHI. Other authors none.

Institutional Review Board Statement: The study was conducted in accordance with the Declaration of Helsinki, and approved by the Institutional Review Board of Toho University Medical Center Omori Hospital (M21153).

Informed Consent Statement: Written informed consent was obtained from all subjects involved in the study.

Data Availability Statement: The data presented in this study are available on request from the corresponding author.

Conflicts of Interest: The authors declare no conflict of interest.

References

1. Raghu, G.; Remy-Jardin, M.; Myers, J.L.; Richeldi, L.; Ryerson, C.J.; Lederer, D.J.; Behr, J.; Cottin, V.; Danoff, S.K.; Morell, F.; et al. Diagnosis of Idiopathic Pulmonary Fibrosis. An Official ATS/ERS/JRS/ALAT Clinical Practice Guideline. *Am. J. Respir. Crit. Care Med.* **2018**, *198*, e44–e68. [CrossRef] [PubMed]
2. Raghu, G.; Rochwerg, B.; Zhang, Y.; Cuello-Garcia, C.; Azuma, A.; Behr, J.; Brozek, J.L.; Collard, H.R.; Cunningham, W.; Homma, S.; et al. An Official ATS/ERS/JRS/ALAT Clinical Practice Guideline: Treatment of Idiopathic Pulmonary Fibrosis. An Update of the 2011 Clinical Practice Guideline. *Am. J. Respir. Crit. Care Med.* **2015**, *192*, e3–e19. [CrossRef] [PubMed]
3. Natsuizaka, M.; Chiba, H.; Kuronuma, K.; Otsuka, M.; Kudo, K.; Mori, M.; Bando, M.; Sugiyama, Y.; Takahashi, H. Epidemiologic Survey of Japanese Patients with Idiopathic Pulmonary Fibrosis and Investigation of Ethnic Differences. *Am. J. Respir. Crit. Care Med.* **2014**, *190*, 773–779. [CrossRef] [PubMed]
4. King, T.E., Jr.; Bradford, W.Z.; Castro-Bernardini, S.; Fagan, E.A.; Glaspole, I.; Glassberg, M.K.; Gorina, E.; Hopkins, P.M.; Kardatzke, D.; Lancaster, L.; et al. A phase 3 trial of pirfenidone in patients with idiopathic pulmonary fibrosis. *N. Engl. J. Med.* **2014**, *370*, 2083–2092. [CrossRef]
5. Richeldi, L.; Costabel, U.; Selman, M.; Kim, D.S.; Hansell, D.M.; Nicholson, A.G.; Brown, K.K.; Flaherty, K.R.; Noble, P.W.; Raghu, G.; et al. Efficacy of a Tyrosine Kinase Inhibitor in Idiopathic Pulmonary Fibrosis. *N. Engl. J. Med.* **2011**, *365*, 1079–1087. [CrossRef]
6. Richeldi, L.; Du Bois, R.M.; Raghu, G.; Azuma, A.; Brown, K.K.; Costabel, U.; Cottin, V.; Flaherty, K.R.; Hansell, D.M.; Inoue, Y.; et al. Efficacy and Safety of Nintedanib in Idiopathic Pulmonary Fibrosis. *N. Engl. J. Med.* **2014**, *370*, 2071–2082. [CrossRef]
7. Aravena, C.; Labarca, G.; Venegas, C.; Arenas, A.; Rada, G. Correction: Pirfenidone for Idiopathic Pulmonary Fibrosis: A Systematic Review and Meta-Analysis. *PLoS ONE* **2015**, *10*, e0140288.
8. Homma, S.; Bando, M.; Azuma, A.; Sakamoto, S.; Sugino, K.; Ishii, Y.; Izumi, S.; Inase, N.; Inoue, Y.; Ebina, M.; et al. Japanese guideline for the treatment of idiopathic pulmonary fibrosis. *Respir. Investig.* **2018**, *56*, 268–291. [CrossRef]
9. Dowman, L.; Hill, C.J.; May, A.; Holland, A.E. Pulmonary rehabilitation for interstitial lung disease. *Cochrane Database Syst Rev.* **2021**, *2*, CD006322. [CrossRef]
10. Yu, X.; Li, X.; Wang, L.; Liu, R.; Xie, Y.; Li, S.; Li, J. Pulmonary Rehabilitation for Exercise Tolerance and Quality of Life in IPF Patients: A Systematic Review and Meta-Analysis. *BioMed Res. Int.* **2019**, *2019*, 8498603. [CrossRef]
11. Kozu, R.; Senjyu, H.; Jenkins, S.C.; Mukae, H.; Sakamoto, N.; Kohno, S. Differences in response to pulmonary rehabilitation in idiopathic pulmonary fibrosis and chronic obstructive pulmonary disease. *Respiration* **2011**, *81*, 196–205. [CrossRef] [PubMed]
12. Noble, P.W.; Albera, C.; Bradford, W.Z.; Costabel, U.; Du Bois, R.M.; Fagan, E.A.; Fishman, R.S.; Glaspole, I.; Glassberg, M.K.; Lancaster, L.; et al. Pirfenidone for idiopathic pulmonary fibrosis: Analysis of pooled data from three multinational phase 3 trials. *Eur. Respir. J.* **2015**, *47*, 243–253. [CrossRef]

13. Kreuter, M.; Wuyts, W.A.; Wijsenbeek, M.; Bajwah, S.; Maher, T.; Stowasser, S.; Male, N.; Stansen, W.; Schoof, N.; Orsatti, L.; et al. Health-related quality of life and symptoms in patients with IPF treated with nintedanib: Analyses of patient-reported outcomes from the INPULSIS® trials. *Respir. Res.* **2020**, *21*, 36. [CrossRef] [PubMed]
14. Igarashi, A.; Iwanami, Y.; Sugino, K.; Gocho, K.; Homma, S.; Ebihara, S. Using 6-Min Walk Distance Expressed as a Percentage of Reference to Evaluate the Effect of Pulmonary Rehabilitation in Elderly Patients With Interstitial Lung Disease. *J. Cardiopulm. Rehabilitation Prev.* **2018**, *38*, 342–347. [CrossRef] [PubMed]
15. Miller, M.R.; Hankinson, J.; Brusasco, V.; Burgos, F.; Casaburi, R.; Coates, A.; Crapo, R.; Enright, P.; Van Der Grinten, C.P.M.; Gustafsson, P.; et al. Standardisation of spirometry. *Eur. Respir. J.* **2005**, *26*, 319–338. [CrossRef]
16. MacIntyre, N.; Crapo, R.O.; Viegi, G.; Johnson, D.C.; Van Der Grinten, C.P.M.; Brusasco, V.; Burgos, F.; Casaburi, R.; Coates, A.; Enright, P.; et al. Standardisation of the single-breath determination of carbon monoxide uptake in the lung. *Eur. Respir. J.* **2005**, *26*, 720–735. [CrossRef]
17. Ley, B.; Ryerson, C.J.; Vittinghoff, E.; Ryu, J.; Tomassetti, S.; Lee, J.S.; Poletti, V.; Buccioli, M.; Elicker, B.M.; Jones, K.D.; et al. A Multidimensional Index and Staging System for Idiopathic Pulmonary Fibrosis. *Ann. Intern. Med.* **2012**, *156*, 684–691. [CrossRef]
18. Natori, H.; Kawayama, T.; Suetomo, M.; Kinoshita, T.; Matsuoka, M.; Matsunaga, K.; Okamoto, M.; Hoshino, T. Evaluation of the Modified Medical Research Council Dyspnea Scale for Predicting Hospitalization and Exacerbation in Japanese Patients with Chronic Obstructive Pulmonary Disease. *Intern. Med.* **2016**, *55*, 15–24. [CrossRef]
19. Dowman, L.; McDonald, C.F.; Hill, C.J.; Lee, A.; Barker, K.; Boote, C.; Glaspole, I.; Goh, N.; Southcott, A.; Burge, A.; et al. Reliability of the hand held dynamometer in measuring muscle strength in people with interstitial lung disease. *Physiotherapy* **2015**, *102*, 249–255. [CrossRef]
20. Ringbaek, T.; Martinez, G.; Lange, P. A comparison of the assessment of quality of life with CAT, CCQ, and SGRQ in COPD patients participating in pulmonary rehabilitation. *COPD J. Chronic Obstr. Pulm. Dis.* **2012**, *9*, 12–15. [CrossRef]
21. Jones, P.W.; Quirk, F.H.; Baveystock, C.M.; Littlejohns, P. A self-complete measure of health status for chronic airflow limitation: The St. George's Respiratory Questionnaire. *Am. Rev. Respir. Dis.* **1992**, *145*, 1321–1327. [CrossRef]
22. Chang, J.A.; Curtis, J.R.; Patrick, D.L.; Raghu, G. Assessment of health-related quality of life in patients with interstitial lung disease. *Chest* **1999**, *116*, 1175–1182. [CrossRef] [PubMed]
23. Nagata, K.; Tomii, K.; Otsuka, K.; Tachikawa, R.; Otsuka, K.; Takeshita, J.; Tanaka, K.; Matsumoto, T.; Monden, K. Evaluation of the chronic obstructive pulmonary disease assessment test for measurement of health-related quality of life in patients with interstitial lung disease. *Respirology* **2012**, *17*, 506–512. [CrossRef] [PubMed]
24. ATS Committee on Proficiency Standards for Clinical Pulmonary Function Laboratories. ATS statement: Guidelines for the six-minute walk test. *Am. J. Respir. Crit. Care Med.* **2002**, *166*, 111–117. [CrossRef] [PubMed]
25. Enright, P.L. The six-minute walk test. *Respir Care* **2003**, *48*, 783–785.
26. Noble, P.W.; Albera, C.; Bradford, W.Z.; Costabel, U.; Glassberg, M.K.; Kardatzke, D.; King, T.E., Jr.; Lancaster, L.; Sahn, S.A.; Szwarcberg, J.; et al. Pirfenidone in patients with idiopathic pulmonary fibrosis (CAPACITY): Two randomised trials. *Lancet* **2011**, *377*, 1760–1769. [CrossRef]
27. Swigris, J.J.; Wamboldt, F.S.; Behr, J.; Du Bois, R.M.; King, T.E.; Raghu, G.; Brown, K.K. The 6 minute walk in idiopathic pulmonary fibrosis: Longitudinal changes and minimum important difference. *Thorax* **2009**, *65*, 173–177. [CrossRef]
28. Eakin, E.G.; Resnikoff, P.M.; Prewitt, L.M.; Ries, A.L.; Kaplan, R.M. Validation of a new dyspnea measure: The UCSD Shortness of Breath Questionnaire. University of California, San Diego. *Chest* **1998**, *113*, 619–624. [CrossRef]
29. Jones, P.W. Health status measurement in chronic obstructive pulmonary disease. *Thorax* **2001**, *56*, 880–887. [CrossRef]
30. Verma, G.; Marras, T.; Chowdhury, N.; Singer, L. Health-related quality of life and 6 min walk distance in patients with idiopathic pulmonary fibrosis. *Can. Respir J.* **2011**, *18*, 283–287. [CrossRef]
31. Brunetti, G.; Malovini, A.; Maniscalco, M.; Balestrino, A.; Carone, M.; Visca, D.; Capelli, A.; Vitacca, M.; Bellazzi, R.; Piaggi, G.; et al. Pulmonary rehabilitation in patients with interstitial lung diseases: Correlates of success. *Respir. Med.* **2021**, *185*, 106473. [CrossRef] [PubMed]
32. Nishiyama, O.; Kataoka, K.; Ando, M.; Arizono, S.; Morino, A.; Nishimura, K.; Ogawa, T.; Shiraki, A.; Watanabe, F.; Kozu, R.; et al. Protocol for long-term effect of pulmonary rehabilitation under nintedanib in idiopathic pulmonary fibrosis. *ERJ Open Res.* **2021**, *7*, 00321–2021. [CrossRef] [PubMed]

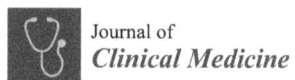
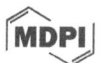

Article

Positive Effect of Manipulated Virtual Kinematic Intervention in Individuals with Traumatic Stiff Shoulder: A Pilot Study

Isabella Schwartz [1,2], Ori Safran [1,3], Naama Karniel [2,4,5], Michal Abel [2,5], Adina Berko [2,5], Martin Seyres [2], Tamir Tsoar [3] and Sigal Portnoy [4,*]

1. Faculty of Medicine, Hebrew University of Jerusalem, Jerusalem 91905, Israel; isabellas@hadassah.org.il (I.S.); oris@hadassah.org.il (O.S.)
2. Department of Physical Medicine & Rehabilitation, Hadassah Medical Center, Jerusalem 9765418, Israel; naamakar@gmail.com (N.K.); micsam@hadassah.org.il (M.A.); badina@hadassah.org.il (A.B.); martin.seyres@mail.huji.ac.il (M.S.)
3. Orthopedic Department, Hadassah Medical Center, Jerusalem 9765418, Israel; tamirt@hadassah.org.il
4. Department of Occupational Therapy, Sackler Faculty of Medicine, Tel Aviv University, Tel Aviv 6997801, Israel
5. Physical Therapy Department, Hadassah Medical Center, Jerusalem 9765418, Israel
* Correspondence: portnoys@tauex.tau.ac.il

Citation: Schwartz, I.; Safran, O.; Karniel, N.; Abel, M.; Berko, A.; Seyres, M.; Tsoar, T.; Portnoy, S. Positive Effect of Manipulated Virtual Kinematic Intervention in Individuals with Traumatic Stiff Shoulder: A Pilot Study. *J. Clin. Med.* **2022**, *11*, 3919. https://doi.org/10.3390/jcm11133919

Academic Editor: Masahiro Kohzuki

Received: 17 June 2022
Accepted: 4 July 2022
Published: 5 July 2022

Publisher's Note: MDPI stays neutral with regard to jurisdictional claims in published maps and institutional affiliations.

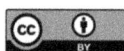

Copyright: © 2022 by the authors. Licensee MDPI, Basel, Switzerland. This article is an open access article distributed under the terms and conditions of the Creative Commons Attribution (CC BY) license (https://creativecommons.org/licenses/by/4.0/).

Abstract: Virtual reality enables the manipulation of a patient's perception, providing additional motivation to real-time biofeedback exercises. We aimed to test the effect of manipulated virtual kinematic intervention on measures of active and passive range of motion (ROM), pain, and disability level in individuals with traumatic stiff shoulder. In a double-blinded study, patients with stiff shoulder following proximal humerus fracture and non-operative treatment were randomly divided into a non-manipulated feedback group (NM-group; $n = 6$) and a manipulated feedback group (M-group; $n = 7$). The shoulder ROM, pain, and disabilities of the arm, shoulder and hand (DASH) scores were tested at baseline and after 6 sessions, during which the subjects performed shoulder flexion and abduction in front of a graphic visualization of the shoulder angle. The biofeedback provided to the NM-group was the actual shoulder angle while the feedback provided to the M-group was manipulated so that 10° were constantly subtracted from the actual angle detected by the motion capture system. The M-group showed greater improvement in the active flexion ROM ($p = 0.046$) and DASH scores ($p = 0.022$). While both groups improved following the real-time virtual feedback intervention, the manipulated intervention provided to the M-group was more beneficial in individuals with traumatic stiff shoulder and should be further tested in other populations with orthopedic injuries.

Keywords: virtual reality; biofeedback; shoulder pain; range of motion; motion capture

1. Introduction

Shoulder stiffness is defined as a restriction of the active and passive range of motion (ROM) of the glenohumeral joint [1]. A limitation in ROM means less than 100° range of motion in forward flexion [1]. Shoulder stiffness prevalence is estimated at 2–5% of the general population [2]. Other upper limb disorders might also limit ROM, e.g., damage following breast cancer treatment [3]. Shoulder stiffness can be secondary to a shoulder affliction, such as rotator cuff disease, osteoarthritis, trauma or surgery. In other cases, when the etiology of the stiffness is unknown, the condition is termed "primary frozen shoulder" or "primary idiopathic stiff shoulder" [1]. The loss of the shoulder's full ROM may lead to significant impairment in functionality that reduces the ability of the patient to accomplish daily activities independently. Furthermore, altered kinematics occur as a compensation mechanism and may lead to the development of subacromial impingement, scapular dyskensia, tendinitis, and degenerative changes [4]. Interventions for this pathology often include physical therapy [5], anti-inflammatory medication, intra-articular hydrocortisone injections, distension arthrography, and surgery [6,7]. Home exercises may also be encouraged [8]. In a recent study that compared the clinical and cost effectiveness of three interventions for adults with frozen shoulder (early structured physiotherapy with a steroid injection, manipulation under anesthesia with a steroid injection followed by post-procedural physiotherapy, and arthroscopic capsular release followed by manipulation and post-procedural physiotherapy) [9], the authors reported that no conclusions regarding the superiority of one intervention over another could be drawn. While physiotherapy with a steroid injection is the most accessible option, manipulation under anesthesia is the most cost-effective option, compared to early structured physiotherapy or arthroscopic capsular release [9]. For all interventions, the main anticipated outcomes are increased ROM and reduced pain levels.

As detailed in a recent review [10], individuals are more interested in leisure activities than in performing repetitive tasks during therapy. Consequently, virtual reality (VR) has been used and shown to induce repetition by enhancing motivation and enjoyment [10]. Since patients with shoulder stiffness might become uninterested in repetitive exercises and abandon them, thereby neglecting their rehabilitation, enriching exercises with newly available technologies may promote their motivation. For example, biofeedback systems have been shown to improve outcome measures in this population. In a recent randomized controlled study of 66 individuals with unilateral adhesive capsulitis, the study group performed shoulder abduction exercises with audible biofeedback provided by a wireless motion sensor [11]. The feedback volume was increased in relation to the elevation of the scapula. Compared to the control group, the study group that used the biofeedback showed increased scapular upward rotation and decreased shoulder pain and disability after two weeks and two months, respectively, and the improvement lasted six months [11]. Telerehabilitation has also evolved in recent years, mainly due to the requirement for social distancing following the outbreak of the COVID pandemic. A recent study showed that using inertial measurement unit-based sensors to track shoulder movements enhanced the three-month rehabilitation outcomes of individuals with stiff shoulder by increasing their compliance with training, thus improving functional recovery [12].

Virtual reality is another means to provide the user with real-time visual feedback of their performance. It has been used extensively for upper limb rehabilitation, e.g., using the Kinect sensor [13]. Different VR systems have been shown to be effective in survivors of stroke [14], as well as in individuals with kinesophobia and fragility in shoulder periarthritis [15]. To the best of our knowledge, it has yet to be applied for individuals with stiff shoulder. However, recently, a system that combines VR with wearable inertial measurement unit sensors was designed to perform motor assessment of shoulder ROM for this population [16]. The system was later utilized as a self-measurement system for shoulder joint mobility during four shoulder joint movements [17]. These systems have been used to provide non-manipulated real-time biofeedback.

Importantly, VR allows influencing of a patient's perception by manipulation of values presented to the user. This unique feature can provide a motivational addition to real-time biofeedback exercises [18,19]. For example, a study showed that when post-stroke individuals ambulated at their own pace on a treadmill connected to a VR visualization of a moving environment, when the VR optic speed was decreased, it promoted an increase in gait speed, although the participants were not consciously aware of it [18]. The authors assumed that if the patient walks faster during the physiotherapy sessions (even unintentionally), then the resulting high intensity exercise will shorten the rehabilitation period. However, the effect of manipulated virtual intervention for rehabilitation of the upper limb, specifically for individuals with traumatic stiff shoulder, is yet to be tested. Therefore, we sought to test the effect of manipulated virtual kinematic intervention on measures of active and passive ROM, pain, and disability level in individuals with traumatic stiff shoulder.

2. Materials and Methods

2.1. Study Design

This was a prospective randomized double-blinded study, in which individuals with stiff shoulder were randomly assigned to two groups, each receiving six sessions of exercises with kinematic biofeedback of shoulder movement. The feedback was manipulated for one group and not manipulated for the other. The group assignment was unknown to both the subjects and the researchers during the data collection.

2.2. Population

We recruited 16 patients with stiff shoulder; however, three dropped out of the study of their own volition (see personal characteristics in Table 1). The inclusion criteria were: age 18 to 70 years, at 6–24 weeks following a fracture of the proximal humerus, with limited flexion and abduction up to 90°, and with normal or corrected eyesight. The exclusion criteria were: neurological pathology that affects the upper body, and previous shoulder injury or degenerative alterations to the shoulder that limit its ROM. Ethical approval was granted by the Hadassah Medical Center Helsinki Committee pretrial (approval number 0321-17-HMO, ClinicalTrials.gov Identifier: NCT03196674). All participants read and signed an informed consent form.

Table 1. Patient characteristics of the non-manipulated feedback treatment group (NM-group) and the manipulated feedback treatment group (M-group).

Characteristic	M-Group (n = 6)	NM-Group (n = 7)	p
Age (years)	60.2 ± 6.1	63.3 ± 7.3	0.518
Sex	5 females, 1 male	7 females	0.261
Injured shoulder	2 left, 4 right	4 left, 3 right	0.391
Weeks from injury	6.2 ± 2.2	8.7 ± 5.1	0.563

2.3. Measurement Tools

A goniometer was used to measure the active and passive ROM of the shoulder (flexion and abduction) before and after the intervention [20,21]. A visual analogue scale (VAS) was used to record shoulder pain [22,23]. In addition, the Disabilities of the Arm, Shoulder and Hand (DASH) questionnaire [24] was administered [25]. The DASH score ranges from '0' (no disability) to '100' (most severe disability). A subjective questionnaire concerning satisfaction with the intervention included nine questions rated from '1' (not at all) to '5' (very much so), including: I was pleased with the exercises, I was motivated by the exercises, the exercises contributed to my self-esteem, I felt comfortable during the exercises, the feedback I received during the exercises was clear, the exercise was easy, I succeeded in the exercises, I enjoyed the exercises, I would have liked to continue with these exercises during the rehabilitation.

2.4. The Intervention

The intervention took place at the Gait and Motion Laboratory at the Hadassah Medical Center in Jerusalem. Each subject received a 6-session treatment plan (2–3 times a week, 30 min per session). Each session included motion exercises of flexion and abduction. In each session, 11 reflective markers were placed on the following anatomic landmarks: right and left acromion, jugular notch, xiphisternal joint, T8 and C7 vertebras, medial and lateral epicondyles of the elbow of the injured limb, and a three-marker cluster placed on the injured humerus in the sagittal plane. Ten infra-red cameras (Qualisys, Gothenburg, Sweden) tracked the coordinates of the markers at a frequency of 120 Hz. The subject sat on a chair with no armrest, 2 m in front of a large screen (42 inch). Real-time visual feedback was provided using Visual 3D (C-motion, Germantown, MD, USA) showing a small skeletal representation of the subject's torso and upper arm and a white moving graph showing advancing time on the X-axis and the 2D shoulder angle currently practiced on the Y-axis, i.e., either flexion or abduction. A yellow horizontal line was set at 90° to serve as a target (Figure 1). The kinematic feedback provided to the NM-group was the actual shoulder angle detected by the motion capture system. The kinematic feedback provided to the M-group was manipulated so that 10° were constantly subtracted from the actual shoulder angle detected by the motion capture system. The rationale for choosing a subtraction of 10° was based on preliminary trial-and-error with healthy individuals, where we surmised that, in the current settings of screen size and distance from the screen, subtraction of less than 5° might not be noticeable on screen, while a subtraction of more than 15° could be detected by the subject and he or she might be aware of a "mistake" in the feedback, so that the subject was not blinded to the manipulation. To achieve blinding of the researcher, four templates were prepared for combinations of flexion/abduction and manipulated/non-manipulated. The templates were named: ABD1, ABD2, Flex1, and Flex2. The subject received either an ABD1 and Flex1 combination or an ABD2 and Flex2 combination. Each combination was either manipulated or not, but this was not disclosed to the researcher collecting the data.

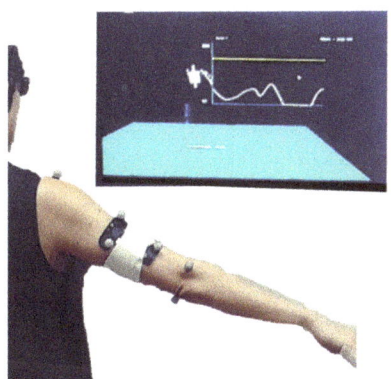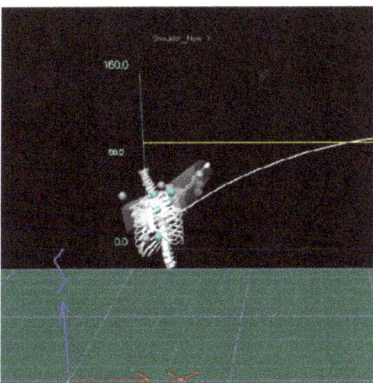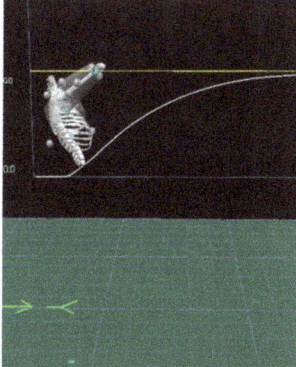

Figure 1. The subject (**left frame**) standing in front of the virtual presentation during shoulder abduction (**middle frame**) and flexion (**right frame**), as presented to the subject. The horizontal yellow line marks the target of 90°. The white line is the shoulder angle, presented in real-time. In these pictures, a healthy volunteer demonstrates a full range of motion.

2.5. Study Protocol

The subjects were randomly divided into two groups. One group received the non-manipulated feedback treatment (NM-group; $n = 6$) and the second group received the manipulated feedback treatment (M-group; $n = 7$). The shoulder passive and active ROM, pain and activity levels were tested at baseline and after the six sessions. The satisfaction questionnaire was filled out by each patient after the sessions.

2.6. Statistical Analysis

Statistical analyses were performed using SPSS 27.0 (SPSS Chicago, IL, USA). We performed a Shapiro–Wilk test and found that most of the parameters were not normally-distributed. We therefore represented descriptive statistics using median and interquartile percentages and chose the Mann–Whitney U test, a non-parametric test, to compare the two groups. The effect size, r, was calculated using the following equation [26]:

$$r = \frac{z}{\sqrt{N}} \qquad (1)$$

Statistical significance was considered at $p < 0.05$.

3. Results

There were no statistically significant between-group differences at baseline in the measures of active and passive ROM, VAS, or DASH scores (Table 2). However, following the intervention, the M-group showed greater improvement in the active flexion ROM and the DASH scores (Table 3). We used the Spearman correlation test to examine correlations between the pain levels and DASH scores before and after the intervention—no statistically significant correlations were found.

Table 2. Baseline active and passive range of motion (ROM) of shoulder flexion and abduction, visual analogue scale (VAS) ratings for pain levels, and Disabilities of the Arm, Shoulder and Hand (DASH) scores. Values are presented as median and interquartile percentages for each of the two groups: the non-manipulated feedback treatment group (NM-group) and the manipulated feedback treatment group (M-group).

Characteristic	M-Group (n = 6)	NM-Group (n = 7)	p	r
Passive flexion ROM (°)	90.0 (70.0–100.0)	97.0 (92.0–105.0)	0.197	−0.358
Passive abduction ROM (°)	64.0 (47.5–75.0)	70.0 (60.0–80.0)	0.428	−0.220
Active flexion ROM (°)	61.5 (38.8–77.5)	82.0 (78.0–85.0)	0.053	−0.536
Active abduction ROM (°)	52.5 (39.5–59.0)	48.0 (44.0–60.0)	0.830	−0.060
VAS (0–10)	3.5 (0.8–5.1)	3.0 (0.0–5.0)	0.942	−0.020
DASH (0–100)	88.6 (72.7–108.6)	96.0 (81.1–104.3)	0.668	−0.119

Table 3. Percent of change (after the intervention/baseline × 100) in active and passive range of motion (ROM) of shoulder flexion and abduction, as well as the Disabilities of the Arm, Shoulder and Hand (DASH) score following 6 treatment sessions. The visual analogue scale (VAS) ratings for pain levels are depicted as difference (after the intervention - baseline). Values are presented as median and interquartile percentages for each of the two groups: the non-manipulated feedback treatment group (NM-group) and the manipulated feedback treatment group (M-group).

Characteristic	M-Group (n = 6)	NM-Group (n = 7)	p	r
Passive flexion ROM (%)	127.8 (113.3–173.2)	125.6 (106.0–152.5)	0.391	−0.238
Passive abduction ROM (%)	134.5 (115.8–191.4)	146.4 (137.3–180.0)	1.000	0
Active flexion ROM (%)	197.1 (140.5–425.0)	142.5 (139.1–151.3)	0.046	−0.555
Active abduction ROM (%)	150.0 (124.8–191.2)	162.5 (129.2–187.5)	1.000	0
VAS (0–10)	75.0 (12.5–106.8)	26.7 (5.0–120.8)	0.916	−0.034
DASH (%)	67.7 (52.8–86.2)	89.7 (83.8–98.3)	0.022	−0.634

As shown in Table 3 and Figure 2, measures of active flexion ROM and DASH scores were improved to a greater extent in the M-group compared to the NM-group. However, all the study population increased their active flexion ROM by at least 16°, which is the minimal clinical difference found for glenohumeral motion of people with a shoulder pathology [27]. However, only four (57.1%) subjects in the NM-group improved their DASH scores by more than 10.8 points, which is the minimal clinically important difference for this evaluation [28], while all of the subjects in the M-group improved their DASH scores by more than 10.8 points.

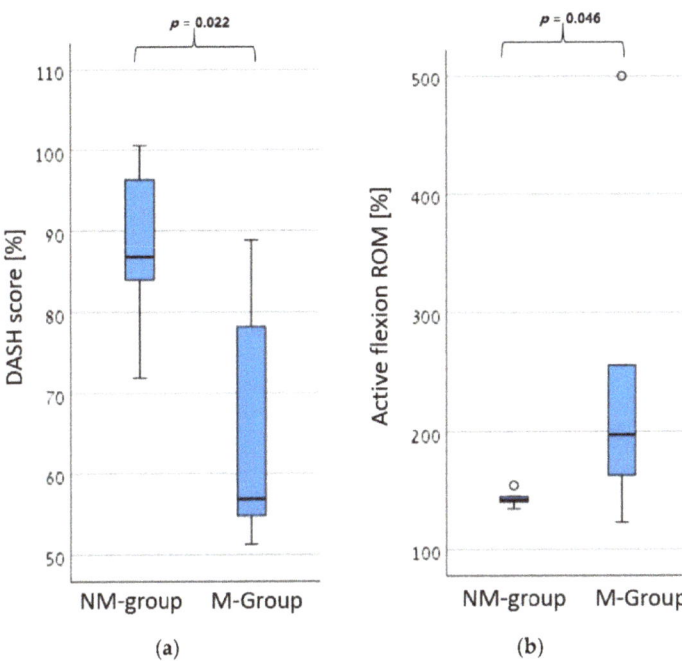

Figure 2. The percentage change (before and after the intervention) in (**a**) the Disabilities of the Arm, Shoulder and Hand (DASH) scores and (**b**) the active flexion range of motion (ROM) for both the non-manipulated feedback treatment group (NM-group; $n = 6$) and the manipulated feedback treatment group (M-group; $n = 7$).

There were no statistically significant between-group differences in the pain VAS scores. Only two subjects (28.6%) in the NM-group and one subject (16.7%) in the M-group improved their VAS score by more than 3 cm, which is the clinically important change in pain VAS score [29].

There was no statistically significant difference in the satisfaction questionnaire scores ($p = 0.712$, $r = -0.111$), as the median and interquartile percentages were 33.0 (25.8–38.0) and 37.0 (29.8–40.5) for the M-group and NM-group, respectively.

4. Discussion

In this double-blinded pilot study, we showed, for the first time, that a manipulated virtual real-time presentation of a subject's movements during shoulder exercises promoted greater active flexion ROM and better DASH scores after six weeks of intervention. These results are consistent with the results of a similar manipulation of gait in stroke survivors [18]. To the best of our knowledge, this is the first study to show an effect of a manipulation-based intervention on functional measures of patients. Our pilot study may serve as a first step towards integrating a perceptual component into designed interventions that incorporate biofeedback to improve rehabilitation outcomes.

The success of the manipulation of visual cues over the proprioceptive cues of the subjects in this study relies on recent findings from an investigation that incorporated a visuo-proprioceptive conflict [30]. In this investigation, reaching movements were viewed in a virtual environment and were altered in time (0.5 s delay). While the subjects were aware of the manipulation, the authors found that precision control determined the influence of separate sensory modalities on behavior, by biasing action towards cues from that modality. In our study, we anticipated that the subjects in the M-group would respond to the virtual visual feedback by increasing the ROM of either flexion or abduction.

The greater improvement observed in active flexion ROM in the M-group is an encouraging finding in support of manipulated real-time kinematic feedback. A recent systematic review [31] concerning shoulder ROM needed for the performance of activities of daily living, showed that a shoulder flexion ROM of more than 90° is required for tasks such as turning a key, combing hair, or putting on a neckless. The majority of the subjects in both groups did not have adequate shoulder ROM to perform these activities. However, the improvement shown by our subjects, especially the significant improvement observed in the M-group, allowed them to extend their daily activities. Unfortunately, there were no between-group differences found in the active abduction ROM and the passive ROM. The baseline measures for the flexion ROM showed a trend for lower ROM of the M-group, although not statistically significant, so that some of the subjects in that group might have had a larger potential for improvement compared to some subjects in the NM-group. However, the highest value of active flexion ROM at baseline in the NM-group was only 92°, which was well below the normal active flexion ROM of 160° reported in a similar age group [32]. Therefore, we believe that the 54.6% median difference in percentage change in the active flexion ROM between the M-group and NM-group indicates an advantage of the manipulated feedback.

While some of the improvement in the active ROM might be attributed to compensation mechanisms via increased scapular upward rotation, clavicular motion, or position alterations [33], the overall results suggests that the M-group achieved improved forward flexion following the intervention, promoting their ability to perform daily activities, as indicated by the higher DASH scores of this group. Since the baseline DASH scores of the two groups were very similar, the statistically significant improvement in DASH scores of the M-group suggests a positive effect of the manipulated intervention. In addition to the improvement in DASH scores, shown by the higher percentage of change following the intervention, it is notable that all the M-group subjects improved these scores by more than the minimal clinically important difference, whereas in the NM-group three out of seven subjects did not improve their scores by more than the minimal clinically important difference. For these three subjects, the intervention was clearly less effective compared to its effect on the rest of the subjects. While there was no between-group difference in pain, we believe that the improvement in active flexion ROM resulted in improved functionality in daily activities, which is a primary outcome measure in patients' rehabilitation. In cases where patients show no improvement in functionality following physical treatment, they become candidates for surgical intervention [34].

There was high between-subject variability in the percentage improvement in pain levels, as measured by the VAS scores. Although both groups showed similar improvement, only three subjects improved their VAS score by more than 3 cm. This might be explained by the use of conventional therapy in our medical center, as the pain level of each patient is respected. In a prospective multi-center study that compared the pain levels of individuals with stiff shoulder, it was found that patients undergoing conventional physiotherapy, where their pain threshold was respected, reported higher pain levels in the first few weeks of the treatment compared to patients who were encouraged to exceed their pain threshold [35]. Since our pilot study lasted only six weeks, the variability in the levels of pain improvement might be related to the effect of physiotherapy exercises conducted under painful conditions. A different method, in which subjects continue to pursue higher levels of ROM, despite their pain threshold being reached, might have produced different results.

Both groups reported similar satisfaction with the intervention. This is an important factor when considering the future integration of manipulated feedback in motor rehabilitation, since it shows that the blinded M-group was not aware of the perceptive alteration imposed by the feedback system. This indicates that the M-group performed non-volitional modulation towards higher intensity exercises, promoted by the reduced kinematics presented to them. This response proved to be advantageous for their rehabilitation. However, since one of the factors influencing patient satisfaction is clinical outcomes [36], the similarity of the satisfaction levels between the two groups seems to contradict the benefits of the

M-group over the NM-group, as found in the active flexion ROM and DASH scores. This might be explained by other factors that can affect patient satisfaction, e.g., characteristics of the physiotherapist, patient features, the physiotherapist-patient relationship, and features of the healthcare setting [36].

The main study limitations are the small sample size and short intervention period. However, the effect sizes for both statistically significant findings, i.e., the active flexion ROM (0.555) and the DASH (0.634) score, exceeded a value of 0.5, which is considered a large effect size [37]. Since effect size is independent of the sample size and was found to be larger than 0.5 in this study, this supports the high impact of the intervention. Moreover, there was high between-subject variability in most measured parameters, which was expected for this population [38]. Future studies of manipulated feedback should involve a longer intervention and examine possible habituation effects of the perception manipulation. In addition, follow up examination to assess lasting effects of the intervention should be added to the protocol.

5. Conclusions

We conclude that manipulated virtual kinematic intervention might be beneficial in individuals with traumatic stiff shoulder and should be further tested for other populations with orthopedic injuries, such as elbow and knee injuries. Furthermore, future system creators should construct VR systems for home-use (personal exercises and/or telerehabilitation exercises), in which kinematic manipulation is included in the exercises. Machine learning algorithms can be applied to negate habituation effects and increase the efficacy of treatment. The positive effect of biofeedback manipulation should also be investigated for other physical measures, such as grip or pinch forces and limb coordination.

Author Contributions: Conceptualization, I.S. and S.P.; methodology, I.S. and S.P.; software, S.P. and M.S.; validation, S.P. and M.S.; formal analysis, S.P.; investigation, S.P.; resources, I.S., O.S. and T.T.; data curation, N.K., M.A. and A.B.; writing—original draft preparation, S.P.; writing—review and editing, S.P., I.S., N.K., M.A., A.B., T.T. and O.S.; visualization, N.K. and S.P.; supervision, I.S., N.K. and S.P.; project administration, M.S., M.A. and A.B.; funding acquisition, I.S. All authors have read and agreed to the published version of the manuscript.

Funding: This research was fully funded by the Hadassah France Association (#6075796).

Institutional Review Board Statement: Ethical approval was granted by the Hadassah Medical Center Helsinki Committee pretrial (approval number 0321-17-HMO, ClinicalTrials.gov Identifier: NCT03196674).

Informed Consent Statement: Informed consent was obtained from all subjects involved in the study.

Data Availability Statement: Data are submitted with the paper.

Conflicts of Interest: The authors declare no conflict of interest.

References

1. Itoi, E.; Arce, G.; Bain, G.I.; Diercks, R.L.; Guttmann, D.; Imhoff, A.B.; Mazzocca, A.D.; Sugaya, H.; Yoo, Y.S. Shoulder Stiffness: Current Concepts and Concerns. *Arthroscopy* **2016**, *32*, 1402–1414. [CrossRef]
2. Pogorzelski, J.; Imhoff, A.B.; Degenhardt, H.; Siebenlist, S. Primary (idiopathic) shoulder stiffness: Definition, disease progression, epidemiology and etiology. *Unfallchirurg* **2019**, *122*, 917–924. [CrossRef] [PubMed]
3. De Groef, A.; Van Kampen, M.; Dieltjens, E.; Christiaens, M.R.; Neven, P.; Geraerts, I.; Devoogdt, N. Effectiveness of postoperative physical therapy for upper-limb impairments after breast cancer treatment: A systematic review. *Arch. Phys. Med. Rehabil.* **2015**, *96*, 1140–1153. [CrossRef] [PubMed]
4. Lin, J.J.; Lim, H.K.; Yang, J.L. Effect of shoulder tightness on glenohumeral translation, scapular kinematics, and scapulohumeral rhythm in subjects with stiff shoulders. *J. Orthop. Res.* **2006**, *24*, 1044–1051. [CrossRef] [PubMed]
5. Chan, H.B.Y.; Pua, P.Y.; How, C.H. Physical therapy in the management of frozen shoulder. *Singap. Med. J.* **2017**, *58*, 685–689. [CrossRef]
6. Donatelli, R.; Ruivo, R.M.; Thurner, M.; Ibrahim, M.I. New concepts in restoring shoulder elevation in a stiff and painful shoulder patient. *Phys. Ther. Sport* **2014**, *15*, 3–14. [CrossRef]
7. Bhargav, D.; Murrell, G.A. Shoulder stiffness: Management. *Aust. Fam. Physician* **2004**, *33*, 149–152.

8. Hanchard, N.C.A.; Goodchild, L.; Brealey, S.D.; Lamb, S.E.; Rangan, A. Physiotherapy for primary frozen shoulder in secondary care: Developing and implementing stand-alone and post operative protocols for UK FROST and inferences for wider practice. *Physiotherapy* **2020**, *107*, 150–160. [CrossRef]
9. Brealey, S.; Northgraves, M.; Kottam, L.; Keding, A.; Corbacho, B.; Goodchild, L.; Srikesavan, C.; Rex, S.; Charalambous, C.P.; Hanchard, N.; et al. Surgical treatments compared with early structured physiotherapy in secondary care for adults with primary frozen shoulder: The UK FROST three-arm RCT. *Health Technol. Assess.* **2020**, *24*, 1–161. [CrossRef]
10. Qian, J.; McDonough, D.J.; Gao, Z. The Effectiveness of Virtual Reality Exercise on Individual's Physiological, Psychological and Rehabilitative Outcomes: A Systematic Review. *Int. J. Environ. Res. Public Health* **2020**, *17*, 4133. [CrossRef]
11. Mohamed, A.A.; Jan, Y.K.; El Sayed, W.H.; Wanis, M.E.A.; Yamany, A.A. Dynamic scapular recognition exercise improves scapular upward rotation and shoulder pain and disability in patients with adhesive capsulitis: A randomized controlled trial. *J. Man. Manip. Ther.* **2020**, *28*, 146–158. [CrossRef]
12. Chen, Y.P.; Lin, C.Y.; Tsai, M.J.; Chuang, T.Y.; Lee, O.K.S. Wearable Motion Sensor Device to Facilitate Rehabilitation in Patients with Shoulder Adhesive Capsulitis: Pilot Study to Assess Feasibility. *J. Med. Internet Res.* **2020**, *22*, e17032. [CrossRef]
13. Muñoz, G.F.; Mollineda, R.A.; Casero, J.G.; Pla, F. A RGBD-Based Interactive System for Gaming-Driven Rehabilitation of Upper Limbs. *Sensors* **2019**, *19*, 3478. [CrossRef]
14. Kiper, P.; Szczudlik, A.; Agostini, M.; Opara, J.; Nowobilski, R.; Ventura, L.; Tonin, P.; Turolla, A. Virtual Reality for Upper Limb Rehabilitation in Subacute and Chronic Stroke: A Randomized Controlled Trial. *Arch. Phys. Med. Rehabil.* **2018**, *99*, 834–842.e4. [CrossRef]
15. Kapşigay, B.; Sari, Z.; Kavlak, B.; Aras, I.; Tanhan, A. Effects of virtual rehabilitation on shoulder periarthritis. *Ann. Rheum. Dis.* **2017**, *76*, 1496.
16. Lee, S.H.; Yeh, S.C.; Chan, R.C.; Chen, S.; Yang, G.; Zheng, L.R. Motor Ingredients Derived from a Wearable Sensor-Based Virtual Reality System for Frozen Shoulder Rehabilitation. *Biomed. Res. Int.* **2016**, *2016*, 7075464. [CrossRef]
17. Cui, J.; Yeh, S.C.; Lee, S.H. Wearable Sensors Integrated with Virtual Reality: A Self-Guided Healthcare System Measuring Shoulder Joint Mobility for Frozen Shoulder. *J. Healthc. Eng.* **2019**, *2019*, 7681237. [CrossRef]
18. Lamontagne, A.; Fung, J.; McFadyen, B.J.; Faubert, J. Modulation of walking speed by changing optic flow in persons with stroke. *J. Neuroeng. Rehabil.* **2007**, *4*, 22. [CrossRef]
19. Adamovich, S.V.; Fluet, G.G.; Tunik, E.; Merians, A.S. Sensorimotor training in virtual reality: A review. *NeuroRehabilitation* **2009**, *25*, 29–44. [CrossRef]
20. Kolber, M.J.; Mdt, C.; Hanney, W.J. The Reliability AND Concurrent Validity of Shoulder Mobility Measurements Using a Digital Inclinometer and Goniometer: A Technical Report. *Int. J. Sports Phys. Ther.* **2012**, *7*, 306.
21. Elgendy, M.H.; El-khalek, W.O.A.A. Validity and Intra-Rater Reliability of Laser Goniometer versus Electro-Goniometer in Measuring Shoulder Range of Motion. *Int. J. Physiother.* **2019**, *6*, 169–176. [CrossRef]
22. Karcioglu, O.; Topacoglu, H.; Dikme, O.; Dikme, O. A systematic review of the pain scales in adults: Which to use? *Am. J. Emerg. Med.* **2018**, *36*, 707–714. [CrossRef]
23. Green, S.; Buchbinder, R.; Hetrick, S.E. Physiotherapy interventions for shoulder pain. *Cochrane Database Syst. Rev.* **2003**, *2003*. [CrossRef]
24. Roy, J.S.; Macdermid, J.C.; Woodhouse, L.J. Measuring shoulder function: A systematic review of four questionnaires. *Arthritis Rheum.* **2009**, *61*, 623–632. [CrossRef]
25. Wajngarten, D.; Campos, J.; Garcia, P. The Disabilities of the Arm, Shoulder and Hand scale in the evaluation of disability—A literature review. *Med. Lav.* **2017**, *108*, 314–323.
26. Fritz, C.O.; Morris, P.E.; Richler, J.J. Effect size estimates: Current use, calculations, and interpretation. *J. Exp. Psychol. Gen.* **2012**, *141*, 2–18. [CrossRef]
27. Susan Muir, C.; Muir, S.W.; Luciak Corea, C.; Beaupre, L. Evaluating Change in Clinical Status: Reliability and Measures of Agreement for the Assessment of Glenohumeral Range of Motion. *N. Am. J. Sports Phys. Ther.* **2010**, *5*, 98.
28. Franchignoni, F.; Vercelli, S.; Giordano, A.; Sartorio, F.; Bravini, E.; Ferriero, G. Minimal clinically important difference of the disabilities of the arm, shoulder and hand outcome measure (DASH) and its shortened version (QuickDASH). *J. Orthop. Sports Phys. Ther.* **2014**, *44*, 30–39. [CrossRef]
29. Lee, J.S.; Hobden, E.; Stiell, I.G.; Wells, G.A. Clinically important change in the visual analog scale after adequate pain control. *Acad. Emerg. Med.* **2003**, *10*, 1128–1130. [CrossRef]
30. Limanowski, J.; Friston, K. Active inference under visuo-proprioceptive conflict: Simulation and empirical results. *Sci. Rep.* **2020**, *10*, 4010. [CrossRef]
31. Oosterwijk, A.M.; Nieuwenhuis, M.K.; Van der Schans, C.P.; Mouton, L.J. Shoulder and elbow range of motion for the performance of activities of daily living: A systematic review. *Physiother. Theory Pract.* **2018**, *34*, 505–528. [CrossRef] [PubMed]
32. Gill, T.K.; Shanahan, E.M.; Tucker, G.R.; Buchbinder, R.; Hill, C.L. Shoulder range of movement in the general population: Age and gender stratified normative data using a community-based cohort. *BMC Musculoskelet. Disord.* **2020**, *21*, 676. [CrossRef] [PubMed]
33. Ludewig, P.M.; Reynolds, J.F. The association of scapular kinematics and glenohumeral joint pathologies. *J. Orthop. Sports Phys. Ther.* **2009**, *39*, 90–104. [CrossRef] [PubMed]
34. Neviaser, A.S.; Neviaser, R.J. Adhesive capsulitis of the shoulder. *J. Am. Acad. Orthop. Surg.* **2011**, *19*, 536–542. [CrossRef]

35. Gleyze, P.; Flurin, P.H.; Laprelle, E.; Katz, D.; Toussaint, B.; Benkalfate, T.; Solignac, N.; Lévigne, C. Pain management in the rehabilitation of stiff shoulder: Prospective multicenter comparative study of 193 cases. *Orthop. Traumatol. Surg. Res.* **2011**, *97*, S195–S203. [CrossRef]
36. Rossettini, G.; Latini, T.M.; Palese, A.; Jack, S.M.; Ristori, D.; Gonzatto, S.; Testa, M. Determinants of patient satisfaction in outpatient musculoskeletal physiotherapy: A systematic, qualitative meta-summary, and meta-synthesis. *Disabil. Rehabil.* **2020**, *42*, 460–472. [CrossRef]
37. Oh-Young, C.; Gordon, H.R.D.; Xing, X.; Filler, J. Meta-Analytic Procedures for Career and Technical Education Post-secondary Researchers and Practitioners. *J. Res. Tech. Careers* **2018**, *2*, 32. [CrossRef]
38. Pease, B.; Ross, M. Defining subgroups of patients with a stiff and painful shoulder: An analytical model using cluster analysis. *Disabil. Rehabil.* **2021**, *43*, 537–544. [CrossRef]

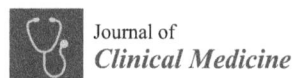 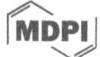

Article

Does Application of Lymphatic Drainage with Kinesiology Taping Have Any Effect on the Extent of Edema and Range of Motion in Early Postoperative Recovery following Primary Endoprosthetics of the Knee Joint?

Magdalena Sobiech, Agata Czępińska *, Grzegorz Zieliński, Magdalena Zawadka and Piotr Gawda

Department of Sports Medicine, Faculty of Health Sciences, Medical University of Lublin, 20-093 Lublin, Poland; magdalena.sobiech@umlub.pl (M.S.); grzegorz.zielinski@umlub.pl (G.Z.); magdalena.zawadka@umlub.pl (M.Z.); piotr.gawda@umlub.pl (P.G.)
* Correspondence: agataczepinska@umlub.pl; Tel.: +48-81448-6760

Abstract: Background: The surgery of knee replacement due to degenerative changes is the last step of the treatment. After surgery, a major problem in patients is pain, swelling, intraarticular hematoma, and the restriction of the mobility of the joint. The aim of this work was to determine the effect of Kinesio Taping (KT) on reducing edema of the subcutaneous tissue and improving the range of motion in the joint. Methods: 82 patients were qualified for the study. After surgery, 42 patients received postoperative edema treatment with KT bands, and 40 patients did not receive the treatment. The swelling thickness and range of mobility were measured on the third and eighth days after the operation. Results: A statistical difference between the longitudinal measurements of the KT group and the group without KT application was shown at the level of the fibula head, 25 mm below the fibula neck, and 50 mm below the fibular neck. There were no statistically significant differences in the change in knee angle between the applied and non-applied patients. Conclusion: The lymphatic application technique KT influences the absorption of subcutaneous edema after primary knee joint replacement surgery but has no influence on mobility.

Keywords: osteoarthritis; rehabilitation; swelling; total knee arthroplasty

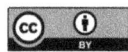

1. Introduction

Osteoarthritis (OA) is a modern-age disease of an unknown etiology and a process including various types of factors, such as genetic, metabolic, inflammatory, and mechanical factors [1–3]. According to specialists, the symptoms of osteoarthritis are revealed in X-Ray imaging in one-third of the world population [4]. Regarding etiology, osteoarthritis can be divided into two types: primary (idiopathic) of unknown etiology and secondary [5]. A knee joint is one of the most vulnerable to overload and the occurrence of degenerative lesions, so-called gonarthrosis [6]. It is related to its structure and the function it serves in transferring heavy loads [7]. The symptoms of gonarthrosis are characterized by pain at the initial stage of motion, flexion deformity of the affected joints, morning stiffness lasting up to 30 min or stiffness after inactivity, crepitus occurring during movement, and joint effusion [8]. In the next stage of the disease, outline thickening and joint instability occur [9]. Conservative treatment of osteoarthritis is based on pain relief, flexion deformity reduction, muscle strength retention preventing joint contractures, tissue swelling reduction, and gait function improvement [10]. Conservative treatment also includes physiotherapy and pharmacological treatment [11]. Surgical treatment of a knee joint is the last part of osteoarthritis treatment. Knee endoprosthesis is a surgical procedure to replace the damaged joint structure with new elements [12]. An artificial knee joint is made of metal elements that imitate distal femoral epiphysis and proximal tibial epiphysis [3,12,13]. They are separated with a spacer made of plastic. The method of surgery and the choice of implant depend on many factors, i.e., degenerative changes in a knee joint, the age of a patient, and their general condition [12,13]. In the first few days after the surgery, a patient may be affected with the following problems: the pain of an operated limb, intra-articular hematoma, subcutaneous edema, and flexion deformity. Long-lasting symptoms may inhibit the process of post-surgical and full recovery [14]. Regarding the growing number of patients undergoing surgery as a result of advanced osteoarthritis, it is legitimate to seek new and effective physiotherapeutic methods applied in the initial phase of a postoperational period) [15,16]. One of the most advanced therapies supporting postoperational recovery, which functions 24 h a day, is the method of dynamic application of Kinesio Taping (KT) [15,16]. Therapeutic knee patching combined with moderate adapted training has been proven to be an effective method for managing pain and disability limitations in patients with knee osteoarthritis [17]. According to the author of this method, it is possible to achieve pain-relieving, anti-swell, corrective, and sensation-improving effects, depending on different types of tensions and applications of the tape [16]. The applied KT lymphatic technique is based on the application of the tape with the tension of 15% with the anchor near the proximal lymph node [15,18–20]. Its aim is to enable the flow of lymph and blood from the place of congestion and lymphedema by a slight elevation of the skin. Tape properties, such as wave pattern, elasticity, thickness, and weight, similar to skin parameters, enable the extension of the space between the dermis and fascia, which improves the uninhibited lymph flow [15,18–20]. A proper application also enables the normalization of muscle and fascial tonus and their corrective positioning. It results in muscle loosening and supports its work during the motion. KT assumes the application of natural self-healing processes of the organism [15,18–20]. The advantage of this method is safety and the low cost of the therapy [21].

On the basis of the above considerations, it can be assumed that in patients who underwent the primary surgery of knee endoprosthetics, the application of the KT lymphatic drainage technique will enhance the subcutaneous edema resorption and improve the range of motion (ROM) in a knee joint in the first days after the surgery.

2. Materials and Methods

In order to obtain a homogenous group, patients qualified for the revision surgery of knee endoprosthetics, patients who suffered or are currently suffering from deep vein thrombosis of the lower limbs, patients qualified for the primary endoprosthetics as a result of post-traumatic osteoarthritis, and patients, after other surgeries carried out on the lower limbs, were excluded from the research. The criterion for entering the group was the qualification for the primary endoprosthetics of a knee joint on the basis of clinical symptoms according to the American College of Rheumatology (ACR) and radiological symptoms according to Kellgren–Lawrence Scale.

After the application of the above criteria, 82 inpatients (17 males and 65 females, median age 67.22 ± 7.14) of the Chair and Department of Rehabilitation and Orthopaedics and Chair and Department of Orthopaedics and Traumatology of the Independent Public Teaching Hospital No.4 in Lublin were qualified, in the period from October 2018 to March 2020 (Table 1). Each qualified patient was provided with an information sheet, and after examining the scope of research, they signed informed consent for participation in the research. The patients were informed about the possibility of withdrawing at any stage of the research. The Bioethical Commission operating at the Medical University of Lublin issued consent for the research to be carried out (Resolution of Ethical Commission, no. KE-0254/288/2018). The group of patients who qualified for the research was divided into two subgroups: a group of 42 members where, in the third 24 h after the surgery, the lymphatic application of Kinesio Taping was introduced into the postoperative edema treatment; and a group of 40 members where dynamic tapes were not applied.

Table 1. Patients characteristics.

	KT	Without KT	Test		p
n	42	40	-	-	-
Age (years)	66.69 ± 6.78	67.78 ± 7.56	T	−0.68	0.51
Sex	M = 33 K = 9	M = 32 F = 8	Z	0.11	0.92
Weight (kg)	81.62 ± 13.57	80.05 ± 15.15	T	0.49	0.62
Height (m)	164.93 ± 6.87	163.20 ± 8.76	Z	1.21	0.23
BMI	30.03 ± 4.85	30.10 ± 5.59	T	−0.06	0.95

2.1. Methods

2.1.1. Clinical Assessment of Disease Activity in Osteoarthritis

The Kellgren–Lawrence scale was applied for the clinical assessment of disease activity in osteoarthritis. It is a five-step grading system allowing for the assessment of radiological changes in patients with osteoarthritis. The radiological assessment of the disease activity was based on radiograms in the anterior-posterior (AP) view that revealed the presence of osteophytes, joint gap narrowing, and subchondral bone sclerosis [22,23]. Patients graded III and IV on the Kellgren–Lawrence scale were qualified for the research.

2.1.2. Assessment of Postoperative Edema

The measurements of edema thickness in the proximity of a knee joint above the fibula were carried out in both groups of patients in the third and eighth 24 h after the surgery by a Simens ACUSON S2000 HELX EVOLUTION (Siemens, Erlangen, Germany) with a linear probe, 18L6 HD. Measurements were taken at the level of the fibula head, 25 mm below the fibular neck, and 50 mm below the fibular neck along the longitudinal axis (Figure 1).

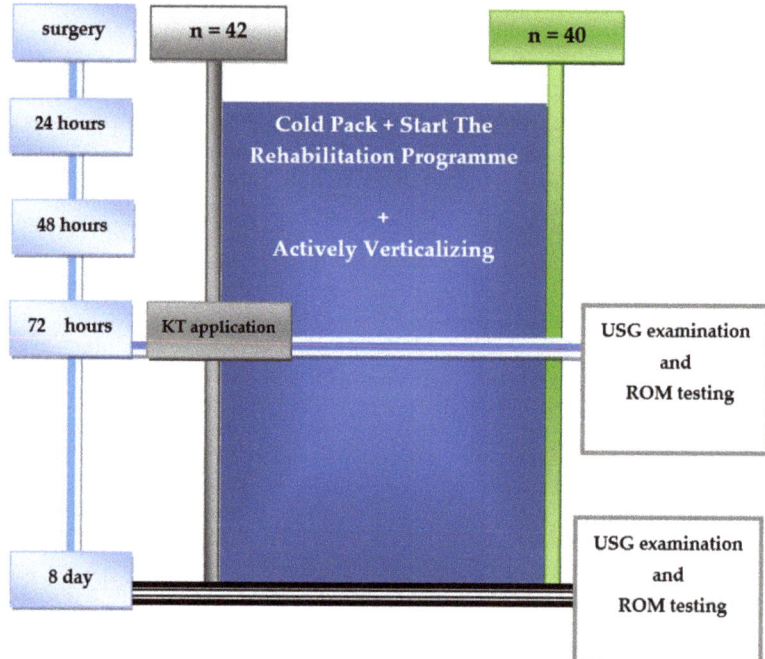

Figure 1. Demonstration of the conduct of a time-divided experiment. ROM—range of motion; KT—Kinesio Taping; USG—ultrasound.

2.1.3. Application of Dynamic Kinesio Tape

In the patients of the research group, in the third 24 h after the surgery, KT 10 mm dynamic tapes in the shape of a fan were applied to the lateral and medial sides of the tibia. The lymphatic drainage technique was introduced. The proximal point, the tip of the tape, i.e., the anchor of the tape, was applied without tension at the level of the popliteal fossa in the proximity of the fibula head lymph nodes on the medial side of a knee. Distal points, or tails, were applied with 15% tension and reached the lateral ankle and medial tibia (Figure 2). The tapes remained on the skin for 5 consecutive days [24,25]. On the eighth 24 h, they were removed, and the skin was cleansed (Figure 3). The application of the tapes was carried out by a qualified physiotherapist with 20-years of experience in rehabilitating patients.

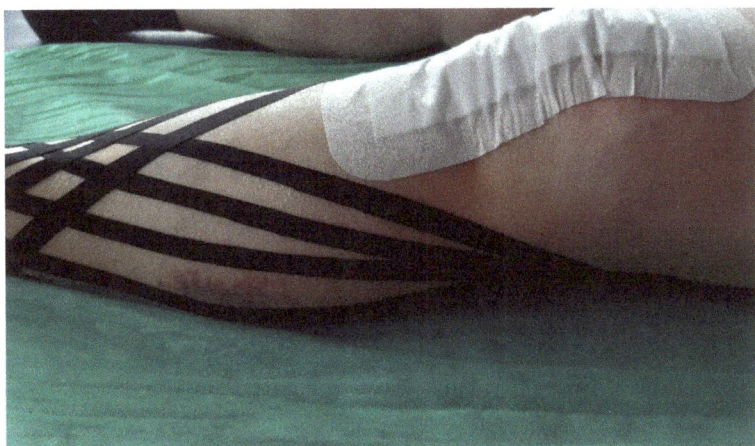

Figure 2. KT Lymphatic application on the lower leg.

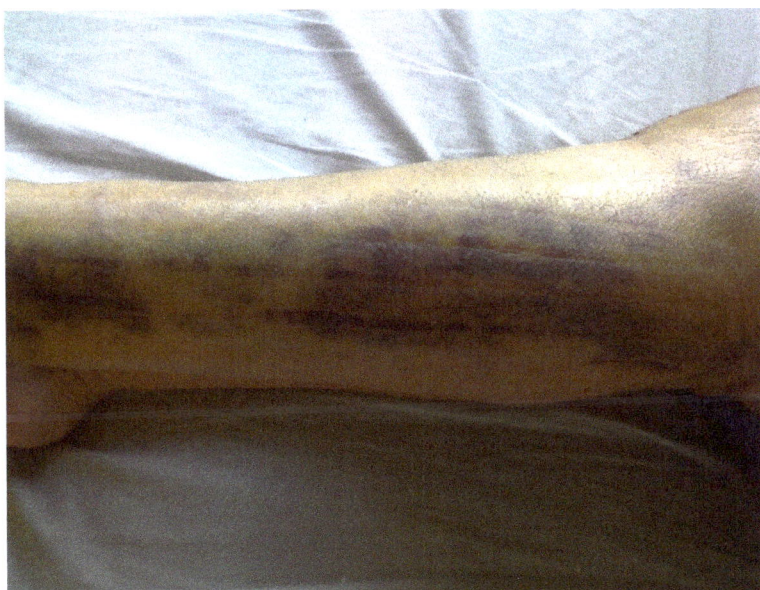

Figure 3. After eighth 24 h, KT Lymphatic application on the lower leg.

2.1.4. ROM Assessment in a Knee Joint

On the third and the eighth 24 h after the surgery, the ROM in the knee joint was tested by the use of a goniometer. The initial position was lying down with straight lower limbs. The goniometer axis was set in the proximity of the fibula head in compliance with the transverse axis of the joint. The fixed arm of the goniometer was aimed at the greater trochanter of the femur, and the mobile arm was aimed at the lateral malleolus [26] (Figure 1).

2.1.5. Postoperational Rehabilitation Programme

The rehabilitation program for all of the 82 patients was equal and introduced in the first 24 h after the surgery. The program included exercises to prevent blood clotting in the lower limbs, inner range quads exercises, isometric gluteus and lower leg exercises, diaphragm breathing exercises, and active slow exercises.

The training was conducted with the application of a passive movement for flexion and extension in the knee joint with the use of CPM within a tolerated painless ROM [27–29]. In the second 24 h after the surgery, the patients were actively verticalized with the use of orthopedic appliances, such as walking frames. In the second or third 24 h, the drains were removed. In both groups, a cold pack compress was applied for the first 24 h after the surgery in order to reduce postoperational edema and pain [28,30,31] (Figure 1).

2.2. Statistical Analysis

In order to present the results in categorical and ordinal scales, methods of descriptive statistics were introduced, i.e., number (N) and percentage (%). The statistical analysis included the test of independence, χ^2, in order to assess the relationship between the examined variables on categorical and ordinal scales. In order to present the results on a quantitative scale, the following methods of descriptive statistics were introduced: arithmetic mean (x), median (Me), standard deviation (SD), minimum (Min), maximum (Max), and interquartile range (IQR). In order to assess the compliance of the distribution of the examined variables with normal distribution, a Shapiro–Wilk test was introduced. In the cases where there was no normal distribution of variables, nonparametric tests were applied, and, in the cases when a normal distribution of variables was revealed, parametric tests were applied. Wilcoxon's signed-ranked test was applied in order to assess the difference between the two measurements. The Student's t-test was applied for the independent trials, and the Mann–Whitney test was applied in order to assess the differences in the values of the variables between the two groups. The assessment of the correlation between the variables was defined by Pearson correlation and Spearman's rank correlation. Statistical inference of 5% and related to its level of statistical significance (α) of 0.05 (α = 0.05) were assumed. On the basis of the results of the analysis, the probability value rules were applied: $p < 0.05$—statistical significance, $p < 0.01$ strong statistical significance, and $p < 0.001$—very strong statistical significance. The statistical analysis was conducted by Statistica v.13.0 software (StatSoft, Tulsa, OK, USA). In order to collect and support statistical analyses, MS Excel 2010 (Microsoft, Redmond, WA, USA) software was used.

3. Results

3.1. Comparison of Differences in Linear Measurement in Ultrasound Scan between 'KT' Group and 'Non-KT' Group

The examination revealed statistically a significant difference in the linear measurements above the fibula head at its peak in patients with KT compared to patients without KT (t = −3.01; $p < 0.01$). In the group of patients with KT, a mean decrease of −1.12 mm was observed, whereas in the group of patients without KT, a mean decrease of −0.18 mm was observed (Table 2).

The research revealed a statistically significant difference in the linear measurements of 2.5 cm from the fibula neck in the group of patients with KT compared to the patients without KT (t = −2.60; $p < 0.05$). In the group of patients with KT, a mean decrease of

−0.9 mm was observed, whereas in the group of patients without KT, a mean increase of 0.02 mm was observed (Table 3).

Table 2. Differences [mm] in linear measurement taken above fibula head at the highest point.

	Group	n	x	Me	Min	Max	IQR	SD	Student's t-Test	
									T	p
Differences in mm	KT	42	−1.12	−1.10	−4.50	1.70	1.90	1.32	−3.01	<0.01 *
Differences in mm	Without KT	40	−0.18	0.00	−3.40	2.70	1.70	1.51		

* Significant difference, IQR—interquartile range, SD—standard deviation, KT—Kinesio Taping.

Table 3. Differences [mm] in linear measurement taken 2.5 cm above fibula neck.

	Group	n	x	Me	Min	Max	IQR	SD	Student's t-Test	
									T	p
Difference in mm	KT	42	−0.90	−0.75	−3.90	2.90	1.40	1.43	−2.60	<0.05 *
Difference in mm	Without KT	40	0.02	−0.05	−4.20	4.40	1.85	1.76		

* Significant difference, IQR—interquartile range, SD—standard deviation, KT—Kinesio Taping.

The research revealed a statistically significant difference in the linear measurement of 5 cm from the fibula neck in the group of patients with KT compared to the patients without KT ($Z = -2.64$; $p < 0.01$). In the group of patients with KT, a mean decrease of −0.82 mm was observed, whereas in the group of patients without KT, the mean value of the change was 0 mm (Table 4).

Table 4. Differences [mm] in linear measurement taken 5 cm above fibula neck.

	Group	n	x	Me	Min	Max	IQR	SD	Mann–Whitney Test	
									Z	p
Difference in mm	KT	42	−0.82	−0.80	−3.60	3.20	1.40	1.34	−2.64	<0.01 *
Difference in mm	Without KT	40	0.00	0.00	−5.20	3.40	2.00	1.79		

* Significant difference, IQR—interquartile range, SD—standard deviation, KT—Kinesio Taping.

3.2. Comparison of Differences in Knee Flexion Angle in the Third and the Eighth 24 Hours in 'KT' Group and 'Non-KT' Group

The research revealed a statistically significant greater knee flexion angle in the patients with KT ($Z = 5.51$; $p < 0.001$). The research revealed a statistically significant greater knee flexion angle in patients without KT ($Z = 5.37$; $p < 0.001$) (Table 5).

Table 5. Measurement of the knee joint angle.

	Group	n	x	Me	Min	Max	IQR	SD	Wilcoxon Test	
									Z	p
3rd 24 h without KT; flexion angle	With KT before	42	44.48	40.00	20.00	80.00	12.00	13.40	5.51	<0.001 *
8th 24 h after KT; flexion angle	With KT after	42	68.64	70.00	40.00	110.00	20.00	15.52		
3rd 24 h without KT; flexion angle	Without KT before	40	41.63	40.00	20.00	75.00	13.50	12.01	5.37	<0.001 *
8th 24 h after KT; flexion angle	Without KT after	40	61.73	60.00	30.00	95.00	20.00	15.97		

* Significant difference, IQR—interquartile range, SD—standard deviation, KT—Kinesio Taping.

The research did not reveal any statistically significant differences in knee flexion angle in patients with KT compared to patients without KT ($t = 1.55$; $p > 0.05$) (Table 6).

Table 6. Difference in knee flexion angle.

	Group	n	x	Me	Min	Max	IQR	SD	Student's t-Test	
									T	p
Difference flexion angle	KT	42	24.17	20.00	0.00	60.00	15.00	13.02	1.55	>0.05

IQR—interquartile range, SD—standard deviation, KT—Kinesio Taping.

The research revealed no statistically significant correlation between the change in ROM in a knee joint and the change of parameters specific to the subcutaneous edema in the group of patients without KT (Table 7).

Table 7. The results of the correlation analysis of the change in improvement in the range of motion (ROM) in the joint with the variables characterizing the level of subcutaneous tissue swelling according to the Spearman and Pearson correlation.

Variable	Group	n	R	p
Difference in mm	KT	42	0.02	>0.05
	without KT	40	0.01	>0.05
Difference in mm	KT	42	0.05	>0.05
	Without KT	40	0.01	>0.05
Difference in mm	KT	42	−0.18	>0.05
	Without KT	40	0.03	>0.05
Circuit difference at the height of the fibula head (cm)	KT	42	−0.22	>0.05
	Without KT	40	−0.11	>0.05
Circuit difference 2.5 cm above fibula neck (cm)	KT	42	−0.08	>0.05
	Without KT	40	−0.06	>0.05
Circuit difference 5 cm above fibula neck (cm)	KT	42	−0.17	>0.05
	Without KT	40	0.09	>0.05

KT—Kinesio Taping.

4. Discussion

The aim of this work was to determine the effect of Kinesio Taping (KT) in reducing edema of the subcutaneous tissue and improving the ROM in the joint. In our study, we saw a positive effect of KT on the amount of swelling. This involves the tape being stuck to the skin to gently lift it, thus removing lymphatic obstructions and reducing pressure by widening the space between the dermis and fascia. It causes an uninhibited flow of lymph and blood. This mechanism results in accelerated tissue healing when lymphatic obstruction and edema are reduced [15,32,33]. In addition, skin elevation elongates the interstitial space, which reduces pressure on subcutaneous nociceptors [33–35]. Previous studies highlight the positive effects of KT on lymphedema [36,37].

Tsai et al. [38] compared traditional arm dressing after breast cancer surgery to the lymphatic drainage application of dynamic tape. In their research paper, the authors stated that in patients with KT, the swelling was reduced faster and with better acceptance than in patients with elastic bandages applied for longer periods [38]. Another example of lymphatic drainage application in postoperational facial skeleton edema was presented by Lietz-Kijak et al. in their research paper. The authors carried out a pilot experiment on 16 patients after orthognathic surgery in which KT was applied twice with a two-day interval in the facial area. The research revealed a statistically significant reduction in edema, which had a substantial influence on further treatment and facial functions [39]. Similar research regarding the efficacy of the lymphatic drainage KT technique after temporomandibular joint surgeries was carried out on a group of 30 patients by Ristow [40]. The aim of his research was to establish if the application of dynamic tape prevents edema, pain, and trismus after the surgery of a broken zygomatic bone and if it improves postoperational quality of life. As in the research of my own, the KT was applied once in the first days after the surgery for a period of 5 days. The growth of facial edema was assessed with linear measurements, and a difference of 60% was revealed compared to a control group in the first two days of application. In the abovementioned research, the KT application had no influence on pain sensation and the ROM in the temporomandibular joints [40,41]. The influence of dynamic KT tapes on postoperational edema was also examined by Białoszewski et al. [42] in patients treated with the Lizarow method in the lower limbs. In their paper, the authors compared the effectiveness of lymphatic drainage application to the application of traditional lymphatic drainage massage.

The application of taping in a sample group resulted in a greater reduction in edema and the reduction in hip and lower leg circumference than after the application of lymphatic drainage [42]. As in the research of my own, V. Donec et al. [43] assessed the influence of anti-swelling KT and other physiotherapeutical treatments used routinely on the reduction in postoperational edema, pain, and ROM improvement after the primary endoprosthetics of a knee joint. The sample group consisted of 94 patients. In all of them, significant improvement was observed regarding pain sensation, measured with a numeric pain rating scale, NPRS, and a statistically significant reduction in limb circumference in patients with KT was revealed. The technique applied in Donec's research had no significant influence on ROM in a knee joint in either of the groups [43]. The abovementioned study revealed results that indicate the positive influence of anti-swelling properties and edema reduction ($t = -3.01$; $p < 0.05$). In Donec's research, KT was also applied on the second 24 h after the surgery and remained attached for up to 28 days, re-applied every fifth day with a one-day interval. Our results are consistent with those of Jarecki, based on a smaller group [20]. In the research of my own, in addition to a centimeter tape measure, an ultrasound scan was also applied, which enabled an objective evaluation of the results and a detailed measure of the subcutaneous tissue. Ultrasound imaging facilitates a detailed assessment of soft tissues surrounding the joint statically and dynamically [44]. Summing up, postoperational subcutaneous edema is a considerable problem in the initial phase of physiotherapy of patients after surgeries. KT dynamic taping is a reliable alternative method, and it supports edema treatment. It should be considered for ongoing therapy for patients with surgical edema. It may accelerate the comfort of hospitalization and surgical sequelae. It is advised to carry out further research in order to prove the effectiveness of the KT method in improving ROM. It should cover a larger number of patients and be extended by the application of dynamic taping after other surgeries in order to enable an objective evaluation of the results of the treatment.

The study presented here has several limitations. The first limitation is the evaluation of therapeutic effects for up to 8 days. Future studies should increase the time to observe treatment effects in subjects. The time of 8 days was related to the average time of patients' discharge from the hospital. This is a crucial time to implement rehabilitation management. Another limitation was the lack of use of an adapted activity protocol, which should be considered in future studies. Another limitation was the lack of consideration of the patients' lifestyle habits before surgery, e.g., alcohol consumption and cigarette smoking.

5. Conclusions

The results indicate that the spread of subcutaneous tissue edema after KT application was significantly reduced, so the extension of postoperative physiotherapy to include KT lymphatic application should be considered. Further research into the possible effects of lymphatic KT on ROM is suggested.

Author Contributions: Conceptualization, M.S., A.C. and G.Z.; methodology, M.S.; formal analysis, M.S.; investigation, M.S.; writing—original draft preparation, M.S., A.C. and G.Z.; writing—review and editing, P.G. and M.Z.; visualization, A.C.; supervision, M.S. and P.G.; funding acquisition, P.G. All authors have read and agreed to the published version of the manuscript.

Funding: This research received no external funding.

Institutional Review Board Statement: The study was conducted according to the guidelines of the Declaration of Helsinki, and approved by the Institutional Ethics Committee of the Medical University in Lublin (KE-0254/288/2018).

Informed Consent Statement: Informed consent was obtained from all subjects involved in the study.

Data Availability Statement: Not applicable.

Conflicts of Interest: The authors declare no conflict of interest.

References

1. Sen, R.; Hurley, J.A. Osteoarthritis. In *StatPearls*; StatPearls Publishing: Treasure Island, FL, USA, 2022.
2. Chen, D.; Shen, J.; Zhao, W.; Wang, T.; Han, L.; Hamilton, J.L.; Im, H.-J. Osteoarthritis: Toward a Comprehensive Understanding of Pathological Mechanism. *Bone Res.* **2017**, *5*, 16044. [CrossRef] [PubMed]
3. Castorina, S.; Guglielmino, C.; Castrogiovanni, P.; Szychlinska, M.A.; Ioppolo, F.; Massimino, P.; Leonardi, P.; Maci, C.; Iannuzzi, M.; Di Giunta, A.; et al. Clinical Evidence of Traditional vs Fast Track Recovery Methodologies after Total Arthroplasty for Osteoarthritic Knee Treatment. A Retrospective Observational Study. *Muscle Ligaments Tendons J.* **2019**, *7*, 504. [CrossRef]
4. Felson, D.T. An Update on the Pathogenesis and Epidemiology of Osteoarthritis. *Radiol. Clin. N. Am.* **2004**, *42*, 1–9. [CrossRef]
5. Altman, R.; Asch, E.; Bloch, D.; Bole, G.; Borenstein, D.; Brandt, K.; Christy, W.; Cooke, T.D.; Greenwald, R.; Hochberg, M.; et al. Development of Criteria for the Classification and Reporting of Osteoarthritis: Classification of Osteoarthritis of the Knee. *Arthritis Rheum.* **1986**, *29*, 1039–1049. [CrossRef] [PubMed]
6. Page, C.J.; Hinman, R.S.; Bennell, K.L. Physiotherapy Management of Knee Osteoarthritis. *Int. J. Rheum. Dis.* **2011**, *14*, 145–151. [CrossRef] [PubMed]
7. Carr, A.J.; Robertsson, O.; Graves, S.; Price, A.J.; Arden, N.K.; Judge, A.; Beard, D.J. Knee Replacement. *Lancet* **2012**, *379*, 1331–1340. [CrossRef]
8. Felson, D.T.; Lawrence, R.C.; Dieppe, P.A.; Hirsch, R.; Helmick, C.G.; Jordan, J.M.; Kington, R.S.; Lane, N.E.; Nevitt, M.C.; Zhang, Y.; et al. Osteoarthritis: New Insights. Part 1: The Disease and Its Risk Factors. *Ann. Intern. Med.* **2000**, *133*, 635–646. [CrossRef]
9. Jordan, K.M.; Arden, N.K.; Doherty, M.; Bannwarth, B.; Bijlsma, J.W.J.; Dieppe, P.; Gunther, K.; Hauselmann, H.; Herrero-Beaumont, G.; Kaklamanis, P.; et al. EULAR Recommendations 2003: An Evidence Based Approach to the Management of Knee Osteoarthritis: Report of a Task Force of the Standing Committee for International Clinical Studies Including Therapeutic Trials (ESCISIT). *Ann. Rheum. Dis.* **2003**, *62*, 1145–1155. [CrossRef]
10. Lim, W.B.; Al-Dadah, O. Conservative Treatment of Knee Osteoarthritis: A Review of the Literature. *World J. Orthop.* **2022**, *13*, 212–229. [CrossRef]
11. Hunter, D.J.; Lo, G.H. The Management of Osteoarthritis: An Overview and Call to Appropriate Conservative Treatment. *Rheum. Dis. Clin. N. Am.* **2008**, *34*, 689–712. [CrossRef]
12. Picard, F.; Deakin, A.; Balasubramanian, N.; Gregori, A. Minimally Invasive Total Knee Replacement: Techniques and Results. *Eur. J. Orthop. Surg. Traumatol. Orthop. Traumatol.* **2018**, *28*, 781–791. [CrossRef] [PubMed]
13. Williamson, L.; Wyatt, M.R.; Yein, K.; Melton, J.T.K. Severe Knee Osteoarthritis: A Randomized Controlled Trial of Acupuncture, Physiotherapy (Supervised Exercise) and Standard Management for Patients Awaiting Knee Replacement. *Rheumatol. Oxf. Engl.* **2007**, *46*, 1445–1449. [CrossRef] [PubMed]
14. Russell, T.G.; Buttrum, P.; Wootton, R.; Jull, G.A. Internet-Based Outpatient Telerehabilitation for Patients Following Total Knee Arthroplasty: A Randomized Controlled Trial. *J. Bone Jt. Surg. Am.* **2011**, *93*, 113–120. [CrossRef]
15. Kase, K.; Wallis, J.; Tsuyoshi, K. *Clinical Therapeutic Applications of the Kinesio Taping Method*, 3rd ed.; Kinesio: Albuquerque, NM, USA, 2013.
16. Kase, K.; Hashimoto, T.; Tomoki, O. Development of Kinesio Tape. In *Kinesio Taping Perfect Manual*; Kinesio Taping Association: Albuquerque, NM, USA, 1996; pp. 117–118.
17. Castrogiovanni, P.; Di Giunta, A.; Guglielmino, C.; Roggio, F.; Romeo, D.; Fidone, F.; Imbesi, R.; Loreto, C.; Castorina, S.; Musumeci, G. The Effects of Exercise and Kinesio Tape on Physical Limitations in Patients with Knee Osteoarthritis. *J. Funct. Morphol. Kinesiol.* **2016**, *1*, 355–368. [CrossRef]
18. Krajczy, M.; Luniewski, J.; Bogacz, K.; Dybek, T.; Kiczyński, P.; Krajczy, E.; Szczegielniak, A.; Szczegielniak, J. Impact of Elastic Therapeutic Tape on Final Effects of Physiotherapy in Patients with Colles' Fracture. *Fizjoterapia Pol.* **2014**, *14*, 42–49.
19. Mostafavifar, M.; Wertz, J.; Borchers, J. A Systematic Review of the Effectiveness of Kinesio Taping for Musculoskeletal Injury. *Phys. Sportsmed.* **2012**, *40*, 33–40. [CrossRef] [PubMed]

20. Jarecki, J.; Sobiech, M.; Turżańska, K.; Tomczyk-Warunek, A.; Jabłoński, M. A Kinesio Taping Method Applied in the Treatment of Postsurgical Knee Swelling after Primary Total Knee Arthroplasty. *J. Clin. Med.* **2021**, *10*, 2992. [CrossRef]
21. Hörmann, J.; Vach, W.; Jakob, M.; Seghers, S.; Saxer, F. Kinesiotaping for Postoperative Oedema—What Is the Evidence? A Systematic Review. *BMC Sports Sci. Med. Rehabil.* **2020**, *12*, 14. [CrossRef]
22. Kohn, M.D.; Sassoon, A.A.; Fernando, N.D. Classifications in Brief: Kellgren-Lawrence Classification of Osteoarthritis. *Clin. Orthop.* **2016**, *474*, 1886–1893. [CrossRef]
23. Schiphof, D.; de Klerk, B.M.; Kerkhof, H.J.M.; Hofman, A.; Koes, B.W.; Boers, M.; Bierma-Zeinstra, S.M.A. Impact of Different Descriptions of the Kellgren and Lawrence Classification Criteria on the Diagnosis of Knee Osteoarthritis. *Ann. Rheum. Dis.* **2011**, *70*, 1422–1427. [CrossRef]
24. Tiffert, M. Kinesiology Taping-Teoria, Metodyka, Przykładowe Aplikacje w Konkretnych Dysfunkcjach. *Prakt. Fizjoterapia Rehabil.* **2010**, *2*, 48–53.
25. Hałas, I. Kinesiology Taping Metoda Wspomagająca Teratpię Tkanek Miękkich. *Praktyczna Fizjoterapia i Rehabilitacja* **2010**, *9/10*, 22–26.
26. Boone, D.C.; Azen, S.P.; Lin, C.M.; Spence, C.; Baron, C.; Lee, L. Reliability of Goniometric Measurements. *Phys. Ther.* **1978**, *58*, 1355–1360. [CrossRef] [PubMed]
27. Artz, N.; Elvers, K.T.; Lowe, C.M.; Sackley, C.; Jepson, P.; Beswick, A.D. Effectiveness of Physiotherapy Exercise Following Total Knee Replacement: Systematic Review and Meta-Analysis. *BMC Musculoskelet. Disord.* **2015**, *16*, 15. [CrossRef]
28. Denis, M.; Moffet, H.; Caron, F.; Ouellet, D.; Paquet, J.; Nolet, L. Effectiveness of Continuous Passive Motion and Conventional Physical Therapy after Total Knee Arthroplasty: A Randomized Clinical Trial. *Phys. Ther.* **2006**, *86*, 174–185. [CrossRef] [PubMed]
29. Herbold, J.A.; Bonistall, K.; Blackburn, M.; Agolli, J.; Gaston, S.; Gross, C.; Kuta, A.; Babyar, S. Randomized Controlled Trial of the Effectiveness of Continuous Passive Motion after Total Knee Replacement. *Arch. Phys. Med. Rehabil.* **2014**, *95*, 1240–1245. [CrossRef]
30. Minns Lowe, C.; Barker, K.; Dewey, M.; Sackley, C. Effectiveness of Physiotherapy Exercise after Knee Arthroplasty for Osteoarthritis: Systematic Review and Meta-Analysis of Randomised Controlled Trials. *BMJ* **2007**, *335*, 812. [CrossRef]
31. Chughtai, M.; Sodhi, N.; Jawad, M.; Newman, J.M.; Khlopas, A.; Bhave, A.; Mont, M.A. Cryotherapy Treatment After Unicompartmental and Total Knee Arthroplasty: A Review. *J. Arthroplast.* **2017**, *32*, 3822–3832. [CrossRef]
32. Dębska, M. Kinesiology Taping Jako Metoda Terapeutyczna I Kosmetyczna W Stłuczeniu Mięśnia—Opis Przypadku. *Polski Przegląd Nauk o Zdrowiu* **2015**, *1*, 42.
33. Osorio, J.A.; Vairo, G.L.; Rozea, G.D.; Bosha, P.J.; Millard, R.L.; Aukerman, D.F.; Sebastianelli, W.J. The Effects of Two Therapeutic Patellofemoral Taping Techniques on Strength, Endurance, and Pain Responses. *Phys. Ther. Sport Off. J. Assoc. Chart. Physiother. Sports Med.* **2013**, *14*, 199–206. [CrossRef]
34. Murray, H.M. Effects of Kinesio Taping® on Muscle Strength after ACL-Repair. *J. Orthop. Sports Phys. Ther.* **2000**, *30*, 1.
35. Kahanov, L. Kinesio Taping®, Part 1: An Overview of Its Use in Athletes. *Athl. Ther. Today* **2007**, *12*, 17–18. [CrossRef]
36. Tantawy, S.A.; Abdelbasset, W.K.; Nambi, G.; Kamel, D.M. Comparative Study between the Effects of Kinesio Taping and Pressure Garment on Secondary Upper Extremity Lymphedema and Quality of Life Following Mastectomy: A Randomized Controlled Trial. *Integr. Cancer Ther.* **2019**, *18*, 1534735419847276. [CrossRef]
37. Bosman, J.; Piller, N. Lymph Taping and Seroma Formation Post Breast Cancer. *J. Lymphoedema* **2010**, *5*, 12–21.
38. Tsai, H.-J.; Hung, H.-C.; Yang, J.-L.; Huang, C.-S.; Tsauo, J.-Y. Could Kinesio Tape Replace the Bandage in Decongestive Lymphatic Therapy for Breast-Cancer-Related Lymphedema? A Pilot Study. *Support. Care Cancer* **2009**, *17*, 1353–1360. [CrossRef]
39. Lietz-Kijak, D.; Kijak, E.; Krajczy, M.; Bogacz, K.; Łuniewski, J.; Szczegielniak, J. The Impact of the Use of Kinesio Taping Method on the Reduction of Swelling in Patients After Orthognathic Surgery: A Pilot Study. *Med. Sci. Monit.* **2018**, *24*, 3736–3743. [CrossRef]
40. Ristow, O.; Pautke, C.; Kehl, V.; Koerdt, S.; Schwärzler, K.; Hahnefeld, L.; Hohlweg-Majert, B. Influence of Kinesiologic Tape on Postoperative Swelling, Pain and Trismus after Zygomatico-Orbital Fractures. *J. Cranio-Maxillofac. Surg.* **2014**, *42*, 469–476. [CrossRef]
41. Ristow, O.; Hohlweg-Majert, B.; Kehl, V.; Koerdt, S.; Hahnefeld, L.; Pautke, C. Does Elastic Therapeutic Tape Reduce Postoperative Swelling, Pain, and Trismus after Open Reduction and Internal Fixation of Mandibular Fractures? *J. Oral Maxillofac. Surg.* **2013**, *71*, 1387–1396. [CrossRef]
42. Białoszewski, D.; Woźniak, W.; Zarek, S. Clinical Efficacy of Kinesiology Taping in Reducing Edema of the Lower Limbs in Patients Treated with the Ilizarov Method—Preliminary Report. *Ortop. Traumatol. Rehabil.* **2009**, *11*, 46–54.
43. Donec, V.; Kriščiūnas, A. The Effectiveness of Kinesio Taping® after Total Knee Replacement in Early Postoperative Rehabilitation Period. A Randomized Controlled Trial. *Eur. J. Phys. Rehabil. Med.* **2014**, *50*, 363–371.
44. Hassan, S. Overview of Musculoskeletal Ultrasound for the Clinical Rheumatologist. *Clin. Exp. Rheumatol.* **2018**, *36* (Suppl. 114), 3–9. [PubMed]

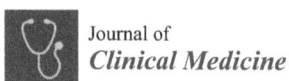 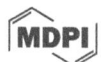

Article

Effects of Electromyographic Biofeedback on Functional Recovery of Patients Two Months after Total Knee Arthroplasty: A Randomized Controlled Trial

Iva Sklempe Kokic [1,*], Matko Vuksanic [2,3], Tomislav Kokic [1,4,5], Ivan Peric [1,6] and Ivana Duvnjak [1]

[1] Faculty of Kinesiology Osijek, Josip Juraj Strossmayer University of Osijek, 31000 Osijek, Croatia; tkokic@gmail.com (T.K.); ivan.peric@kifos.hr (I.P.); ivana.duvnjak@kifos.hr (I.D.)
[2] Bizovacke Toplice Rehabilitation Hospital, 31222 Bizovac, Croatia; matko.vuksanic@bizovacke-toplice.hr
[3] Department of Health Studies, College of Applied Sciences "Lavoslav Ruzicka" in Vukovar, 32000 Vukovar, Croatia
[4] Faculty of Medicine, Josip Juraj Strossmayer University of Osijek, 31000 Osijek, Croatia
[5] County General Hospital Vinkovci, 32100 Vinkovci, Croatia
[6] Faculty of Dental Medicine and Health, Josip Juraj Strossmayer University of Osijek, 31000 Osijek, Croatia
* Correspondence: iva.sklempe.kokic@kifos.hr; Tel.: +385-915082854

Citation: Sklempe Kokic, I.; Vuksanic, M.; Kokic, T.; Peric, I.; Duvnjak, I. Effects of Electromyographic Biofeedback on Functional Recovery of Patients Two Months after Total Knee Arthroplasty: A Randomized Controlled Trial. *J. Clin. Med.* **2022**, *11*, 3182. https://doi.org/10.3390/jcm11113182

Academic Editors: Masahiro Kohzuki and Yuichi Hoshino

Received: 8 May 2022
Accepted: 1 June 2022
Published: 2 June 2022

Publisher's Note: MDPI stays neutral with regard to jurisdictional claims in published maps and institutional affiliations.

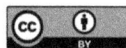

Copyright: © 2022 by the authors. Licensee MDPI, Basel, Switzerland. This article is an open access article distributed under the terms and conditions of the Creative Commons Attribution (CC BY) license (https://creativecommons.org/licenses/by/4.0/).

Abstract: The incidence of total knee arthroplasty (TKA) is steadily increasing worldwide. Therefore, it is crucial to develop efficient rehabilitation protocols and investigate the innovations in medical technology, which could improve rehabilitation outcomes. The aim of the study was to investigate the effect of adding electromyographic biofeedback (EMG-BF) to the conventional program of rehabilitation after TKA on quality of life, intensity of pain, and functional performance. The study was designed as a randomized controlled trial. A total of 131 patients were randomly assigned to two groups: an experimental group ($n = 67$; median age 70 (IQR 10)), and a control group ($n = 64$; median age 69 (IQR 9)). Both groups participated in an inpatient program of 21 days of rehabilitation, including land-based and aquatic exercise therapy, electrotherapy, and education. In the experimental group, a portion of land-based exercise therapy was supplemented by EMG-BF. A numeric rating scale (NRS), Knee Injury and Osteoarthritis Outcome Score (KOOS), use of mobility aids, 30 s chair stand test (CST), and timed up and go (TUG) test were used to measure outcomes. Both groups improved their functional abilities from day 1 to day 21 of rehabilitation. A higher proportion of participants did not use a walking aid ($p < 0.002$), and their NRS, KOOS, 30 s CST and TUG scores improved ($p < 0.001$). There were no significant differences between the groups in the outcomes. EMG-BF did not provide additional benefits to the conventional rehabilitation after TKA.

Keywords: biofeedback; knee replacement; rehabilitation; quality of life; physical functional performance

1. Introduction

Knee osteoarthritis is one of the most frequent musculoskeletal degenerative disorders in older age. The knee joint has an important role in mobility and activities of daily life, and pain and lack of knee function greatly affect the quality of life [1]. In advanced stages of osteoarthritis, patients face progressive disability and lowered quality of life, and the healthcare system faces higher costs [2]. Established conservative treatments for knee osteoarthritis include exercise therapy [3], knee bracing [4], physical modalities [5], and pharmacotherapy [6], but their long-term effectiveness is limited; thus, total knee replacement is ultimately needed for the majority of patients with knee osteoarthritis.

Therefore, many older adults undergo total knee arthroplasty (TKA) to restore their ability to walk, independence, and quality of life. TKA has become one of the most common orthopedic procedures [7], and its incidence has increased steadily since the introduction of the procedure and continues to increase in all age groups with the goal of relieving symptoms of osteoarthritis and restoring function [8].

Efficient rehabilitation is crucial for restoring function following TKA [9]. Patients after TKA often experience pain and impaired muscle strength, especially of m. quadriceps femoris and decreased neuromuscular control [10], which is dealt with during the postoperative rehabilitation. These problems affect patients' function and satisfaction. Restoring m. quadriceps femoris strength is a common goal following TKA. Most rehabilitation protocols include therapeutic exercise and physical agents such as cryotherapy and electrotherapy [11,12].

Despite significant efforts to improve the outcomes after TKA, many patients following TKA experience persistent muscle weakness, functional impairment, and pain in the long term [13–15]. Therefore, investigating the efficiency of innovations in medical technology which could improve rehabilitation outcomes for this group of patients is rather important. Recent innovations in rehabilitation technology have to be verified to prove their clinical meaningfulness and justify their cost. One of the recent innovations in medical rehabilitative technology is electromyographic biofeedback (EMG-BF), which could hypothetically improve m. quadriceps femoris strength and therefore positively impact functional outcomes after TKA and offer additional benefits to these patients. Its usefulness after TKA is still rather unexplored.

Electromyographic biofeedback is an additional treatment modality that can be used to modulate muscle contraction by bringing the muscular tension to the level of consciousness [16]. It is the technique of providing biological information to patients in real-time that otherwise would be unknown [17]. EMG-BF is used in combination with conventional rehabilitation with the goal of improving strength and functionality for various orthopedic conditions. The evidence regarding its efficacy after TKA is still limited, but a recent systematic review showed its potential in controlling pain and improving m. quadriceps femoris strength and functionality after TKA [16].

The objective of this study was to examine the effects of adding EMG-BF to the conventional program of rehabilitation after TKA, consisting of therapeutic exercise and electrotherapy, on objective and subjective functional outcomes, including pain, patient-reported measure of quality of life, lower body strength, mobility, and functional performance. This would add new evidence to the body of scientific knowledge regarding the optimal design of rehabilitation protocols after TKA and improve patients' outcomes. If EMG-BF is found to have significant effects on patients' recovery, then its use could be justified in postoperative rehabilitation after TKA. We hypothesized that adding EMG-BF to the conventional rehabilitation program would improve the objective and subjective functional outcomes of patients.

2. Materials and Methods

2.1. Study Design and Population

The study was carried out as a prospective, parallel-group, single-blinded, randomized controlled trial on patients after TKA attending inpatient postoperative rehabilitation at Bizovacke Toplice Rehabilitation Hospital, Bizovac, Croatia, between November 2018 and December 2019. The study was not blinded to participants because of its nature. However, the assessors were blinded.

Patients were recruited by direct contact after checking into a rehabilitation institution. Inclusion criteria were as follows: (1) patients of both genders after TKA without previous postoperative inpatient postoperative rehabilitation; (2) age between 18 and 79 years; and (3) ability to read, understand, and speak Croatian language.

Exclusion criteria were: (1) patients after revision TKA, (2) patients with comorbidities that did not allow normal mobility due to other causes (e.g., hemiparesis, severe diseases, and conditions affecting internal organs), (3) non-ambulatory patients before TKA where surgery was performed only for pain relief, and (4) patients not able to follow standard institutional rehabilitation protocol.

Ethical approval was obtained from the Ethics Committee of the Bizovacke Toplice Rehabilitation Hospital, Bizovac, Croatia (no. 71/2018/I), and the trial was registered with

The Australian New Zealand Clinical Trials Registry (ACTRN12618001782224). Participants gave their written informed consent. The trial was conducted in accordance with the Declaration of Helsinki.

2.2. Randomization

When patients satisfied all inclusion criteria and gave their written informed consent, they were randomly assigned into 2 groups: experimental (EG) and control (CG). We used a computerized randomization stratification procedure with the 1:1 ratio in permuted blocks of four to ensure a similar number of participants between groups. The assessors were blinded to the group allocation of participants.

2.3. Sample Size and Power Analysis

Before conducting the study, the sample size was calculated using G*Power Software [18], considering timed up and go test (TUG) as one of the primary outcome measures, based on the results of studies published by Yuksel et al. [19] and Mizner et al. [20]. Considering a power of 80%, an effect size of 0.05, a one-sided 0.05 significance level, and a 15% dropout rate, 117 patients would be necessary to detect a 2.27 s difference between the two groups, which is a minimal clinically important difference for this outcome measure.

2.4. Rehabilitation Protocol

Both groups participated in an inpatient program, which included 21 days of postoperative rehabilitation after TKA according to standard institution's protocol, which consists of daily sessions of land-based exercise therapy, application of physical agents (interferential current therapy and electrostimulation), group aquatic exercise, and individual education.

Each of the 21 days of rehabilitation followed the same protocol, except on Sundays when patients did not receive physiotherapy. On average, there were three Sundays during the patients' stay at the rehabilitation institution, and there were 18 days of rehabilitation consisting of 50 min of land-based exercise, 30 min of aquatic exercise, 10 min of interferential current therapy, and 10 min of electrostimulation. All interventions were performed on a daily basis, except individual education, which was performed once. The intervention was provided once per day, face to face, by a physiotherapist in a special hospital for rehabilitation. Adherence to the treatment was monitored by the physiotherapist in charge.

Program of land-based exercise consisted of 20 exercises. Patients performed 7 variations of isometric exercises for thigh muscles and 13 dynamic exercises for lower limbs, which include active straight leg raise (upward and combined upward and into hip abduction) from a long-sitting position with and without elastic band, hip abduction straight leg raise (and in combination with hip flexion and extension), hip flexion in long-sitting position, leg extension in sitting position with an elastic band, hip abduction from sitting position, hip flexion from sitting position, hip flexion and leg extension exercise on a Swiss ball, and pelvic lift exercise. Isometric exercises were performed in sets of 1, with 5 repetitions with a maximal effort lasting 5 s. Dynamic exercises were performed in 1–2 sets, with 10 repetitions. Progression of the dynamic exercise was achieved with an elastic band, and during the last 6 days of rehabilitation, ankle weights (1 kg) were included.

Interferential current therapy was provided using Myomed 632 device (Enraf-Nonius B. V., Rotterdam, The Netherlands) for a duration of 10 min using symmetrical waves, phase duration of 100 μs, phase interval 0 μs, impulse frequency 80 Hz, modulation frequency 0 Hz, modulation program 1/1 s, with intensity in mA according to patient's tolerance.

Electrostimulation was provided using Myomed 632 device (Enraf-Nonius B. V., Rotterdam, The Netherlands) for a duration of 10 min using symmetrical waves, phase duration of 500 μs, phase interval 0 μs, impulse frequency 1 Hz, modulation frequency 0 Hz, modulation program 1/1 s, with intensity in mA according to patient's tolerance.

Group aquatic exercise included 13 exercises for range of motion and strength (standing toe raise, standing heel raise, semi-squats, hip flexion, extension and abduction in standing position and while floating in the water, knee flexion and extension in standing position and while floating in water).

Individual education was mainly targeted to the long-term care of the prosthesis regarding how to return to activities of daily life, recommended and non-recommended activities, coping with postoperative pain, and prevention of blood clots by regular physical activity. It was provided by physiotherapists once, at the start of the rehabilitation, with additional explaining as necessary (if patients had questions) during further rehabilitation sessions.

2.4.1. Experimental Biofeedback-Assisted Exercise Therapy

In the experimental group, a portion of land-based exercise therapy was biofeedback-assisted (Myomed 632, Enraf-Nonius B. V., Rotterdam, The Netherlands), with individually adjusted targets for muscular isometric contraction, according to the manufacturer's instruction. Biofeedback was provided by superficial electromyography (EMG) unit, e.g., electrical activity of a muscle is registered and passed on as quantitative information (feedback) to the patient and the physiotherapist in real-time, during exercise. That way, the patients were able to monitor the strength of the contraction on screen and try to achieve adequate intensity of the muscular isometric contraction.

The device was attached to the patient via three electrodes, two EMG electrodes, and one reference electrode. The EMG electrodes were placed on the muscle belly of the m. quadriceps femoris according to manufacturer's instruction. The reference electrode was placed on the anterior portion of the tibia of the opposite leg. At the beginning of the biofeedback-assisted exercise, the patient performed maximal isometric contraction of the m. quadriceps femoris to establish the threshold, e.g., the target intensity of the muscular contraction. The sensitivity of the EMG signal was set to 200 μV to achieve good visibility to the patient, e.g., to achieve a good graphical representation of the muscle's electrical activity on the screen of the device. After the patient performed maximal isometric contraction, this was recorded by the device.

The physiotherapist in charge set the threshold, which was the value of the muscular contraction the patient should accomplish during the exercise, e.g., during periods of active muscular contraction. The patient should have contracted the muscle above the threshold, which was visible on the screen. The threshold was set to 80% of the maximal isometric contraction achieved at the start of the session. The biofeedback-assisted exercise consisted of isometric contractions of the m. quadriceps femoris for 15 min (10 s periods of contraction and 10 s periods of relaxation between contractions).

2.4.2. Conventional Rehabilitation Protocol

The control group was given the same rehabilitation protocol except for biofeedback-assisted exercise. They performed this portion of isometric exercises without biofeedback assistance.

2.5. Outcome Measures

Baseline information, taken at the initial interview on the first day of rehabilitation, included demographic data, medical history, height and body mass, side of the operated knee, level of the constraint of TKA, surgical technique and approach, place of the surgery and whether it was performed at the university hospital or general hospital, postoperative day, and mobility aid currently in use (one crutch, two crutches, walker or no mobility aid used).

Body mass index (BMI) was calculated according to the standard equation. Both groups had their assessments and measurements taken on their 1st and 21st day of inpatient rehabilitation. They included the self-reported functional status of the knee using Knee Injury and Osteoarthritis Outcome Score (KOOS), Croatian version LK1.0, pain intensity measured by numeric rating scale (NRS), functional status of the lower extremity using 30 s chair stand test (CST), and patients' mobility using TUG.

2.5.1. Knee Injury and Osteoarthritis Outcome Score

KOOS is a self-reported questionnaire consisting of 42 items in 5 separate subscales of pain, other symptoms, function in daily living (ADL), function in sport and recreation, and knee-related quality of life with acceptable psychometric properties [21–23]. Standardized options are given, and each question is assigned a score from 0 to 4. A normalized score (where 100 indicates no symptoms and 0 indicates extreme symptoms) was calculated for each subscale.

2.5.2. Numeric Rating Scale

NRS is a reliable and valid method of measuring pain intensity [24]. Common 11-item NRS was used in which the participant selects a whole number between 0 (no pain) and 10 (worst pain imaginable) that best reflects the intensity of their pain.

2.5.3. Thirty-Second Chair Stand Test

Thirty-second CST is measured as a number of stands where the participants are encouraged to complete as many full stands from a chair as possible within a 30 s time limit. The score is the total number of stands executed correctly within 30 s. This test provides a reasonably reliable and valid indicator of lower body strength in older adults [25,26].

2.5.4. Timed Up and Go Test

TUG measures the time that a person needs to rise from a chair, walk 3 m, turn around, walk back to the chair, and sit down [27]. It has acceptable reliability and has a reasonable predictive value of functional performance following TKA [25,28,29].

2.6. Statistical Analyses

Statistical analyses were performed using SPSS 25.0 (IBM, Armonk, NY, USA). The normality of data was checked using the Shapiro–Wilk test, and the homogeneity of variances was checked with Levene's test. Descriptive statistics were performed for all variables of interest and expressed as median and interquartile ranges.

The distribution of data was not normal except for the variables of body height and body mass index, and we used the Mann–Whitney U test, Fisher's exact test, and Chi-square test for between-group analyses

For within-group analyses of dependant variables (pre- and post-intervention comparisons), we used Wilcoxon signed-rank test, Fisher's exact test, and Chi-square test. Results were considered significant for $p < 0.05$. All the analyses included all participants for which data were available.

3. Results

A total of 131 participants admitted to inpatient rehabilitation were finally enrolled in the trial and randomized into two groups: 67 to the EG and 64 to the CG. Fourteen participants (10.7%) dropped out of the trial, eight from the EG (11.9%), and six from the CG (9.4%) (Figure 1). Data from 117 participants were included for the final analysis, 59 from the EG and 58 from the CG. The EG and CG were well matched, without differences in the baseline variables (Table 1) ($p > 0.05$). Both groups were comparable in terms of age, sex, body height, body mass, BMI, level of education, operated side of the body, level of the constraint of TKA, surgical technique and approach, place of the surgery, postoperative day, use of walking aid, KOOS, NRS, and functional tests at the beginning of their inpatient rehabilitation. All patients received posterior-stabilized implants using the medial parapatellar surgical approach. The alignment was mechanical in all but six (three from EG and three from CG) patients where kinematic alignment was used. The level of expertise of the surgeons exceeded 50 TKA per year.

Patients in both groups spent 21(0) days hospitalized, and they had 18(0) days of active rehabilitation.

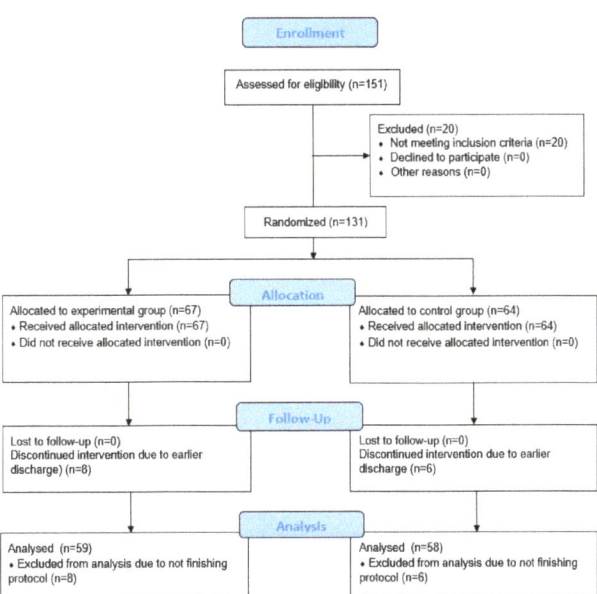

Figure 1. Consolidated Standards of Reporting Trials (CONSORT) flowchart of the study showing recruitment of participants.

Table 1. Baseline characteristics for the experimental and control group.

Variable	EG (N = 59)	CG (N = 58)
Age (years; median (IQR))	70 (10)	69 (9)
Body height (cm; median (IQR))	168 (13)	165 (12)
Body mass (kg; median (IQR))	87 (20)	84 (18)
Body mass index (kg/m^2; median (IQR))	30.8 (9.3)	30.3 (7.1)
Sex (N (%))		
Male	17 (29)	24 (41)
Female	42 (71)	34 (59)
Education (N (%))		
Secondary level	49 (83)	52 (90)
Tertiary level	10 (17)	6 (10)
Side of the operated knee (N (%))		
Left	25 (42)	32 (55)
Right	34 (58)	26 (45)
Place of the surgery (N (%))		
University hospital	13 (22)	15 (26)
General hospital	46 (78)	43 (74)
Postoperative day at the beginning of the inpatient rehabilitation (day; median (IQR))	64 (84)	70.5 (84)
Use of walking aid upon admission (N (%))		
One crutch	21 (36)	17 (30)
Two crutches	29 (49)	32 (55)
Walker	0 (0)	0 (0)
No use of walking aid	9 (15)	9 (15)
KOOS score (0–100 scale; median (IQR))		
Pain	25 (22)	29.5 (30.8)
Symptoms	32 (32)	32 (33)
ADL function	16 (17)	21.5 (31)
Sport and recreation function	5 (25)	5 (26.3)
Quality of life	44 (31)	38 (34)
NRS (0–10 scale; median (IQR))	2 (5)	3 (5)
30 s chair stand test (no. of stands; median (IQR))	9 (2)	9 (3)
TUG (seconds; median (IQR))	13.8 (5.5)	15 (6.9)

EG—experimental group; CG—control group; IQR—interquartile range; N—Sample size; KOOS—Knee Injury and Osteoarthritis Outcome Score; ADL—activities of daily living; NRS—numeric rating scale; TUG—timed up and go test.

3.1. Within-Group Analyses

Both groups improved their functional abilities from 1st day of rehabilitation until the 21st day of rehabilitation when final assessments were done. A higher proportion of participants did not use walking aid at the end of rehabilitation in both groups ($p < 0.05$) (Figure 2). In the EG, 85% needed some form of walking aid at the beginning of the rehabilitation, but only 49% of the patients needed walking aid on their 21st day of rehabilitation ($p < 0.002$). Likewise, 85% of the patients from the CG used walking aid on their 1st day of rehabilitation compared to 53% of them on their 21st day of rehabilitation ($p < 0.001$).

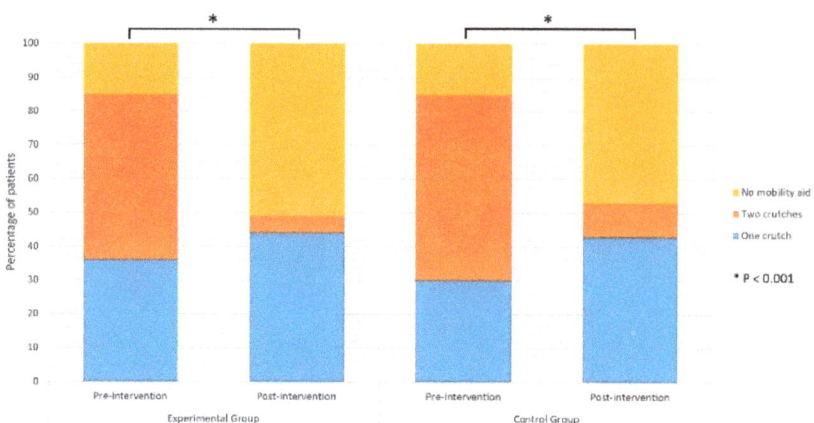

Figure 2. Use of walking aids pre-intervention (day 1) and post-intervention (day 21).

KOOS scores improved in both groups when pre-intervention and post-intervention values in all subscales were compared ($p < 0.001$) (Figure 3). Pain subscale improved by 61 points in the EG, and by 56.5 points in the CG. Symptoms score improved by 61 in both groups. ADL function subscale improved by 77 points in the EG, and by 68.5 points in the CG. Sport and recreation function improved by 15 points in both groups. Improvement of the quality-of-life subscale was by 6 points in both groups.

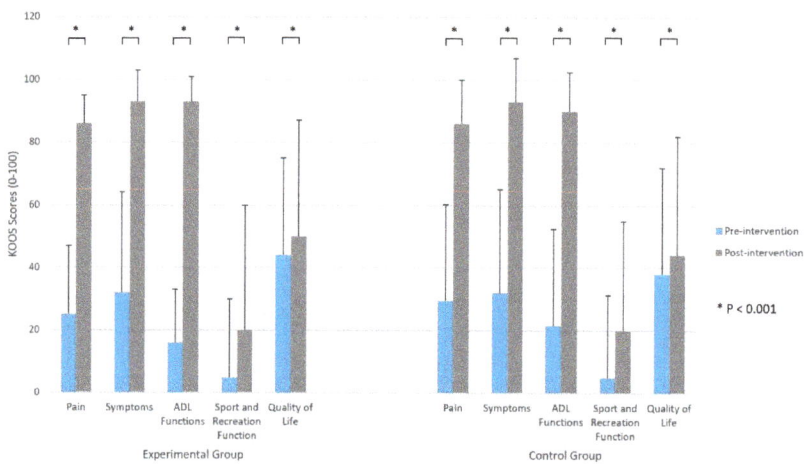

Figure 3. Knee Injury and Osteoarthritis Outcome Score (KOOS) pre-intervention (day 1) and post-intervention (day 21).

NRS scores lowered significantly ($p < 0.001$), on average, by two points in both groups (Figure 4). Both groups improved their 30 s CST result ($p < 0.001$) (Figure 4). The average difference was the addition of three stands in the EG and two stands in the CG in comparison with the pre-intervention number of stands. The time needed to perform the TUG test was significantly shorter in both groups ($p < 0.001$) (Figure 4). In the EG, the average time period was shorter by 3.8 s, and in the CG, it was shorter by 4 s on average.

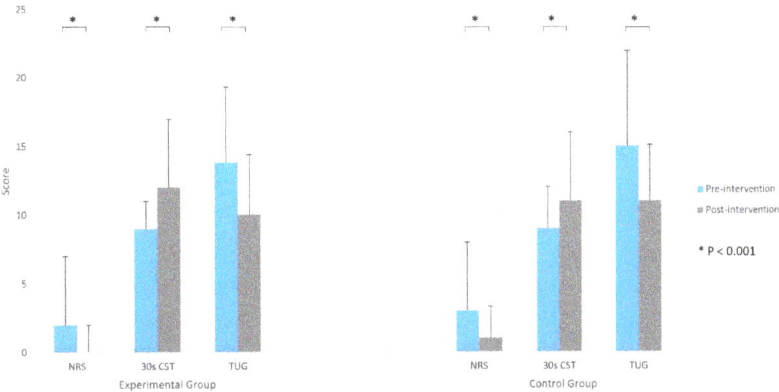

Figure 4. Numeric rating scale (NRS), 30 s chair stand test (CST), and timed up and go test (TUG) scores pre-intervention (day 1) and post-intervention (day 21).

3.2. Between-Group Analyses

Table 2 shows walking aid use, KOOS and NRS scores, as well as 30 s CST and TUG results on the 21st day of rehabilitation. There were no significant differences between the EG and CG on 21st day of rehabilitation regarding walking aid use (Figure 2). Furthermore, no differences were reported between groups in KOOS and NRS scores at the end of the rehabilitation (Figures 3 and 4). Although the results of KOOS subscales ADL function ($p = 0.07$) and Quality of life ($p = 0.06$) were borderline, there were below the determined level of significance. Additionally, there were no significant differences between groups in their 30 s CST nor TUG test results on their final assessment (Figure 4).

Table 2. Walking aid use, KOOS, NRS, 30 s chair stand test and TUG results on 21st day of rehabilitation.

Variable	EG (N = 59)	CG (N = 58)	
Use of walking aid (N (%))			
One crutch	26 (44)	25 (43)	
Two crutches	3 (5)	6 (10)	0.557 [a]
Walker	0 (0)	0 (0)	
No use of walking aid	30 (51)	27 (47)	
KOOS score (0–100 scale; median (IQR))			
Pain	86 (9)	86 (14)	0.212 [b]
Symptoms	93 (10)	93 (14)	0.488 [b]
ADL function	93 (8)	90 (12.5)	0.073 [b]
Sport and recreation function	20 (40)	20 (35)	0.660 [b]
Quality of life	50 (37)	44 (38)	0.055 [b]
NRS (0–10 scale; median (IQR))	0 (2)	1 (2.3)	0.298 [b]
30 s chair stand test (no. of stands; median (IQR))	12 (5)	11 (5)	0.129 [b]
TUG (seconds; median (IQR))	10 (4.4)	11 (4.1)	0.143 [b]

EG—experimental group; CG—control group; IQR—interquartile range; N—Sample size; KOOS—Knee Injury and Osteoarthritis Outcome Score; ADL—activities of daily living; NRS—numeric rating scale; TUG—timed up and go test. [a] Chi-Square test; [b] Mann–Whitney U test.

4. Discussion

This study aimed to examine the effects of adding EMG-BF to the conventional program of rehabilitation after TKA on the objective and subjective functional outcomes of the patients. The results did not confirm the beneficial effects of adding EMG-BF to the regimen of rehabilitation that consisted of therapeutic exercise performed on land and in the water, education, and electrotherapy, which consisted of interferential current therapy and electrostimulation. There were no significant differences between the EG and the CG regarding pain intensity, patient-reported measure of quality of life, or results of 30 s CST and TUG at the end of the rehabilitation. We were not able to confirm our hypothesis. To the best of our knowledge, only two previous studies have examined the effects of EMG-BF in smaller samples of the TKA population, which makes the comparison of our study with other studies difficult.

EMG-BF is a relatively new method of retraining muscles in orthopedic rehabilitation. It converts myoelectrical signals in the muscle by using surface electrodes which detect a change in muscle activity and feedback this information to the user by visual or auditory signals [17]. Its main use in orthopedic rehabilitation is to increase activity in weak muscles and to improve awareness regarding the contraction and relaxation of the muscle.

One of the previous studies comparing the effects of EMG-BF on a sample of the TKA population was performed by Shanb et al. [30]. They evaluated the effects of adding EMG-BF to active exercise training on m. quadriceps femoris torque, voluntary activation, and functional activity in 45 patients with unilateral TKA. Beneficial effects of adding EMG-BF to the exercise program were found only for The Western Ontario and McMaster Universities Osteoarthritis Index in favor of the EG. The authors did not report significant differences in m. quadriceps femoris torque and voluntary activation between groups. Their sample was younger than ours, with an average age of 60.6 and 60 years for the EG and CG, respectively. Furthermore, Shanb et al. excluded patients with BMI > 30 kg/m^2, and the BMI of their patients was, on average, 26 and 25 kg/m^2, respectively. In our study, the median of patients' BMI was 30.7 kg/m^2. Additionally, their intervention was different, and it included exercise training sessions performed twice per week for 4 months.

Another previous study, conducted by Wang et al. [31], examined the effects of biofeedback training performed twice daily for 5 days in the early postoperative period after TKA on pain levels. Patients in both groups received continuous passive motion (CPM) therapy; however, those in the EG received 30 min of biofeedback-assisted progressive muscle relaxation during the CPM sessions. Patients in the EG reported less pain caused by CPM than the CG. The study provided support for biofeedback relaxation for pain management in the early postoperative period.

Some other studies investigated the use of EMG-BF on different orthopedic conditions affecting the knee joint. Draper and Ballard [32] reported that EMG-BF is more effective than electrical stimulation in the facilitation of the recovery of peak torque of the quadriceps femoris in patients after anterior cruciate ligament reconstruction. Furthermore, EMG-BF has superior effects regarding m. quadriceps femoris strength and Lysholm Knee Scoring Scale in comparison to home exercise and electrical stimulation after partial meniscectomy [33]. On the other hand, no significant additive effect of EMG-BF on regular strengthening exercise programs in participants with knee osteoarthritis was reported by Yilmaz et al. [34]. Few studies investigated the use of EMG-BF for patellofemoral pain syndrome. Yip and Ng [35], as well as Ng et al. [36], suggested that EMG-BF coupled with exercise provides effective treatment for patellofemoral pain syndrome. On the contrary, Dursun et al. [37] did not find any beneficial effect of adding EMG-BF to the conventional exercise program for patellofemoral pain syndrome.

While the use of EMG-BF seems promising in the rehabilitation of knee disorders, further work is required to justify its use in patients after TKA. Voluntary activation and strength of the m. quadriceps femoris are usually reduced after TKA and m. quadriceps femoris strength in some patients can drop up to 62% of preoperative levels from three to four weeks after surgery [20,38]. This negatively affects the quality of life, mobility, and balance, as well as increases the risk of falling [39]. Conventional strengthening exercise programs used after TKA have limited success in long-term improvements of m. quadriceps function [40], and up to 17% of patients are dissatisfied with the outcome after TKA [41].

Significant efforts to improve patient outcomes after TKA, including implant design, patient optimization, perioperative pain management, and rehabilitation, have been undertaken [12]. Postoperative rehabilitation has a significant contribution to patient outcomes. Despite many rehabilitation modalities available, optimal rehabilitation strategy has yet to be determined, and there is a scarcity of evidence-based practice guidelines and recommendations for postoperative rehabilitation after TKA [12]. Therefore, it is extremely important to investigate the factors that could improve patients' outcomes after TKA and to identify therapeutic interventions which could be added to the conventional rehabilitation programs to further improve functional outcomes and patient satisfaction scores. Still, their use should be evidence-based, and the cost of providing them should be justified. New equipment, methods, and devices intended to improve patient outcomes arrive on the market and in rehabilitation facilities, but their comparative effectiveness and clinical meaningfulness to the standard of care often remain unknown or uncertain [42].

This study has clinical relevance for patients after TKA. It confirmed that both groups had significant improvements after intensive inpatient rehabilitation. However, the use of EMG-BF did not justify the cost of the device, which could be taken into account when planning to purchase expensive equipment with often uncertain clinical benefits. Expensive equipment does not always give the best results.

The current study has some limitations. First, our period of intervention was only 21 days, which could be possibly too short a period to realize the full potential of EMG-BF on the muscle function. Furthermore, we only did one final assessment on the participants' final, 21st day of hospital stay. Follow-up after an additional month could have shown some long-term effects of EMG-BF not visible on the 21st day of hospital stay. Additionally, we did not measure m. quadriceps femoris torque and voluntary activation, but we relied only on functional tests to assess the quadriceps strength and function. Quantitative measurements of m. quadriceps femoris torque and voluntary activation would add to the quality of the study. Likewise, our patients started the use of EMG-BF rather late in their rehabilitation, and their BMI was above 30 kg/m^2 on average. Thus, we cannot generalize our results to the wider population of patients after TKA.

The impact of our research will facilitate further research regarding the use of EMG-BF technology by seeking other modalities of its use that could be more clinically meaningful and efficient. Future research should aim to investigate the long-term effects of EMG-BF in various regimens, including different combinations of biofeedback-assisted isometric and dynamic exercise during longer periods. Additionally, apart from using EMG-BF only on m. quadriceps femoris, it should also be used on the m. gluteus medius since its strength is also diminished in patients after TKA.

In conclusion, data suggest that EMG-BF proves no additional benefits to the rehabilitation after TKA. Conventional rehabilitation consisting of therapeutic exercise, education, and electrotherapy yielded comparable results in terms of patient-reported quality of life, pain intensity, and tests for lower body strength, mobility, and functional performance. Further studies are needed to confirm these findings.

Author Contributions: Conceptualization, I.S.K., M.V. and T.K.; methodology, I.S.K., M.V., I.D. and I.P.; validation, I.S.K. and M.V.; formal analysis, I.S.K., I.P. and I.D.; investigation, I.S.K. and M.V.; resources, I.S.K. and M.V.; data curation, I.S.K. and M.V.; writing—original draft preparation, I.S.K., T.K. and M.V.; writing and editing, I.S.K., I.P. and I.D.; visualization, T.K.; supervision, I.S.K. All authors have read and agreed to the published version of the manuscript.

Funding: This research received no external funding.

Institutional Review Board Statement: The study was conducted in accordance with the Declaration of Helsinki and approved by the Ethics Committee of the Bizovacke Toplice Rehabilitation Hospital, Bizovac, Croatia (protocol code 71/2018/I), and the trial was registered with The Australian New Zealand Clinical Trials Registry (ACTRN12618001782224).

Informed Consent Statement: Informed consent was obtained from all subjects involved in the study.

Data Availability Statement: The data presented in this study are available on request from the corresponding author.

Conflicts of Interest: The authors declare no conflict of interest.

References

1. Vitaloni, M.; Botto-van Bemden, A.; Sciortino Contreras, R.M.; Scotton, D.; Bibas, M.; Quintero, M.; Monfort, J.; Carné, X.; de Abajo, F.; Oswald, E.; et al. Global Management of Patients with Knee Osteoarthritis Begins with Quality of Life Assessment: A Systematic Review. *BMC Musculoskelet. Disord.* **2019**, *20*, 493. [CrossRef] [PubMed]
2. Litwic, A.; Edwards, M.H.; Dennison, E.M.; Cooper, C. Epidemiology and Burden of Osteoarthritis. *Br. Med. Bull.* **2013**, *105*, 185–199. [CrossRef] [PubMed]
3. Vincent, K.R.; Vincent, H.K. Resistance Exercise for Knee Osteoarthritis. *PMR* **2012**, *4*, S45–S52. [CrossRef] [PubMed]
4. Cudejko, T.; van der Esch, M.; Schrijvers, J.; Richards, R.; van den Noort, J.C.; Wrigley, T.; van der Leeden, M.; Roorda, L.D.; Lems, W.; Harlaar, J.; et al. The Immediate Effect of a Soft Knee Brace on Dynamic Knee Instability in Persons with Knee Osteoarthritis. *Rheumatology* **2018**, *57*, 1735–1742. [CrossRef] [PubMed]
5. Cherian, J.J.; Kapadia, B.H.; Bhave, A.; McElroy, M.J.; Cherian, C.; Harwin, S.F.; Mont, M.A. Use of Transcutaneous Electrical Nerve Stimulation Device in Early Osteoarthritis of the Knee. *J. Knee Surg.* **2015**, *28*, 321–327. [CrossRef] [PubMed]
6. Steinmeyer, J.; Bock, F.; Stöve, J.; Jerosch, J.; Flechtenmacher, J. Pharmacological Treatment of Knee Osteoarthritis: Special Considerations of the New German Guideline. *Orthop. Rev.* **2018**, *10*, 7782. [CrossRef]
7. Li, J.-W.; Ma, Y.-S.; Xiao, L.-K. Postoperative Pain Management in Total Knee Arthroplasty. *Orthop. Surg.* **2019**, *11*, 755–761. [CrossRef]
8. Singh, J.A.; Vessely, M.B.; Harmsen, W.S.; Schleck, C.D.; Melton, L.J.; Kurland, R.L.; Berry, D.J. A Population-Based Study of Trends in the Use of Total Hip and Total Knee Arthroplasty, 1969–2008. *Mayo Clin. Proc.* **2010**, *85*, 898–904. [CrossRef]
9. Wang, S.-Q.; Gao, Y.-Q.; Zhang, C.; Xie, Y.-J.; Wang, J.-X.; Xu, F.-Y. A Bibliometric Analysis Using CiteSpace of Publications from 1999 to 2018 on Patient Rehabilitation After Total Knee Arthroplasty. *Med. Sci. Monit.* **2020**, *26*, e920795. [CrossRef]
10. Mizner, R.L.; Petterson, S.C.; Stevens, J.E.; Vandenborne, K.; Snyder-Mackler, L. Early Quadriceps Strength Loss after Total Knee Arthroplasty. The Contributions of Muscle Atrophy and Failure of Voluntary Muscle Activation. *J. Bone Jt. Surg.* **2005**, *87*, 1047–1053. [CrossRef]
11. Fortier, L.M.; Rockov, Z.A.; Chen, A.F.; Rajaee, S.S. Activity Recommendations After Total Hip and Total Knee Arthroplasty. *J. Bone Jt. Surg.* **2021**, *103*, 446–455. [CrossRef]
12. Dávila Castrodad, I.M.; Recai, T.M.; Abraham, M.M.; Etcheson, J.I.; Mohamed, N.S.; Edalatpour, A.; Delanois, R.E. Rehabilitation Protocols Following Total Knee Arthroplasty: A Review of Study Designs and Outcome Measures. *Ann. Transl. Med.* **2019**, *7*, S255. [CrossRef]
13. Bade, M.J.; Kohrt, W.M.; Stevens-Lapsley, J.E. Outcomes before and after Total Knee Arthroplasty Compared to Healthy Adults. *J. Orthop. Sports Phys. Ther.* **2010**, *40*, 559–567. [CrossRef]
14. Mizner, R.L.; Snyder-Mackler, L. Altered Loading during Walking and Sit-to-Stand Is Affected by Quadriceps Weakness after Total Knee Arthroplasty. *J. Orthop. Res.* **2005**, *23*, 1083–1090. [CrossRef]
15. Walsh, M.; Woodhouse, L.J.; Thomas, S.G.; Finch, E. Physical Impairments and Functional Limitations: A Comparison of Individuals 1 Year after Total Knee Arthroplasty with Control Subjects. *Phys. Ther.* **1998**, *78*, 248–258. [CrossRef] [PubMed]
16. Karaborklu Argut, S.; Celik, D.; Yasacı, Z. Effectiveness of Therapeutic Electromyographic Biofeedback after Orthopedic Knee Surgeries: A Systematic Review. *Disabil. Rehabil.* **2021**, 1–9. [CrossRef]
17. Giggins, O.M.; Persson, U.M.; Caulfield, B. Biofeedback in Rehabilitation. *J. Neuroeng. Rehabil.* **2013**, *10*, 60. [CrossRef]
18. Faul, F.; Erdfelder, E.; Lang, A.-G.; Buchner, A. G*Power 3: A Flexible Statistical Power Analysis Program for the Social, Behavioral, and Biomedical Sciences. *Behav. Res. Methods* **2007**, *39*, 175–191. [CrossRef]
19. Yuksel, E.; Kalkan, S.; Cekmece, S.; Unver, B.; Karatosun, V. Assessing Minimal Detectable Changes and Test-Retest Reliability of the Timed Up and Go Test and the 2-Minute Walk Test in Patients with Total Knee Arthroplasty. *J. Arthroplast.* **2017**, *32*, 426–430. [CrossRef]
20. Mizner, R.L.; Petterson, S.C.; Snyder-Mackler, L. Quadriceps Strength and the Time Course of Functional Recovery after Total Knee Arthroplasty. *J. Orthop. Sports Phys. Ther.* **2005**, *35*, 424–436. [CrossRef]
21. Roos, E.M.; Roos, H.P.; Lohmander, L.S.; Ekdahl, C.; Beynnon, B.D. Knee Injury and Osteoarthritis Outcome Score (KOOS)—Development of a Self-Administered Outcome Measure. *J. Orthop. Sports Phys. Ther.* **1998**, *28*, 88–96. [CrossRef] [PubMed]
22. Peer, M.A.; Lane, J. The Knee Injury and Osteoarthritis Outcome Score (KOOS): A Review of Its Psychometric Properties in People Undergoing Total Knee Arthroplasty. *J. Orthop. Sports Phys. Ther.* **2013**, *43*, 20–28. [CrossRef]

23. Alviar, M.J.; Olver, J.; Brand, C.; Tropea, J.; Hale, T.; Pirpiris, M.; Khan, F. Do Patient-Reported Outcome Measures in Hip and Knee Arthroplasty Rehabilitation Have Robust Measurement Attributes? A Systematic Review. *J. Rehabil. Med.* **2011**, *43*, 572–583. [CrossRef]
24. Downie, W.W.; Leatham, P.A.; Rhind, V.M.; Wright, V.; Branco, J.A.; Anderson, J.A. Studies with Pain Rating Scales. *Ann. Rheum. Dis.* **1978**, *37*, 378–381. [CrossRef] [PubMed]
25. Dobson, F.; Hinman, R.S.; Roos, E.M.; Abbott, J.H.; Stratford, P.; Davis, A.M.; Buchbinder, R.; Snyder-Mackler, L.; Henrotin, Y.; Thumboo, J.; et al. OARSI Recommended Performance-Based Tests to Assess Physical Function in People Diagnosed with Hip or Knee Osteoarthritis. *Osteoarthr. Cartil.* **2013**, *21*, 1042–1052. [CrossRef] [PubMed]
26. Jones, C.J.; Rikli, R.E.; Beam, W.C. A 30-s Chair-Stand Test as a Measure of Lower Body Strength in Community-Residing Older Adults. *Res. Q. Exerc. Sport* **1999**, *70*, 113–119. [CrossRef] [PubMed]
27. Podsiadlo, D.; Richardson, S. The Timed "Up & Go": A Test of Basic Functional Mobility for Frail Elderly Persons. *J. Am. Geriatr. Soc.* **1991**, *39*, 142–148. [CrossRef]
28. Yeung, T.S.M.; Wessel, J.; Stratford, P.W.; MacDermid, J.C. The Timed up and Go Test for Use on an Inpatient Orthopaedic Rehabilitation Ward. *J. Orthop. Sports Phys. Ther.* **2008**, *38*, 410–417. [CrossRef]
29. Bade, M.J.; Kittelson, J.M.; Kohrt, W.M.; Stevens-Lapsley, J.E. Predicting Functional Performance and Range of Motion Outcomes after Total Knee Arthroplasty. *Am. J. Phys. Med. Rehabil.* **2014**, *93*, 579–585. [CrossRef]
30. Shanb, A.; Youssef, E. Effects of Adding Biofeedback Training to Active Exercises after Total Knee Arthroplasty. *J. Musculoskelet. Res.* **2014**, *17*, 1450001. [CrossRef]
31. Wang, T.-J.; Chang, C.-F.; Lou, M.-F.; Ao, M.-K.; Liu, C.-C.; Liang, S.-Y.; Wu, S.-F.V.; Tung, H.-H. Biofeedback Relaxation for Pain Associated with Continuous Passive Motion in Taiwanese Patients after Total Knee Arthroplasty. *Res. Nurs. Health* **2015**, *38*, 39–50. [CrossRef]
32. Draper, V.; Ballard, L. Electrical Stimulation versus Electromyographic Biofeedback in the Recovery of Quadriceps Femoris Muscle Function Following Anterior Cruciate Ligament Surgery. *Phys. Ther.* **1991**, *71*, 455–461; discussion 461–464. [CrossRef]
33. Akkaya, N.; Ardic, F.; Ozgen, M.; Akkaya, S.; Sahin, F.; Kilic, A. Efficacy of Electromyographic Biofeedback and Electrical Stimulation Following Arthroscopic Partial Meniscectomy: A Randomized Controlled Trial. *Clin. Rehabil.* **2012**, *26*, 224–236. [CrossRef]
34. Yilmaz, O.O.; Senocak, O.; Sahin, E.; Baydar, M.; Gulbahar, S.; Bircan, C.; Alper, S. Efficacy of EMG-Biofeedback in Knee Osteoarthritis. *Rheumatol. Int.* **2010**, *30*, 887–892. [CrossRef]
35. Yip, S.L.M.; Ng, G.Y.F. Biofeedback Supplementation to Physiotherapy Exercise Programme for Rehabilitation of Patellofemoral Pain Syndrome: A Randomized Controlled Pilot Study. *Clin. Rehabil.* **2006**, *20*, 1050–1057. [CrossRef]
36. Ng, G.Y.F.; Zhang, A.Q.; Li, C.K. Biofeedback Exercise Improved the EMG Activity Ratio of the Medial and Lateral Vasti Muscles in Subjects with Patellofemoral Pain Syndrome. *J. Electromyogr. Kinesiol.* **2008**, *18*, 128–133. [CrossRef]
37. Dursun, N.; Dursun, E.; Kiliç, Z. Electromyographic Biofeedback-Controlled Exercise versus Conservative Care for Patellofemoral Pain Syndrome. *Arch. Phys. Med. Rehabil.* **2001**, *82*, 1692–1695. [CrossRef]
38. Stevens, J.E.; Mizner, R.L.; Snyder-Mackler, L. Quadriceps Strength and Volitional Activation before and after Total Knee Arthroplasty for Osteoarthritis. *J. Orthop. Res.* **2003**, *21*, 775–779. [CrossRef]
39. Ikezoe, T.; Asakawa, Y.; Tsutou, A. The Relationship between Quadriceps Strength and Balance to Fall of Elderly Admitted to a Nursing Home. *J. Phys. Ther. Sci.* **2003**, *15*, 75–79. [CrossRef]
40. Magan, A.A.; Ahmed, S.S.; Paton, B.; Konan, S.; Haddad, F.S. Does Multimodal Therapy Influence Functional Outcome After Total Knee Arthroplasty? *Orthop. Clin. N. Am.* **2020**, *51*, 453–459. [CrossRef]
41. Choi, Y.-J.; Ra, H.J. Patient Satisfaction after Total Knee Arthroplasty. *Knee Surg. Relat. Res.* **2016**, *28*, 1–15. [CrossRef] [PubMed]
42. DeJong, G.; Hsieh, C.J.; Vita, M.T.; Zeymo, A.; Boucher, H.R.; Thakkar, S.C. Innovative Devices Did Not Provide Superior Total Knee Arthroplasty Outcomes in Post-Operative Rehabilitation: Results from a Four-Arm Randomized Clinical Trial. *J. Arthroplast.* **2020**, *35*, 2054–2065. [CrossRef] [PubMed]

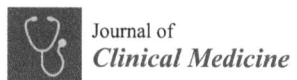

Article

Improving Upper Extremity Bradykinesia in Parkinson's Disease: A Randomized Clinical Trial on the Use of Gravity-Supporting Exoskeletons

Loredana Raciti [1], Loris Pignolo [2], Valentina Perini [3], Massimo Pullia [4], Bruno Porcari [4], Desiree Latella [4], Marco Isgrò [4], Antonino Naro [5] and Rocco Salvatore Calabrò [4,*]

[1] GCA-Centro Spoke AO Cannizzaro, Catania, IRCCS Centro Neurolesi Bonino-Pulejo, 98124 Messina, Italy; loredana.raciti@irccsme.it
[2] S. Anna Institute, Research in Advanced Neurorehabilitation, 88900 Crotone, Italy; lpignolo@gmail.com
[3] Spoke Centre of Palermo, IRCCS Centro Neurolesi Bonino-Pulejo, 98124 Messina, Italy; valentina.pirini@irccsme.it
[4] Behavioral and Robotic Neurorehabilitation Unit, IRCCS Centro Neurolesi Bonino Pulejo, 98124 Messina, Italy; massimo.pullia@irccsme.it (M.P.); bruno.porcari@irccsme.it (B.P.); desiree.latella@irccsme.it (D.L.); marco.isgro@irccsme.it (M.I.)
[5] Department of Clinical and Experimental Medicine, University of Messina, 98122 Messina, Italy; g.naro11@alice.it
* Correspondence: salbro77@tiscali.it; Fax: +39-9060128950

Abstract: Hand movements are particularly impaired in patients with Parkinson's Disease (PD), contributing to functional disability and difficulties in activities of daily living. Growing evidence has shown that robot-assisted therapy may be considered an effective and reliable method for the delivery of the highly repetitive training that is needed to trigger neuroplasticity, as intensive, repetitive and task-oriented training could be an ideal strategy to facilitate the relearning of motor function and to minimize motor deficit. The purpose of this study is to evaluate the improvement of hand function with semi-autonomous exercises using an upper extremity exoskeleton in patients with PD. A multicenter, parallel-group, randomized clinical trial was then carried out at the IRCCS Centro Neurolesi Bonino-Pulejo (Messina, Italy). Thirty subjects with a diagnosis of PD and a Hoehn–Yahr score between 2 and 3 were enrolled in the study. Patients were 1:1 randomized into either the experimental group (ERT), receiving 45 min training daily, 6 days weekly, for 8 weeks with Armeo®Spring (Volketswil, Switzerland) (a gravity-supporting device), or the control group (CPT), which was subjected to the same amount of conventional physical therapy. Motor abilities were assessed before and after the end of the training. The main outcomes measures were the Nine-hole peg test and the motor section of the UPDRS. All patients belonging to ERT and 9 out of 15 patients belonging to the CPT completed the trial. ERT showed a greater improvement in the primary outcome measure (nine-hole peg test) than CPT. Moreover, a statistically significant improvement was found in ERT concerning upper limb mobility, and disease burden as compared to CPT. Using an upper extremity exoskeleton (i.e., the Armeo®Spring) for semi-autonomous training in an inpatient setting is a new perspective to train patients with PD to improve their dexterity, executive function and, potentially, quality of life.

Keywords: gravity-supporting device; hand bradykinesia; Parkinson's disease; upper-limb rehabilitation; neurodegenerative diseases

1. Introduction

Bradykinesia and hypo-akinesia are the clinical hallmarks of Parkinson's disease (PD), mostly impairing the sequentiality and dexterity of upper extremities (UE) movements [1]. Notably, the motor impairment degree in PD patients has been shown to inversely correlate with movement velocity and directly with task difficulty [2,3]. Indeed, UE functionality impairment is usually characterized by aberrant timing and force modulation, resulting in a poor quality of hand movements [4]. These alterations contribute to the impairments of body functions and structures and the difficulty in activities and participation [5,6], leading to a lack of independence and poor quality of life [7,8].

Whether motor control deficits in PD are related to the slowness of movements rather than to impairments in movement selection is still controversial, as the nature of bradykinesia is still under investigation [9,10]. Initially, some authors suggested that bradykinesia is due to an inability to generate appropriate muscle activity before and during voluntary movements for the completion of the intended movement [11]. This was likely related to executive function deficit and reduced motor information-processing in PD [11], resulting in hypometric and increasingly impaired movements when the difficulty of a sequential motor task increases [11]. Additionally, a decreased ability in thumb–index maximum torque generation was found in PD patients [12]. Moreover, the basal ganglia have been recently described to have a pivotal role in the pathogenesis of the disorder. Then, PD is considered the consequence of the disruption of the excitability and plasticity of the basal ganglia circuits, specifically of the M1 and other non-primary motor areas [9,13].

Some therapies have proven to be effective in the improvement of motor function, enhancing the impact of non-motor symptoms and improving quality of life, even though a poor response has been demonstrated concerning hand movement dexterity [14]. To date, only a few studies focused on intervention strategies on UE and hand movements, particularly regarding fully adaptive, assist-as-needed exercises of the traditional rehabilitation [15].

Indeed, most of the existing data have focused on gait using either robotics [16] or other less expensive devices to improve the different gait parameters in patients with PD [17].

Innovative technologies are widely used in many neurological diseases, including stroke, multiple sclerosis, and spinal cord injury, with the paramount effort to increase the active range of motion and muscle strength [18,19]. Moreover, it has been shown that better outcomes could be achieved when robotics is coupled to virtual reality, resulting in a potentiation of body function and activities [20]. Such promising results depend on the fact that conjugating robotics and virtual reality allows maximizing neural, motor and functional recovery, by providing patients with lasting, challenging, repetitive, task-oriented, motivating, salient, and intensive motor exercises; furthermore, virtual reality may also provide patients with a potentiation of motor and cognitive functions [20–23].

There is an increasing interest in robotic rehabilitation in PD. Some studies showed that the use of robot-assisted rehab is useful for gait training [15,24], improve freezing of gait [25] to reduce the muscular activity requirements of PD patients [26], balance [27], and reduce the amplitude of tremors [28]. Then, the use of advanced and computerized technologies could provide a better rehabilitation in patients with PD [29,30]. However, no data are available about the use of specific robotic devices to recover arm impairment in PD patients.

The aim of this pilot study is to evaluate the efficacy of a gravity-supporting exoskeleton apparatus (i.e., the Armeo Spring; Hocoma, Zurich, Switzerland) on hand dexterity and overall motor functions in PD patients (experimental robotic therapy-ERT) as compared to conventional physical therapy (CPT).

2. Materials and Methods

2.1. Study Design and Population

We carried out a parallel-group, single-blinded, randomized controlled trial on the PD patients attending either the Movement Disorders Clinic of the IRCCS Centro Neurolesi Bonino-Pulejo (Messina, Italy) or its Spoke Centre (Palermo, Italy) between July 2019 and March 2020. Indeed, the enrollment period was interrupted due to the COVID-19 pandemic and some patients abandoned the study (Figure 1).

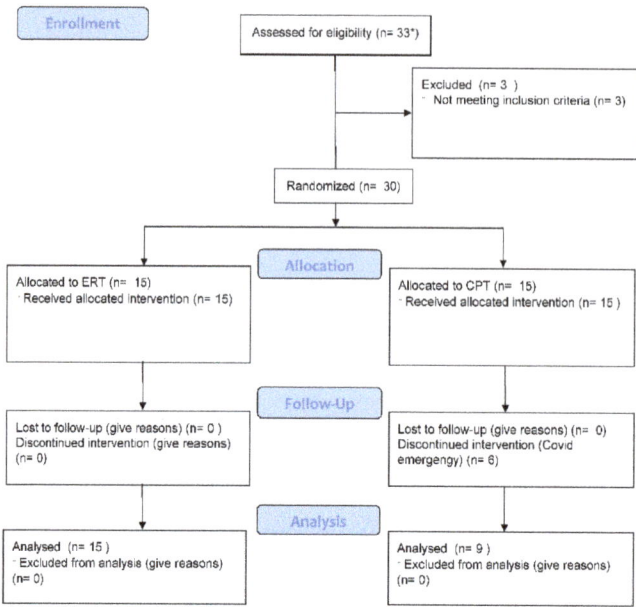

* 31 patients from the Department of Movement Disorders of the IRCCS Centro Neurolesi Bonino Pulejo (Messina, Italy); 4 patients from the Villa delle Ginestre Hospital (Palermo, Italy)

Figure 1. Patients' diagram flow.

The inclusion criteria were as follows: (i) history of idiopathic PD diagnosed according to the UK Brain Bank criteria [31]; (ii) a Hoehn–Yahr stage between 2 and 3 determined in the "on" phase [32]; and (iii) age between 50 and 80 years old. The exclusion criteria were: (1) moderate to severe cognitive deficits potentially limiting comprehension of the experimental task (i.e., a Mini-Mental State Examination < 20) [33]; (2) severe dyskinesia or severe on–off motor fluctuations; (3) stereotaxic brain surgery for PD; (4) changes in dopamine therapy dose (as per levodopa equivalent daily dose, LEDD) within 3 months prior to baseline; (5) unstable cardiac or respiratory illness potentially interfering with the training; and (6) any other medical condition that could compromise the training, including severe osteoarthritis or peripheral neuropathies.

Written informed consent was obtained from all participants. The study was conducted according to the laws, regulations, and administrative provisions relating to the implementation of good clinical practice in the conduct of clinical trials on medicinal products for human use, as applicable by national legislation and the Declaration of Helsinki. The protocol (No. U0074917/11110) was approved by the Ethical Committee of the IRCCS Centro Neurolesi Bonino Pulejo (Messina, Italy) and was registered at ClinicalTrials.gov (NCT02721212).

2.2. Randomization

After the screening session, when patients satisfied all inclusion criteria, they were randomly assigned to ERT or CPT. To this end, we adopted a computerized randomization stratification approach. The randomization scheme (1:1 ratio) was set up in permuted blocks of three to ensure a similar number of participants between groups. Additionally, participants were stratified by their degree of disability and impairment (Unified Parkinson's Disease Rating Scale score, UPDRS) [34] to obtain a balance between groups regarding the baseline physical capacity. The assessors were blinded to the group allocation of participants.

2.3. Sample Size and Power Analysis

The sample size, in relation to the clinically significant changes in the primary outcome, was calculated by means of a 2-sided, 2-sample t-test, and estimated in 60 patients (30 per arm). More specifically, this sample size was required to maintain a type I error rate of 0.05 and an 80% power to detect a significant between-group difference of 5.65 s [35] (including a 10% dropout rate or loss to follow-up).

2.4. Experimental Robotic Therapy

The Armeo®Spring (Figure 2) is a mechanical device (Hocoma Inc., Zurich, Switzerland) characterized by an adaptable suspension system for the upper limb that offers support from the shoulder to the wrist ending with a grasping system for the hand.

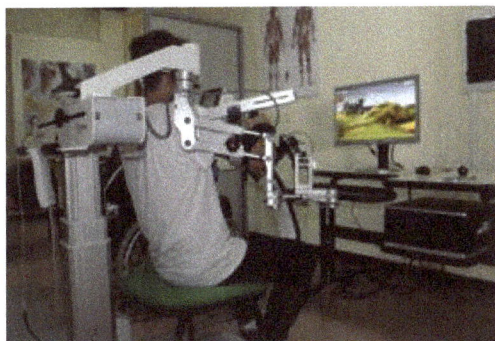

Figure 2. A patient with PD receiving the experimental training with the Armeo©Spring device.

System sensitivity can be adjusted depending on the patient's condition. The system gives information about movement parameters, such as resistance, strength, range of motion, and coordination. Based on the patient's active mobility, the system allows to calibrate the working space and level of difficulty during the entire training period. The device expands any movement, allowing reinforcement and facilitation of the arm by visual feedback (2D virtual reality) with a three-dimensional space [36].

The training was supervised by a physiotherapist expert in robot-assisted therapy. After the device was adjusted for the patient's arm size and angle of suspension, the workspace and exercises were selected. Exercise difficulties were modified during the following sessions. Each training session consisted of 45 min per session for each arm with Armeo®Spring, 6 days per week, for 8 weeks.

2.5. Conventional Physical Therapy

Patients in the control group received the same global treatment time of the ERT. Patients were submitted to conventional rehabilitation, such as passive- and active-assisted mobilization of the upper limbs, traditional training for neuromuscular facilitation, proprioception exercises, and reducing joints and muscles stiffness. Active exercises of reaching and picking objects were also performed.

2.6. Outcome Measures

We provided the patients with the motor section of the UPDRS and the Motricity Index for Upper Extremity (MI-UE) to test motor impairment, the nine-hole peg test (9HPT) [37] to objectively evaluate hand dexterity, the Fugl-Meyer Assessment for the upper extremity (FMA-UE) to test the UE motor ability to perform selective movements, the Functional Independence Measure (FIM) to estimate the disability burden, and the numerical rating scale of pain (P-NRS) to measure the range of pain intensity. The primary outcome was the change of the 9HPT from baseline (T0) to post-treatment (T1). The secondary outcomes were the changes of UPDRS, FMA-UE, FIM, P-NRS, and MI-UE from T0 to T1.

2.6.1. Primary Outcome Measure

The 9HPT test was used to assess hand dexterity, by asking the patients to take nine pegs from a container and place them into nine holes on a board and vice versa as quickly as possible. Score was the time taken to complete the test activity [38].

2.6.2. Secondary Outcome Measures

The UPDRS is the most used screening tool to detect disease severity and motor and non-motor complications in PD [34,38]. It consists of three subscales: part I: evaluation of mentation, behavior, and mood by an interview; part II: the activities of daily life by self-evaluation; part III or motor section is a clinician-scored motor evaluation; and part IV is the evaluation of long-term levodopa complications, such as dyskinesia and motor fluctuations.

The FMA-UE was used to evaluate upper limb motor ability to perform selective movements. Of the motricity scales, the most popular used scale in PD is the Fugl-Meyer Motor Assessment Scale [39,40].

The 33-item scale consists of 3 response categories (scores 0–2) for each item, with a maximum score of 66 (indicating no impairment) with sub-scores of 36 for the upper arm, 10 for the wrist, 14 for the hand, and 6 for coordination and speed of movement [39,41].

The FIM measures the level of a patient's disability burden and indicates how much assistance is required for the individual to carry out activities of daily living. Each task is rated on a 7-point ordinal scale that ranges from 1 = total assistance (or complete dependence) to 7 = complete independence [42].

The P-NRS typically consists of a series of numbers with verbal anchors representing the entire possible range of pain intensity. Generally, patients rate their pain from 0 to 10, from 0 to 20, or from 0 to 100. Zero represents "no pain", whereas 10, 20, or 100 represent the opposite end of the pain continuum (e.g., "the most intense pain imaginable", "pain as intense as it could be", and "maximum pain") [43].

The MI-UE can be used to assess motor impairment. MI is a feasible measure that can demonstrate the overall patients' impairment. It is a simple, brief measure of general motor function that can predict mobility outcomes post-stroke [44]. All motor assessment and motor training sessions were performed bilaterally, in the affected and unaffected side.

2.7. Statistical Analysis

Between-group T0 differences were estimated using the Mann–Whitney test. The significance of the changes in each outcome measure was calculated by conducting a repeated-measure ANOVA for continuous numerical variables (using time, two levels, and group, two levels, as factors) or a Wilcoxon signed-rank test for ordinal or nominal variables. Depending on the significance of the main interactions and effects, Bonferroni corrected pairwise comparisons using *t*-tests, Wilcoxon test, or Mann–Whitney test, where appropriate, were tested. For all statistical tests, the significance level was set at $\alpha < 0.05$. All the analyses included all participants for which data were available.

3. Results

3.1. Baseline (T0)

Thirty-three patients were consecutively screened for study inclusion. Three failed the inclusion criteria. Therefore, 30 patients were randomized to ERT or CPT. There were no differences at baseline between the groups concerning age, disease duration, and LEDD (Table 1; all $p > 0.2$).

Table 1. Clinical-demographic features at baseline (T0). Data are reported as mean (SD) or median (interquartile range), and *p*-value of Mann–Whitney test.

	ERT (*n* = 15)	CPT (*n* = 9)	*p*-Value
Age (years)	65.7 (7)	62.7 (10.1)	0.1
Disease Duration (years)	5.3 (3.4)	6.2 (4.6)	0.6
LEDD (mg/day)	544 (198)	583 (191)	0.7
H&Y	2 (2–3)	2 (2–3)	0.4

Legend: CPT, conventional physical therapy; ERT, experimental robotic therapy; H&Y, Hoehn–Yahr stage determined in the "on" phase; LEDD, levodopa equivalent daily dose.

Particularly, both groups had a Hoehn–Yahr stage between 2 and 3, which corresponded to an on-average moderate impairment of body functions and structure and a moderate difficulty impairment in activities and participation (i.e., present <50% of time, with intensity that interferes with day-to-day lift, occurring occasionally over last 30 days). The 9HPT, MI-UE, and FIM data were not available for three subjects belonging to the ERT group (Tables 2 and 3).

Table 2. Outcome measure scores at T0 (baseline) and T1 (post-treatment) in the ERT (*n* = 15; * *n* = 12) and CPT (*n* = 9) group. Data are reported as mean (SD) or median (interquartile range), and *p*-value of within-group (using *t*-test or Wilcoxon test) and between-group comparison (using *t*-test or Mann–Whitney test).

		T0	T1	Within-Group Comparison	Between-Group Comparison
9HPT	ERT	42.2 (17)	34.1 (14)	0.006	0.004
	CPT	35.1 (6.8)	31.4 (5.4)	0.9	
UPDRS-III	ERT	28 (23–33)	21 (16–26)	0.06	0.5
	CPT	37 (31.5–41)	32 (23.25;40)	0.9	
P-NRS	ERT	2.5 (0.5–3.5)	1.1 (0.3–1.8)	0.007	0.9
	CPT	4 (3–5)	1 (0–1.5)	0.01	
MI-UE	ERT	72 (65–80) *	89 (83–94) *	0.04	0.0001
	CPT	77 (73.25–82)	82 (79.25;88.5)	0.8	
FIM	ERT	104 (98–109) *	110 (105–115) *	0.6	0.6
	CPT	100 (99–103)	101 (100–106)	0.9	
FMA-UE	ERT	48 (45–52)	53 (5–56)	0.007	0.009
	CPT	53 (51–55)	56 (52.5–59.5)	0.9	

Legend: 9HPT, nine-hole peg test; UPDRS, Unified Parkinson's Disease Rating Scale; P-NRS, numerical rating scale of pain; MI-UE, Motricity Index for Upper Extremity; FIM, Functional Independence Measure; FMA-UE, Fugl-Meyer Assessment for Upper Extremity.

3.2. Post-Treatment (T1)

Six patients belonging to the CPT dropped out (Figure 1). Therefore, 15 patients belonging to ERT and 9 to CPT were analyzed. No adverse events were reported, apart from the worsening of Pisa Syndrome in one patient. The analyses showed that ERT achieved a greater improvement in 9HPT than CPT (Table 2). Furthermore, ERT showed a greater improvement in UPDRS III, MI-UE, and FMA-UE (Table 2). On the other hand, both ERT and CPT equally improved in P-NRS (Table 2). Most of the patients reported an improvement in FIM; for instance, a patient started to work at the crochet again. When considering the most affected UE (Table 3), greater changes were appreciable concerning P-NRS, MI-UE, and FIM in ERT than in CPT, whereas both groups equally improved in 9HPT and FMA-UE.

Table 3. Affected side assessment at T0 (baseline) and T1 (post-treatment) in the ERT (n = 15; * n = 12) and CPT (n = 9) group. Data are reported as mean (SD) or median (interquartile range), and p-value of within-group (using t-test or Wilcoxon test) and between-group comparison (using t-test or Mann–Whitney test).

		T0	T1	Within-Group Comparison	Between-Group Comparison
9HPT	ERT	42.2 (17.3) *	34.1 (13.9)	0.001	0.7
	CPT	35.1 (6.8)	31.4 (5.4)	0.003	
UPDRS-III	ERT	28 (23.25–32)	21 (15–22.5)	0.07	0.7
	CPT	28 (26.25–31)	24 (23.25–26)	0.1	
P-NRS	ERT	2.1 (1.1–4.1)	1.3 (1.2–1.4)	0.01	0.001
	CPT	1.7 (1.6–1.9)	1.5 (1.4–1.6)	0.3	
MI-UE	ERT	69 (64.25–76) *	87 (82.25–94)	0.001	0.002
	CPT	84 (78–91.5)	82 (78.25–90.5)	0.4	
FIM	ERT	103 (100.25–106.5) *	109 (104.25–112.5)	0.0001	0.4
	CPT	86 (82.25–90)	122 (118.25–124)	0.0001	
FMA-UE	ERT	48 (45.25–51)	52 (50.25–54)	0.001	0.008
	CPT	56 (50–57.5)	57 (52.26–59)	0.08	

Legend: 9HPT, nine-hole peg test; UPDRS, Unified Parkinson's Disease Rating Scale; P-NRS, numerical rating scale of pain; MI-UE, Motricity Index for Upper Extremity; FIM, Functional Independence Measure; FMA-UE, Fugl-Meyer Assessment for Upper Extremity.

4. Discussion

The PD patients included in the study complained of altered UE functions (including impaired timing and force modulation), with a compromised quality of hand movement. Furthermore, all patients complained of a mild to moderate motor impairment and ability to perform selective movements (UPDRS, MI-UE, and FMA-UE), disability burden (FIM), and very mild pain rating (P-NRS). Overall, they thus complained of a moderate impairment of body functions and structures and a moderate difficulty in activities and participation consistently with the International Classification of Functioning, Disability and Health [6].

To the best of our knowledge, this is the first study preliminarily evaluating the efficacy of an exoskeleton-based rehabilitation strategy in potentiating UE functions in PD patients as compared to CPT [4]. Actually, there are not available specific rehabilitation protocols or approaches to improve UE dexterity learning in PD. Both rehabilitation approaches were able to provide PD patients with a significant improvement in UE functions. However, ERT offered patients with specific benefits in terms of hand dexterity, overall UE movement, and disability burden as compared to CPT.

This finding is consistent with a pilot study by Picelli et al. [14], which showed the efficacy of the Bi-Manu-Track (Reha-Stim, Berlin, Germany) training in PD patients. In particular, ten sessions of bilateral (mirror-like) passive and active, computer-controlled, repetitive practice of forearm pronation/supination and wrist extension/flexion improved 9HPT and the FMA-UE. Despite the results of our study and those by Picelli et al. not being directly comparable due to the different devices used, both studies suggest that repetitive, robot-assisted UE training would be a promising tool to improve motor outcomes in PD patients. Furthermore, our results are in line with those by Lee et al., who observed significant improvements of UE fine and gross motor performance after several, repetitive treatment sessions by constraint-induced movement therapy in twenty patients with PD [32].

The superiority of gravity-supporting device as compared to CPT in reducing the impairment of, at least, some motor outcomes in PD patients is likely to depend on the intensive, repetitive, assisted-as-needed, and task-oriented motor practice provided by the mechanical device [45]. It has been proposed that such an approach allows exploiting the brain neural plasticity mechanisms both within affected and intact brain structures through the stimulation of motor learning processes and a reshape of the "inter-hemispheric inhibition" mechanisms by means of repetitive sessions of robot-assisted therapy, as demonstrated by UE dexterity improvement in post-stroke patients [46–48]. This extends to the case of basal ganglia impairment, where an intensive, continual, and contextual training allows facilitating the relearning of motor functions and minimizing motor deficit by acting on the internal regulator mechanisms of movement flow and programming [17,45,49]. Particularly, the improvement in motor outcomes following ERT sessions could be considered the expression of a relearning process resulting from the stimulation and the activation of the mirror neuron system, inducing profound cortical and subcortical changes at both the cellular and synaptic levels [50]. The role of the cerebellum in motor and reinforcement learning has been recognized. Recently, it has been shown that the cerebellum may have a compensatory and adaptive role concerning gait function recovery by favoring the precise timing of motor actions along the gait cycle phases. This probably occurs by compensating the deficient internal timing clock within the basal ganglia [51]. These results have been obtained in PD patients receiving gait training plus music (i.e., a repetitive exercise with an external cue). It is then hypothesizable that UL robotic rehabilitation with VR may have boosted neural plasticity also at the cerebellar level, further improving motor recovery.

In addition, UE training benefitted from the adjunction of virtual reality treatment. This is thought to increase the motor learning of well-defined motor tasks and improve motivation due to the feedback provided by the device itself [18–23,48–50,52–54]. Overall, these motor improvements allowed the patients to achieve a significant improvement in UE functions and disability burden. For instance, a patient was able to do a crochet work carried out after a 25% of ERT sessions. Such activity was referred to as difficult to carry out for about two years by the patient.

Although we have not specifically investigated quality of life, it is possible that the improvement in disability burden has also improved patients' health-related quality of life, as suggested by other chronic diseases [55].

Strengths and Limitations

Our data suggest that UE training using a gravity-supporting device could be considered a safe and effective approach for the recovery of UE motor functions in PD patients. Additionally, the rehabilitation technology is a cost-effective practice to reduce the need for one-to-one skilled interventions. The training sessions can be performed with minimal supervision once the therapist has set up the exercises. The attention of the patient is triggered by the visual and acoustic feedback while the exercise is performed. Moreover, the training is reproducible and essentially safe and can be easily conducted in the hospital setting. However, our study is limited by the small sample size (we were able to enroll only 30 patients compared to the estimated 60 because of the onset of COVID-19 pandemic). This could have had relevant consequences on the results, considering that an intention-to-treat analysis was not performed. It is true that an intention-to-treat approach tends to under-estimate an effect, being thus a more conservative approach in a clinical superiority trial. Nevertheless, a per-protocol approach is a reasonable analysis strategy for sensitivity analyses. Actually, a per-protocol approach is suitable when the exclusion of patients from the analysis due to major protocol deviations (which can of course cause a tendency to wrong estimations of a treatment effect) tends to vary among the study groups. However, it is not straightforward to pre-guess the direction of a wrong estimation and the general claim that a per-protocol analysis tends to overestimate an effect that cannot be mathematically proven [56–58]. Studies with larger and homogeneous samples could allow for a more accurate statistical analysis, including multivariate data analysis or more advanced tools, such as machine learning, aimed to point out predictive marker of recovery.

Another main limitation of our study is the lack of evaluation of long-term efficacy of the ERT (also due to COVID-19 pandemic restrictions). Nonetheless, previous studies have shown a persistent efficacy of robotic rehabilitation after two weeks only for the 9HPT [15]. Moreover, Taveggia et al. recorded a stability of motor assessment after 6 weeks from the end of treatment in stroke patients [59]; lastly, the improvement in the functional capacity outcome measures were found at 2-month follow-up in multiple sclerosis patients [60]. Last, one could criticize that the use of MI-UE is not usual in evaluating clinical impairment in PD, compared to the FMA-UE [61]. In fact, MI-UE assesses the motor impairment in a patient who has had a stroke evaluating the ability of the patient to hold a cube against gravity, the capacity to flex the elbow from 90° (so that the arm touches the shoulder) and the capacity of the shoulder to abduct to more than 90° beyond the horizontal against gravity. Rigidity in PD refers to increased muscular tone with more resistance than normal when the limb is passively moved, experienced by the patients as a sense of feeling stiff and uncomfortable. Then, even though the physiopathology of abnormal movements in PD are different from strokes [59], similar difficulties in achieving MI-UE goals are seen in PD patients. Then, further validation studies are needed to confirm the possibility to use the scale even in Parkinsonism. Larger sample size RCTs are, notwithstanding, needed to address this concern.

5. Conclusions

Our data suggest that exoskeleton-assisted therapy, such as the Armeo©Spring, may represent a safe and effective strategy for delivering a highly intensive and repetitive training, which is necessary to trigger the neuroplasticity mechanisms subtending UE motor function improvement. Few studies are however available on the UE rehabilitation of patients with PD, particularly regarding technology-enhanced physical therapy, except for gait training. Therefore, further investigations with larger sample sizes are needed to confirm our results and to optimize PD-specific rehabilitation protocols.

Author Contributions: Conceptualization, R.S.C. and V.P.; methodology, A.N., V.P., R.S.C., L.R. and L.P.; software, L.P.; validation, D.L., M.I., B.P. and M.P.; formal analysis, A.N.; investigation, D.L., M.I., B.P. and M.P.; resources, L.R.; data curation, A.N. and L.R.; writing—original draft preparation, L.R. and A.N.; writing—review and editing, A.N. and R.S.C.; visualization, D.L., M.I., B.P. and M.P.; supervision, R.S.C. and L.P. All authors have read and agreed to the published version of the manuscript.

Funding: This research received no external funding.

Institutional Review Board Statement: The study was conducted in accordance with the Declaration of Helsinki and approved by the Ethics Committee of the IRCCS Centro Neurolesi Bonino Pulejo (Messina, Italy) (protocol code No. U0074917/11110) and was registered at ClinicalTrials.gov (NCT02721212).

Informed Consent Statement: Informed consent was obtained from all subjects involved in the study.

Data Availability Statement: Data could be requested on demand to the corresponding author.

Conflicts of Interest: The authors declare no conflict of interest.

References

1. Ponsen, M.M.; Daffertshofer, A.; Wolters, E.C.; Beek, P.J.; Berendse, H.W. Impairment of complex upper limb motor function in de novo Parkinson's disease. *Parkinsonism Relat. Disord.* **2008**, *14*, 199–204. [CrossRef] [PubMed]
2. Fitts, P.M. The information capacity of the human motor system in controlling the amplitude of movement. *J. Exp. Psychol.* **1954**, *47*, 381–391. [CrossRef] [PubMed]
3. Sanes, J.N. Information processing deficits in Parkinson's disease during movement. *Neuropsychologia* **1985**, *23*, 381–392. [CrossRef]
4. Quinn, L.; Busse, M.; Dal Bello-Haas, V. Management of upper extremity dysfunction in people with Parkinson disease and Huntington disease: Facilitating outcomes across the disease lifespan. *J. Hand Ther.* **2013**, *26*, 148–155. [CrossRef] [PubMed]

5. Rocchi, L.; Chiari, L.; Horak, F.B. Effects of deep brain stimulation and levodopa on postural sway in Parkinson's disease. *J. Neurol. Neurosurg. Psychiatry* **2002**, *73*, 267–274. [CrossRef]
6. Raggi, A.; Leonardi, M.; Ajovalasit, D.; Carella, F.; Soliveri, P.; Albanese, A.; Romito, L. Disability and profiles of functioning of patients with Parkinson's disease described with ICF classification. *Int. J. Rehabil. Res.* **2011**, *34*, 141–150. [CrossRef]
7. Diederich, N.J.; Moore, C.G.; Leurgans, S.E.; Chmura, T.A.; Goetz, C.G. Parkinson disease with old-age onset: A comparative study with subjects with middle-age onset. *Arch. Neurol.* **2003**, *60*, 529–533. [CrossRef]
8. Soh, S.E.; McGinley, J.L.; Watts, J.J.; Iansek, R.; Murphy, A.T.; Menz, H.B.; Huxham, F.; Morris, M.E. Determinants of health-related quality of life in people with Parkinson's disease: A path analysis. *Qual. Life Res.* **2013**, *22*, 1543–1553. [CrossRef]
9. Berardelli, A.; Rothwell, J.C.; Thompson, P.D.; Hallett, M. Pathophysiology of bradykinesia in Parkinson's disease. *Brain* **2001**, *124*, 2131–2146. [CrossRef]
10. Espay, A.J.; Beaton, D.E.; Morgante, F.; Gunraj, C.A.; Lang, A.E.; Chen, R. Impairments of speed and amplitude of movement in Parkinson's disease: A pilot study. *Mov. Disord.* **2009**, *24*, 1001–1008. [CrossRef]
11. Hallett, M.; Khoshbin, S. A physiological mechanism of bradykinesia. *Brain* **1980**, *103*, 301–314. [CrossRef] [PubMed]
12. Oliveira, M.A.; Rodrigues, A.M.; Caballero, R.M.; Petersen, R.D.; Shim, J.K. Strength and isometric torque control in individuals with Parkinson's disease. *Exp. Brain Res.* **2008**, *184*, 445–450. [CrossRef] [PubMed]
13. Bologna, M.; Paparella, G.; Fasano, A.; Hallett, M.; Berardelli, A. Evolving concepts on bradykinesia. *Brain* **2020**, *143*, 727–750. [CrossRef] [PubMed]
14. Vercruysse, S.; Gilat, M.; Shine, J.M.; Heremans, E.; Lewis, S.; Nieuwboer, A. Freezing beyond gait in Parkinson's disease: A review of current neurobehavioral evidence. *Neurosci. Biobehav. Rev.* **2014**, *43*, 213–227. [CrossRef] [PubMed]
15. Picelli, A.; Tamburin, S.; Passuello, M.; Waldner, A.; Smania, N. Robot-assisted arm training in patients with Parkinson's disease: A pilot study. *J. Neuroeng. Rehabil.* **2014**, *11*, 28. [CrossRef]
16. Calabrò, R.S.; Cacciola, A.; Bertè, F.; Manuli, A.; Leo, A.; Bramanti, A.; Naro, A.; Milardi, D.; Bramanti, P. Robotic gait rehabilitation and substitution devices in neurological disorders: Where are we now? *Neurol. Sci.* **2016**, *37*, 503–514. [CrossRef]
17. Brognara, L.; Navarro-Flores, E.; Iachemet, L.; Serra-Catalá, N.; Cauli, O. Beneficial Effect of Foot Plantar Stimulation in Gait Parameters in Individuals with Parkinson's Disease. *Brain Sci.* **2020**, *10*, 69. [CrossRef]
18. Mehrholz, J.; Hädrich, A.; Platz, T.; Kugler, J.; Pohl, M. Electromechanical and robot-assisted arm training for improving generic activities of daily living, arm function, and arm muscle strength after stroke. *Cochrane Database Syst. Rev.* **2012**, *6*, CD006876. [CrossRef]
19. Bonanno, L.; Russo, M.; Bramanti, A.; Calabrò, R.S.; Marino, S. Functional connectivity in multiple sclerosis after robotic rehabilitative treatment: A case report. *Medicine* **2019**, *98*, e15647. [CrossRef]
20. Maggio, M.G.; Russo, M.; Cuzzola, M.F.; Destro, M.; Rosa, G.L.; Molonia, F.; Bramanti, P.; Lombardo, G.; Luca, R.D.; Calabrò, R.S. Virtual reality in multiple sclerosis rehabilitation: A review on cognitive and motor outcomes. *J. Clin. Neurosci.* **2019**, *65*, 106–111. [CrossRef]
21. Clark, W.E.; Sivan, M.; O'Connor, R.J. Evaluating the use of robotic and virtual reality rehabilitation technologies to improve function in stroke survivors: A narrative review. *J. Rehabil. Assist. Technol. Eng.* **2019**, *6*, 2055668319863557. [CrossRef]
22. Baur, K.; Schättin, A.; de Bruin, E.D.; Riener, R.; Duarte, J.E.; Wolf, P. Trends in robot-assisted and virtual reality-assisted neuromuscular therapy: A systematic review of health-related multiplayer games. *J. Neuroeng. Rehabil.* **2018**, *15*, 107. [CrossRef] [PubMed]
23. Park, J.; Chung, Y. The effects of robot-assisted gait training using virtual reality and auditory stimulation on balance and gait abilities in persons with stroke. *NeuroRehabilitation* **2018**, *43*, 227–235. [CrossRef]
24. Smania, N.; Picelli, A.; Geroin, C.; Munari, D.; Waldner, A.; Gandolfi, M. Robot-assisted gait training in patients with Parkinson's disease. *Neurodegener. Dis. Manag.* **2013**, *3*, 321–330. [CrossRef]
25. Capecci, M.; Pournajaf, S.; Galafate, D.; Sale, P.; Pera, D.L.; Goffredo, M.; Pandis, M.F.D.; Andrenelli, E.; Pennacchioni, M.; Ceravolo, M.G.; et al. Clinical effects of robot-assisted gait training and treadmill training for Parkinson's disease. A randomized control. *Trial. Ann. Phys. Rehabil. Med.* **2019**, *62*, 303–312. [CrossRef]
26. Cifuentes, C.A.; Frizera, A. Human-Robot Interaction for Assisting. In *Human-Robot Interaction Strategies for Walker-Assisted Locomotion*; Locomotion, H., Ed.; Springer: Berlin/Heidelberg, Germany, 2016; pp. 17–31.
27. Scaletta, T.; Komada, S.; Oboe, R. Development of a human assistive robot to support hip joint movement during sit-to-stand using non-linear springs. *IEEJ J. Ind. Appl.* **2016**, *5*, 261–266. [CrossRef]
28. Huen, D.; Liu, J.; Lo, B. An integrated wearable robot for tremor suppression with context aware sensing. In Proceedings of the 2016 IEEE 13th International Conference on Wearable and Implantable Body Sensor Networks (BSN), San Francisco, CA, USA, 14–17 June 2016.
29. Voiculescu, I.; Cameron, S.; Zabarauskas, M.; Kozlowski, P. Towards Robot-Assisted Rehabilitation of Upper Limb dysfunction. In *Advances in Robot Design and Intelligent Control: Advances in Intelligent Systems and Computing*; Borangiu, T., Ed.; Springer: Berlin/Heidelberg, Germany, 2016; pp. 347–355.
30. Asakawa, T.; Sugiyama, K.; Nozaki, T.; Sameshima, T.; Kobayashi, S.; Wang, L.; Hong, Z.; Chen, S.; Li, C.; Namba, H. Can the Latest Computerized Technologies Revolutionize Conventional Assessment Tools and Therapies for a Neurological Disease? The Example of Parkinson's Disease. *Neurol. Med.-Chir.* **2019**, *59*, 69–78. [CrossRef]

31. Hughes, A.J.; Daniel, S.E.; Kilford, L.; Lees, A.J. Accuracy of clinical diagnosis of idiopathic Parkinson's disease: A clinico-pathological study of 100 cases. *J. Neurol. Neurosurg. Psychiatry* **1992**, *55*, 181–184. [CrossRef]
32. Hoehn, M.M.; Yahr, M.D. Parkinsonism: Onset, progression and mortality. *Neurology* **1967**, *17*, 427–442. [CrossRef]
33. Folstein, M.F.; Folstein, S.E.; McHugh, P.R. "Mini-mental state". A practical method for grading the cognitive state of patients for the clinician. *J. Psychiatr. Res.* **1975**, *12*, 189–198. [CrossRef]
34. Movement Disorder Society Task Force on Rating Scales for Parkinson's Disease. The Unified Parkinson's Disease Rating Scale (UPDRS): Status and recommendations. *Mov. Disord.* **2003**, *18*, 738–750. [CrossRef] [PubMed]
35. Proud, E.L.; Bilney, B.; Miller, K.J.; Morris, M.E.; McGinley, J.L. Measuring Hand Dexterity in People with Parkinson's Disease: Reliability of Pegboard Tests. *Am. J. Occup. Ther.* **2019**, *73*, p1–p7304205050. [CrossRef] [PubMed]
36. Colomer, C.; Baldoví, A.; Torromé, S.; Navarro, M.D.; Moliner, B.; Ferri, J.; Noé, E. Efficacy of Armeo® Spring during the chronic phase of stroke. *Study Mild Moderate Cases Hemiparesis Neurol.* **2013**, *28*, 261–267. [CrossRef]
37. Oxford Grice, K.; Vogel, K.A.; Le, V.; Mitchell, A.; Muniz, S.; Vollmer, M.A. Adult norms for a commercially available Nine Hole Peg Test for finger dexterity. *Am. J. Occup. Ther.* **2003**, *57*, 570–573. [CrossRef] [PubMed]
38. Raciti, L.; Nicoletti, A.; Mostile, G.; Bonomo, R.; Contrafatto, D.; Dibilio, V.; Luca, A.; Sciacca, G.; Cicero, C.E.; Vasta, R.; et al. Validation of the UPDRS section IV for detection of motor fluctuations in Parkinson's disease. *Parkinsonism Relat. Disord.* **2016**, *27*, 98–101. [CrossRef]
39. Fugl-Meyer, A.R.; Jääskö, L.; Leyman, I.; Olsson, S.; Steglind, S. The post-stroke hemiplegic patient. 1. a method for evaluation of physical performance. *Scand. J. Rehabil. Med.* **1975**, *7*, 13–31. [PubMed]
40. Opara, J.; Małecki, A.; Małecka, E.; Socha, T. Motor assessment in Parkinson's disease. *Ann. Agric. Environ. Med.* **2017**, *24*, 411–415. [CrossRef]
41. Lee, K.S.; Lee, W.H.; Hwang, S. Modified constraint-induced movement therapy improves fine and gross motor performance of the upper limb in Parkinson disease. *Am. J. Phys. Med. Rehabil.* **2011**, *90*, 380–386. [CrossRef]
42. Keith, R.A.; Granger, C.V.; Hamilton, B.B.; Sherwin, F.S. The functional independence measure: A new tool for rehabilitation. *Adv. Clin. Rehabil.* **1987**, *1*, 6–18.
43. Childs, J.D.; Piva, S.R.; Fritz, J.M. Responsiveness of the numeric pain rating scale in patients with low back pain. *Spine* **2005**, *30*, 1331–1334. [CrossRef]
44. Demeurisse, G.; Demol, O.; Robaye, E. Motor evaluation in vascular hemiplegia. *Eur. Neurol.* **1980**, *19*, 382–389. [CrossRef] [PubMed]
45. Calabrò, R.S.; Naro, A.; Russo, M.; Leo, A.; Luca, R.D.; Balletta, T.; Buda, A.; Rosa, G.L.; Bramanti, A.; Bramanti, P. The role of virtual reality in improving motor performance as revealed by EEG: A randomized clinical trial. *J. Neuroeng. Rehabil.* **2017**, *14*, 53. [CrossRef] [PubMed]
46. Raciti, L.; Pizzurro, R.; Occhipinti, F.; Manuli, A.; Corallo, F.; Calabrò, R.S. A multidisciplinary advanced approach in central pontine myelinolysis recovery: Considerations about a case report. *Disabil. Rehabil. Assist. Technol.* **2020**, 1–12. [CrossRef] [PubMed]
47. Maggio, M.G.; Torrisi, M.; Buda, A.; Luca, R.D.; Piazzitta, D.; Cannavò, A.; Leo, A.; Milardi, D.; Manuli, A.; Calabro, R.S. Effects of robotic neurorehabilitation through lokomat plus virtual reality on cognitive function in patients with traumatic brain injury: A retrospective case-control study. *Int. J. Neurosci.* **2020**, *130*, 117–123. [CrossRef]
48. Calabrò, R.S.; Russo, M.; Naro, A.; Milardi, D.; Balletta, T.; Leo, A.; Filoni, S.; Bramanti, P. Who May Benefit from Armeo Power Treatment? A Neurophysiological Approach to Predict Neurorehabilitation Outcomes. *PM R.* **2016**, *8*, 971–978. [CrossRef]
49. Bruni, M.F.; Melegari, C.; De Cola, M.C.; Bramanti, A.; Bramanti, P.; Calabrò, R.S. What does best evidence tell us about robotic gait rehabilitation in stroke patients: A systematic review and meta-analysis. *J. Clin. Neurosci.* **2018**, *48*, 11–17. [CrossRef]
50. Moon, S.; Huang, C.K.; Sadeghi, M.; Akinwuntan, A.E.; Devos, H. Proof-of-Concept of the Virtual Reality Comprehensive Balance Assessment and Training for Sensory Organization of Dynamic Postural Control. *Front. Bioeng. Biotechnol.* **2021**, *9*, 678006. [CrossRef]
51. Naro, A.; Pignolo, L.; Bruschetta, D.; Calabrò, R.S. What about the role of the cerebellum in music-associated functional recovery? A secondary EEG analysis of a randomized clinical trial in patients with Parkinson disease. *Parkinsonism Relat. Disord.* **2022**, *96*, 57–64. [CrossRef]
52. Straudi, S.; Benedetti, M.G.; Venturini, E.; Manca, M.; Foti, C.; Basaglia, N. Does robot-assisted gait training ameliorate gait abnormalities in multiple sclerosis? A pilot randomized-control trial. *NeuroRehabilitation* **2013**, *33*, 555–563. [CrossRef]
53. Masiero, S.; Armani, M.; Rosati, G. Upper-limb robot-assisted therapy in rehabilitation of acute stroke patients: Focused review and results of new randomized controlled trial. *J. Rehabil. Res. Dev.* **2011**, *48*, 355–366. [CrossRef]
54. Maggio, M.G.; Luca, R.D.; Manuli, A.; Buda, A.; Cuzzola, M.F.; Leonardi, S.; D'Aleo, G.; Bramanti, P.; Russo, M.; Calabrò, R.S. Do patients with multiple sclerosis benefit from semi-immersive virtual reality? A randomized clinical trial on cognitive and motor outcomes. *Appl. Neuropsychol. Adult* **2022**, *29*, 59–65. [CrossRef]
55. López-López, D.; Pérez-Ríos, M.; Ruano-Ravina, A.; Losa-Iglesias, M.E.; Becerro-de-Bengoa-Vallejo, R.; Romero-Morales, C.; Calvo-Lobo, C.; Navarro-Flores, E. Impact of quality of life related to foot problems: A case-control study. *Sci. Rep.* **2021**, *11*, 14515. [CrossRef]
56. Mazzoni, P.; Shabbott, B.; Cortés, J.C. Motor control abnormalities in Parkinson's disease. *Cold Spring Harb. Perspect. Med.* **2012**, *2*, a009282. [CrossRef]

57. Intention to treat analysis and per protocol analysis: Complementary information. *Prescrire Int.* **2012**, *21*, 304–306.
58. Tripepi, G.; Chesnaye, N.C.; Dekker, F.W.; Zoccali, C.; Jager, K.J. Intention to treat and per protocol analysis in clinical trials. *Nephrology* **2020**, *25*, 513–517. [CrossRef]
59. Taveggia, G.; Borboni, A.; Salvi, L.; Mule, C.; Fogliaresi, S.; Villafañe, J.H.; Casale, R. Efficacy of robot-assisted rehabilitation for the functional recovery of the upper limb in post-stroke patients: A randomized controlled study. *Eur. J. Phys. Rehabil. Med.* **2016**, *52*, 767–773.
60. Gijbels, D.; Lamers, I.; Kerkhofs, L.; Alders, G.; Knippenberg, E.; Feys, P. The Armeo Spring as training tool to improve upper limb functionality in multiple sclerosis: A pilot study. *J. Neuroeng. Rehabil.* **2011**, *8*, 5. [CrossRef]
61. Ishikuro, K.; Dougu, N.; Nukui, T.; Yamamoto, M.; Nakatsuji, Y.; Kuroda, S.; Matsushita, I.; Nishimaru, H.; Araujo, M.F.P.; Nishijo, H. Effects of Transcranial Direct Current Stimulation (tDCS) Over the Frontal Polar Area on Motor and Executive Functions in Parkinson's Disease; A Pilot Study. *Front. Aging Neurosci.* **2018**, *10*, 231. [CrossRef]

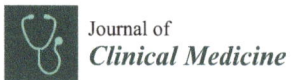

Review

Renal Rehabilitation: Present and Future Perspectives

Masahiro Kohzuki [1,2,3,4]

[1] President and Chairman, Department of Health Sciences, Yamagata Prefectural University of Health Sciences, Yamagata 990-2212, Japan; kohzuki@med.tohoku.ac.jp; Tel./Fax: +81-23-686-6601
[2] Professor Emeritus, Department of Health Sciences, Tohoku University Graduate School of Medicine, Sendai 980-8575, Japan
[3] Chairman of the Board of Directors, International Society of Renal Rehabilitation, Sendai 980-8575, Japan
[4] Former Chairman of the Board of Directors, Japanese Society of Renal Rehabilitation; Tokyo 150-0043, Japan

Abstract: Chronic kidney disease (CKD) is a global health problem. In patients with CKD, exercise endurance is decreased, especially as renal dysfunction advances. This is due to the combined effects of protein-energy wasting, uremic acidosis, and inflammatory cachexia, which lead to sarcopenia and are aggravated by a sedentary lifestyle, resulting in a progressive downward spiral of deconditioning. Renal rehabilitation (RR) is a coordinated, multifaceted intervention designed to optimize a patient's physical, psychological, and social functioning, as well as to stabilize, slow, or even reverse the progression of renal deterioration, improving exercise tolerance and preventing the onset and worsening of heart failure, thereby reducing morbidity and mortality. This review focused on the history and benefits of RR in patients with CKD. Based on current evidence, RR is an effective, feasible, and safe secondary prevention strategy in CKD. RR is a promising model for a new field of rehabilitation. Therefore, efforts to increase RR implementation rates are urgently needed.

Keywords: chronic kidney disease; exercise; rehabilitation; renal protection; cardio-renal syndrome; Japanese Society of Renal Rehabilitation; International Society of Renal Rehabilitation

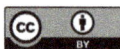

1. Introduction

Chronic kidney disease (CKD) is a global health problem. For example, the number of CKD patients in Japan is more than 11% of the total population. The number of patients undergoing hemodialysis (HD) in Japan is 349,700, corresponding to 1 in 359 of the total population in 2021 [1].

Further, CKD is associated with premature aging. Patients with CKD are characterized by frailty, osteoporosis, muscle wasting, cardiovascular hypertrophy, and vascular calcification [2]. Patients with CKD with dialysis have a very high mortality risk due to cardiovascular diseases such as chronic heart failure, and sedentary patients with CKD undergoing dialysis have an even higher mortality risk [3]. An independent, graded association has been found between a reduced glomerular filtration rate (GFR) and the risk of cardiovascular events, hospitalization, and death [4]. In addition to being a strong cardiovascular risk factor, physical inactivity is associated with an increased risk of rapid decline in renal function in patients with CKD [5].

In patients with CKD, exercise endurance is decreased, and this becomes more distinct as renal dysfunction advances. This is due to the combined effects of protein-energy wasting (PEW), uremic acidosis, and inflammatory cachexia, which lead to sarcopenia and are aggravated by a sedentary lifestyle. Collectively, these factors result in a progressive downward spiral of deconditioning [2].

Renal rehabilitation (RR) is a coordinated, multifaceted intervention designed to optimize a patient's physical, psychological, and social functioning, as well as to stabilize, slow, or even reverse the progression of renal deterioration, improving exercise tolerance and preventing the onset and worsening of heart failure, thereby reducing morbidity and mortality. [6,7]. This review focused on the history and benefits of RR in patients with CKD.

2. CKD and Physical Inactivity

Physical inactivity is a major health problem. Regular exercise is important for maintaining good health and preventing chronic diseases. Moreover, an association between physical inactivity and poor outcomes in patients with CKD has been well established [7–9]. Patients with CKD typically engage in lower levels of physical activity than the general population, which can induce a catabolic state, including reduced neuromuscular functioning, exercise tolerance, and cardiorespiratory fitness.

In addition to physical inactivity, cardiorespiratory (CR) fitness is an important consideration, as a strong predictor of mortality [10,11]. Low CR fitness has a particularly high risk of death compared to that for other common risk factors, such as dyslipidemia, hypertension, and diabetes. [12]. CR fitness is defined as the ability of the respiratory and circulatory systems to supply oxygen during physical activity, and is usually expressed as the maximal oxygen uptake (VO_2 max) or peak oxygen uptake (peak VO_2) during exercise testing [13]. VO_2 max is the maximum rate of oxygen consumption attainable during physical exertion. A similar measure is peak VO_2, which is the measurable value from a session of physical exercise. Be it incremental or otherwise, it could match or underestimate the actual VO_2 max. Figure 1 shows the five major determinants of VO_2 max, peak VO_2, and their relationships in CKD [14]. The gears in Figure 1 represent the functional interdependence of the physiological components of the system. Pulmonary diffusion capacity, cardiac output, oxygen-carrying capacity, renal function, and other peripheral limitations such as capillary density, muscle diffusion capacity, and mitochondrial enzymes are all examples of VO_2 determinants.

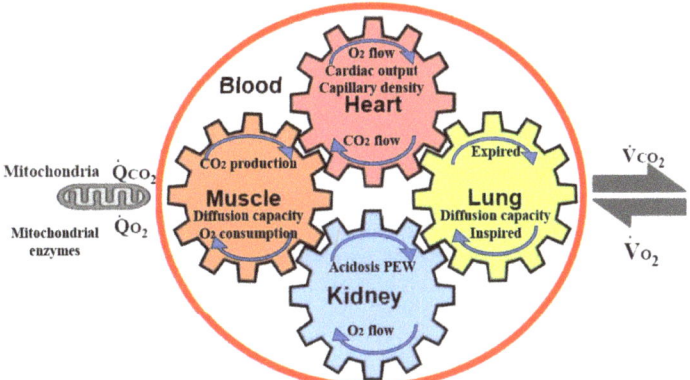

Figure 1. The five major determinants of VO_2 max, peak VO_2, and their relationships in CKD (based on [14]). The gears represent the functional interdependence of the physiological components of the system. Cardiac output, pulmonary diffusion capacity, oxygen-carrying capacity, renal function, metabolic acidosis, and other peripheral limitations, such as muscle diffusion capacity, mitochondrial enzymes, and capillary density, are all examples of VO_2 max determinants. VO_2, O_2 uptake; VCO_2, CO_2 output; QCO_2, CO_2 production; QO_2, O_2 consumption by cells.

An increase in O_2 utilization by the muscles (QO_2) is achieved by an increase in ventilation, an increase in pulmonary blood flow by recruitment and vasodilatation of pulmonary blood vessels, an increase in cardiac output (stroke volume and heart rate), dilatation of selected peripheral vessels, and increased extraction of O_2 from the blood perfusing the muscles. O_2 is taken up from the alveoli (VO_2) in proportion to the pulmonary blood flow and degree of O_2 desaturation of hemoglobin in the pulmonary capillary blood. Metabolic acidosis in CKD patients promotes protein-energy wasting (PEW) [15], muscle protein wasting, and reducing protein synthesis [16,17]. In addition to sarcopenia by physical inactivity, PEW, metabolic acidosis, angiotensin II accumulation, and myostatin overexpression in uremia also contribute to the pathogenesis of muscle wasting, especially in CKD [18]. Erythropoietin can increase VO_2 max in humans [19].

3. Chronic Effects of Exercise in CKD Animal Models

Evidence of the benefits of regular exercise in long-term conditions is accumulating. Further, the influence of chronic exercise on renal function must be considered, as acute exercise causes proteinuria, reduction in renal blood flow, and reduction in GFR. As it is shown clinically, sudden severe exercise decreases renal function [20,21]. However, such intense exercise cannot be performed for long. In other words, it is important to look at the effects of exercise over the long term. However, there is insufficient information regarding the influence of chronic exercise on renal function and the effect of exercise in pre-dialysis patients with CKD. For instance, the optimal duration and intensity of exercise for CKD patients with pre-dialysis has not yet been determined.

Since the late 1990s, my colleagues and I have published several papers in this field. We assessed the renal effects of moderate treadmill chronic exercise in several CKD rat models and found that exercise does not worsen renal function and had renoprotective effects in some rat models, such as a remnant kidney model of genetic hypertensive rats [22], 5/6-nephrectomized rats [23], diabetic nephropathy rats [24], and Zucker diabetic rats [25].

4. Chronic Effect of Exercise in Patients with CKD Undergoing Dialysis

In the Dialysis Outcomes and Practice Patterns Study, patients with CKD undergoing dialysis who were regular exercisers had higher health-related quality of life (HR-QOL), sleep quality scores, and physical functioning; the study also reported fewer limitations in physical activities than those who were not regular exercisers [8]. Regular exercise was also correlated with more positive patient effects and fewer depressive symptoms [8]. Further, in models extensively adjusted for demographics and comorbidities, the mortality risk was lower with regular exercise and at facilities with more regular exercisers [8].

Meta-analyses of randomized controlled trials (RCTs) have reported that regular exercise training in patients with CKD undergoing dialysis (HD) has benefits in physical function, aerobic capacity, dialysis adequacy, depressive symptoms, and HR-QOL [26–30]. Additionally, a meta-analysis of combined aerobic and resistance exercises (CARE) performed during HD by Liu et al. [31] found that CARE improved the peak oxygen uptake; performance on the six-minute walking test; 60-s and 30-s sit-to-stand tests; dialysis adequacy; scores on five (out of eight) domains and the physical component summary for HR-QOL on the Medical Outcomes Study Short Form-36; blood pressure; and hemoglobin levels in patients on maintenance HD compared to those with usual care. Further, subgroup analysis showed that intradialytic CARE resulted in the amelioration of more evaluated outcomes than non-intradialytic CARE, with the exception of handgrip strength and hemoglobin levels [31]. The authors concluded that CARE is an effective way to improve physical function, aerobic capacity, HR-QOL, and dialysis adequacy in patients on maintenance HD [31].

5. Chronic Effect of Exercise in Pre-Dialysis Patients with CKD

In the first RCT on the effect of exercise in CKD patients with pre-dialysis, reported by Baria et al. [32], sedentary pre-dialysis men with CKD (creatine-based estimated GFR) were randomly assigned to home-based exercise group, a center-based exercise group, or control group. In the exercise group, aerobic exercise was done three times per week for 12 weeks. During the study period, eGFRcreat was increased by 3.6 ± 4.6 mL/min ($p = 0.03$) in the center-based group, but remained unchanged in the control group [32]. Further, in a single-blind randomized controlled study of the effects of moderate-intensity regular exercise on renal function and indices of cardiovascular risk in patients with stages 3–4 CKD by Greenwood et al., there was a significant difference in the rate of change in eGFRcreat between exercise and usual care groups, with the exercise group showing a slower decline in function [33].

Chen et al. reported the associations between walking, mortality, and renal replacement therapies (RRTs), such as peritoneal dialysis, HD, and kidney transplantation, in patients with stages 3–5 CKD [34]. Among 6363 patients (mean age, 70 years), 1341 (21.1%) reported walking as their most common form of exercise. The rate of mortality was lower in walking patients than in non-walking patients (2.7 vs. 5.4 per 100 person-years). Similarly, the incidence of RRT was significantly lower in walking patients than in non-walking patients (22 vs. 32.9 per 100 person-years) [34]. Further, walking was associated with lower mortality and RRT risk on multivariate regression. The adjusted sub-distribution hazard ratio (SHR) of walking was 0.67 ($p < 0.001$) for overall mortality and 0.79 ($p < 0.001$) for the risk of RRT. Further, the SHRs of overall mortality were 0.83, 0.72, 0.42, and 0.41. Thus, walking is the most popular form of exercise for patients with CKD and is associated with a lower risk of mortality and RRT. [34].

Recently, Ma et al. reported a meta-analysis of 12 RCTs, comprising 410 patients with CKD; the results indicated that regular aerobic exercise significantly improves the estimated GFR (eGFR), and the levels of serum creatinine, daily urinary protein excretion, and serum urea nitrogen in CKD patients. Further, a single exercise session of more than 30 min was associated with significantly improved eGFR ($p < 0.01$), including walking and running, but not cycling, as exercise modalities were associated with significantly improved serum creatinine levels ($p < 0.05$) in CKD patients (Figures 2 and 3) [35]. Thus, regular aerobic exercise has beneficial effects on the eGFR (especially with durations longer than 30 min), serum creatinine (especially with walking or running as the modality), daily urinary protein excretion, and blood urea nitrogen levels in CKD patients [35].

Study	Exercise Mean	SD	Total	Control Mean	SD	Total	Weight	Std. Mean Difference IV, Random, 95% CI
Leehey et al., 2009	39.00	22.00	7	41.00	5.30	4	5.5%	-0.10 [-1.33; 1.13]
Leehey et al., 2009	45.00	31.00	7	36.00	14.00	4	5.4%	0.31 [-0.93; 1.55]
Straznicky et al., 2010	109.80	1.00	13	106.90	1.20	13	6.6%	2.54 [1.47; 3.62]
Toyama et al., 2010	55.20	16.90	10	44.60	8.20	9	7.7%	0.75 [-0.19; 1.69]
Shi et al., 2014	51.00	6.50	11	43.00	7.80	10	7.8%	1.07 [0.15; 2.00]
Liang et al., 2016	69.65	11.23	29	60.68	11.22	29	12.2%	0.79 [0.25; 1.32]
Liang et al., 2018	66.80	6.40	20	61.00	6.30	20	10.7%	0.90 [0.24; 1.55]
Miele et al., 2017	52.40	19.10	25	50.10	16.20	21	11.7%	0.13 [-0.45; 0.71]
Craenenbroeck et al., 2015	38.60	14.20	19	39.20	15.20	21	11.1%	-0.04 [-0.66; 0.58]
Rahmy et al., 2016	31.47	10.62	30	24.57	11.39	20	11.7%	0.62 [0.04; 1.20]
Aoike et al., 2014	31.90	13.70	14	23.90	12.20	15	9.6%	0.60 [-0.15; 1.35]
Total (95% CI)			**185**			**166**	**100.0%**	**0.65 [0.30; 1.00]**

Heterogeneity: Tau^2 = 0.1859; Chi^2 = 23.02, df = 10 (P = 0.01); I^2 = 57%
Test for overall effect: Z = 3.65 (P < 0.01)

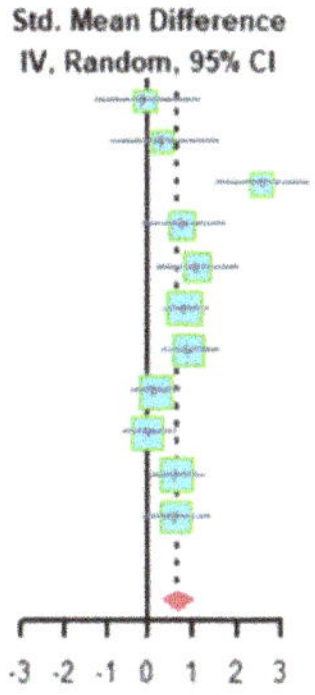

Figure 2. Meta-analysis of the effect of aerobic exercise on eGFR (adapted from [35]). The results indicate that regular aerobic exercise significantly improves the eGFR. eGFR, estimated glomerular filtration rate; CI, confidence interval; SD, standard deviation.

Study	Exercise Mean	SD	Total	Control Mean	SD	Total	Weight	Std. Mean Difference IV, Fixed, 95% CI
Leehey et al., 2009	821.00	1010.00	7	490.00	237.00	4	5.5%	0.36 [-0.88; 1.60]
Leehey et al., 2009	891.00	831.00	7	383.00	256.00	4	5.2%	0.67 [-0.61; 1.95]
Straznicky et al., 2010	15.00	5.00	4	16.00	8.00	8	5.9%	-0.13 [-1.33; 1.07]
Liang et al., 2016	4.30	1.72	29	5.58	1.64	29	29.9%	-0.75 [-1.29; -0.22]
Zhou et al., 2017	4.19	2.39	35	5.35	3.07	35	37.9%	-0.42 [-0.89; 0.06]
Aoike et al., 2014	4.12	0.34	14	4.27	0.31	15	15.6%	-0.45 [-1.19; 0.29]
Total (95% CI)			**96**			**95**	**100.0%**	**-0.41 [-0.70; -0.11]**

Heterogeneity: Tau^2 = 0.0307; Chi^2 = 6.02, df = 5 (P = 0.30); I^2 = 17%
Test for overall effect: Z = -2.72 (P < 0.01)

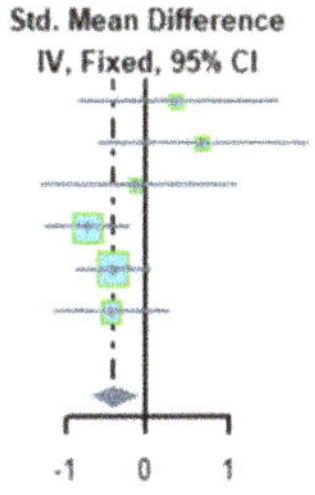

Figure 3. Meta-analysis of the effect of aerobic exercise on 24-h urinary protein excretion (adapted from [35]). The results indicate that regular aerobic exercise significantly improves the 24-h urine protein volume in patients with chronic kidney disease. CI, confidence interval; SD, standard deviation.

6. Chronic Effect of Exercise in Pre-Dialysis CKD Patients with Acute Myocardial Infarction (AMI)

CKD is common in patients with diabetes mellitus, occurring in approximately 40% of cases. Diabetes mellitus is also an important risk factor for cardiovascular diseases; however, CKD is an important mediator of this risk [36]. Kidney function is closely linked to heart function. Renal dysfunction/disease may initiate, accentuate, or precipitate cardiac dysfunction/disease, and vice versa [37].

Combined, renal dysfunction worsens the prognosis after AMI. My colleagues and I investigated the association between physical activity levels and renal function changes in AMI patients [38]. Renal function was measured using the cystatin C-based eGFR (eGFRcys), which is independent of muscle mass. Patients were stratified into a low exercise group (2335 ± 1219 steps/day) and a high exercise group (7102 ± 2365 steps/day). eGFRcys was significantly increased after 3 months of exercise in the high exercise group, whereas no significant change was observed in the low exercise group. Further, the change in eGFRcys was greater in the high exercise group (+6.7 mL/min/1.73 m^2) than in the low exercise group (−2.9 mL/min/1.73 m^2) [38]. The physical activity level was positively associated with renal function changes, demonstrating that high physical activity levels may suppress renal function decline in AMI patients. Figure 4 indicates the association between the number of steps and eGFRcys or eGFRcreat [38]. Pearson's correlation analysis revealed significant correlations between the number of daily steps and both eGFR parameters. Furthermore, the coefficient was greater for the correlation between ΔeGFRcys and the number of daily steps ($r = 0.55$, $p < 0.001$) than between ΔeGFRcreat and the number of daily steps ($r = 0.38$, $p = 0.015$). As previously indicated, changes in serum creatinine levels can be caused by changes in skeletal muscles through exercise, highlighting the importance of using eGFRcys as an indicator of renal function [39,40]. A recent prospective study verified the association between physical activity levels and renal function in patients with CKD [39]. The results were similar to those in the above-mentioned study and indicated that maintaining a high level of physical activity in daily life leads to the suppression of renal function deterioration [41]. However, our study was the first to show an association between physical activity level and changes in renal function after the onset of AMI using an accelerometer and eGFRcys. Our findings support the importance of interventions to maintain a high physical activity level as a strategy for renal protection in patients with AMI. Future research should verify the long-term effects of physical activity on renal function in patients with AMI.

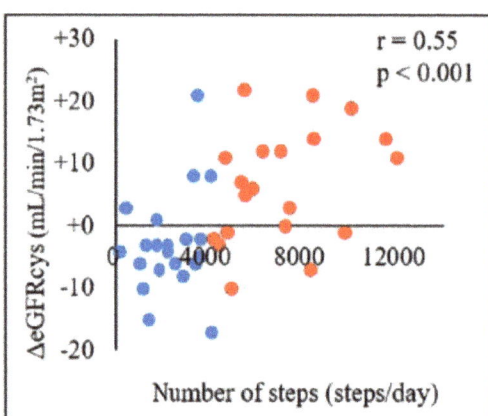 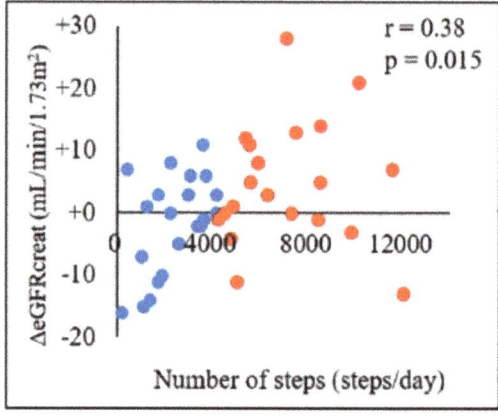

Figure 4. Association between the number of steps and ΔeGFRcys or ΔeGFRcreat (adapted from [38]). The association between the number of steps and eGFRcys or eGFRcreat in all patients is shown [38].

Pearson's correlation analysis revealed significant correlations between the number of steps and both eGFR parameters, with a higher correlation between ΔeGFRcys and the number of steps than between ΔeGFRcreat and the number of steps. eGFRcreat, creatine-based estimated glomerular filtration rate; eGFRcys, cystatin C-based estimated glomerular filtration rate.

There is immense potential for research in the field of cardio-nephrology, in terms of diagnosis, prognosis, complication risk evaluation, and the utilization of novel therapeutic approaches for CKD patients and associated cardiovascular complications. However, significant advancements have been made to improve patient care and outcomes in patients with CKD [42].

7. Mechanisms of Renal Protection by Chronic Exercise

Increasing evidence indicates that chronic exercise has beneficial effects on chronic inflammation, muscle and bone strength, CR fitness, and metabolic markers in patients with CKD or kidney transplants [43]. However, the mechanisms underlying these benefits have received little attention, and the available clinical evidence is mainly from small, short-duration (<12 weeks) exercise studies [43]. Bishop et al. summarized that the available data, suggest exercise results in shifts towards a less inflammatory immune cell profile, reduced monocyte infiltration into the adipose tissue, and enhanced activity of the NRF2 pathway, may underlie improvements in inflammatory biomarkers [43]. Exercise-mediated increases in nitric oxide release and bioavailability, left ventricular remodeling, myocardial fibrosis, and reductions in angiotensin II accumulation in the heart may contribute to improvements in left ventricular hypertrophy. Although exercise stimulates an anabolic response in skeletal muscles in CKD, satellite cell activation and increases in mitochondrial mass seem to be impaired in this population. Exercise-mediated activation of the canonical "Wnt" pathway may lead to bone formation and improvements in the levels of the bone-derived hormones, Klotho, and fibroblast growth factor 23 (FGF23) [43].

The musculoskeletal and cardiopulmonary systems are the predominant organ systems typically considered in exercise studies. The importance of renal physiology in physical activity and exercise can be easily overlooked. However, over the past 30 years, research has revealed the relevance of renal function in regulating physiological responses to exercise, providing insights on how exercise can alter the pathophysiology of kidney diseases [44]. In support of this, the editors of the American Journal of Physiology-Renal Physiology have encouraged submissions to the Call for Papers on "Exercise and the Kidney in Health and Disease" [44].

8. Barriers to Exercise Participation among Patients with CKD

Unfortunately, the role of physical activity in CKD has been largely overlooked, and the provision of rehabilitation and exercise for CKD patients lags behind that for cardiac and pulmonary services. The Kidney Disease Outcomes Quality Initiative (K/DOQI) clinical practice guidelines comment that all dialysis patients should be counseled and regularly encouraged by nephrology and dialysis staff to increase their physical activity [45].

Delgado et al. reported the survey on exercise counseling to nephrologists [46]. On multivariate analysis, older nephrologists (odds ratio 3.3) and more physically active nephrologists (odds ratio: 5.5) were more likely to counsel CKD patients about exercise [46]. Responses related to less counseling behavior included a lack of confidence in the ability to discuss physical activity.

Delgado and colleagues also reported that patients with CKD undergoing dialysis were interested in exercise [47]. However, 92% of participants reported at least one barrier to physical activity. The most commonly reported barriers were shortness of breath and fatigue on non-dialysis and dialysis days. On multivariate analysis, a greater number of barriers was associated with a lower level of physical activity. Additionally, a lack of motivation was associated with a lower physical activity level. Endorsement of too many medical problems and insufficient time on dialysis days were also associated with lower physical activity levels in an adjusted analysis [47].

The location of exercise is also an important factor that influences adherence. In CKD patients with dialysis, exercise during dialysis programs have been found to achieve higher adherence rates than home exercise or supervised programs on non-dialysis days [48].

9. Present Status of RR

9.1. Societies and Meetings

Several international working groups have been established to address the physical inactivity contributes to the burden of disease in CKD patients [49–52]. The Japanese Society of Renal Rehabilitation (JSRR) was established in 2011 to promote and disseminate RR in Japan. I was the first president of the board of directors from 2011–2020. The number of members in the JSRR has increased annually; as of 1 April 2023, the number of individual members was 3005, and the number of facilities or supporting members was 170. Annual scientific meetings of the JSRR are held, and approximately 300 papers are presented every year. The number of participants in seminars for RR professionals is expected increase to over 8000 in 2023.

In the JSRR, we consider RR to include five major components: exercise training, diet and fluid management, medication and medical surveillance, education, and psychological and vocational counseling [6,7]. The JSRR uses a comprehensive approach to RR, including physical exercise and psychological, vocational, and dietary counselling. The JSRR has a newsletter, an official English journal (Renal Replacement Therapy), and an official Japanese journal (The Japanese Journal of Renal Rehabilitation).

In March 2018, in order to improve the quality of RR and educate RR professionals in Japan, the JSRR established a certification program for a Registered Instructor of RR (RIRR). The minimum requirements for candidates of the RIRR certification examination are as follows: (1) possess a certification or degree for any of the following positions: physician, nurse, physical therapist, occupational therapist, medical engineer, clinical psychologist, clinical laboratory technician, and exercise trainer; (2) be a member of the JSRR for more than 2 years; (3) have a minimum of 1 year of experience in a RR program or equivalent; and (4) submit 10 case reports on rehabilitation for patients with CKD. To date, 738 members have undergone this examination. Those who qualify for RIRR can provide exercise therapy and RR to dialysis patients and claim medical fees for exercise therapy during dialysis. Therefore, obtaining the RIRR would give the instructor an advantage in finding employment at dialysis facilities and rehabilitation facilities.

In November 2019, the Global Renal Exercise Network (GREX) held a meeting in Canada which was attended by international clinicians and researchers, including myself. Taking a global perspective, the meeting highlighted Japanese, Canadian, and other regional examples of policies developed regarding exercise and rehabilitation [53]. In the meeting, it was noticed that Japan leads the field of RR in four ways: Japan has a national society (JSRR), certification for RR (RIRR), guidelines for RR, and a National Health Insurance Reimbursement program for RR.

I was invited to give a lecture on "Rehabilitation for Visceral Impairment (Renal rehabilitation)" at the ISPRM2020 meeting in Orlando, Florida; viewing this lecture was mandatory for a specialist renewal from the Association of Academic Physiatrist Rehabilitation from 1 July 2020 to 1 July 2023.

Finally, as there was no international society for RR, the International Society of Renal Rehabilitation (ISRR) was established in 2020 to promote and disseminate RR. An annual scientific meeting of the ISRR is held every March.

9.2. Guidelines of RR

The American College of Sports Medicine and KDIGO have published guidelines for exercise testing and prescription, as well as for specific methods and cautions regarding exercise therapy for patients with CKD [54,55].

I first edited and published a book titled "Renal Rehabilitation" [6]. In order to clarify the programs and effectiveness of RR, the Renal Rehabilitation Guideline Preparation Committee was launched in 2016 under JSRR, which created a guideline in accordance with the "Minds Handbook for Clinical Practice Guideline Development 2014" [54,55]. Six recommendations were created for various kidney disorders, with groups addressing CKD, nephritis, nephrosis, dialysis, and kidney transplantation [56,57]. All the recommendation grades were determined through a consensus conference. The exercise prescriptions for individuals with kidney disease which are recommended by JSRR are shown [55,56]. In brief, the exercise prescription consists of three exercises: an aerobic exercise, a resistance exercise, and a flexibility exercise. The frequency (F), intensity (I), time (T), and type (T) of each exercise is as follows.

In aerobic training, F (3–5 d·wk^{-1}), I (moderate intensity (40–59% VO$_2$R (oxygen uptake reserve), RPE 12–13 on a scale of 6–20), T (20–60 min of continuous activity; however, if this cannot be tolerated, use 3–5 min bouts of intermittent exercise, aiming to accumulate 20–60 min·d^{-1}), T (prolonged, rhythmic activities using large muscle groups (e.g., walking, cycling, swimming)) [55,56].

In the resistance exercise, F (2–3 d·wk^{-1}), I (65–75% 1-RM (one repetition maximum). The performance of 1-RM is not recommended; estimate 1-RM from a ≥3-RM test), T (a minimum of one set of 10–15 repetitions, with a goal in most patients to achieve multiple sets. Choose 8–10 different exercises targeting the major muscle groups) and T (machines, free weights, or bands) [55,56].

In the flexibility exercise, F (2–3 d·wk^{-1}), I (static: stretch to the point of tightness or slight discomfort; PNF (proprioceptive neuromuscular facilitation): 20–75% of the maximum voluntary contraction), T (60 s per joint for static (10–30 s hold per stretch); 3–6 s contraction followed by 10–30 s assisted stretch for PNF), and T (static or PNF) [55,56].

9.3. National Health Insurance Reimbursement

Infrastructure and reimbursement systems for cardiac rehabilitation exist in many countries. In contrast, heath care systems in most countries have no or limited coverage of for exercise training for CKD patients. Therefore, CKD patients are often unable to overcome barriers to exercise and are unable to find appropriate exercise facilities [58].

To our knowledge, Japan is the only country in the world with a national health insurance system for RR [59,60]. In April 2016, Japan's Ministry of Health, Labor and Welfare decided to expand the scope of rehabilitation to diabetic patients with CKD stages 4 to 5 through the world's first national health insurance reimbursement system. Each hospital or clinic can receive one additional medical fee per month for each CKD patients with RR. Eligible conditions include: 50% or more of patients suppressing the increase in serum creatinine or serum cystatin, a 20% or more decrease in daily urine protein excretion, or a 30% reduction in the slope of 1/creatinine or 1/cystatin. The content of the exercise should be in accordance with JSRR guidelines [55,56], and it is desirable to have RIRR qualifications. Nature Review in Nephrology introduced Japan's national health insurance system for JSRR and RR [59].

Additionally, from April 2018, exercise training for diabetic patients with CKD stage 3b is covered by the National Health Insurance. Furthermore, from April 2022, exercise training for CKD patients with HD is covered by the National Health Insurance. Under this system, if a patient receives exercise therapy instructions for 20 min or more during dialysis, a medical fee is allowed for up to 90 days from the start of the fee. The conditions are that the instructor has an RIRR (valid forever), or if the instructor is without an RIRR, they must attend a JSRR seminar and pass the examination (valid for 3 years). A qualified physician, physical therapist, or an occupational therapist can supervise 15 inpatients and 20 outpatients at a time, and a qualified nurse can supervise 5 inpatients and 8 outpatients at a time.

10. Future perspectives of RR: Adding Life to Years and Years to Life

Evidence regarding the effectiveness of components other than exercise therapy in renal rehabilitation, such as education, is still emerging. However, in order to encourage inactive CKD patients to exercise, education about the effects of exercise is a prerequisite. In addition, the importance of dietary therapy that increases the effectiveness of exercise therapy, the importance of dietary therapy that does not cause sarcopenia or frailty, and how to continue exercise are very important when performing RR. JSRR's annual scientific meeting features many presentations on these topics. In the future, it is expected that more effective educational methods, more effective dietary therapy menus, and more effective exercise therapy menus will be established regarding RR. The next RR guideline by JSRR will include a comprehensive list of factors beyond exercise therapy.

As a super-aged society has emerged, the number of individuals with multiple morbidities and disabilities who require rehabilitation has increased more rapidly than expected [60]. Medical science basically aims to add years to life by increasing life expectancy. Rehabilitation generally aims to add life to years by helping patients with impairment achieve and use their full physical, mental, and social potential. However, accumulating evidence suggests that rehabilitation for patients with visceral impairments, such as renal, cardiac, and pulmonary impairments, can not only improve exercise performance and HR-QOL, but can also increase survival (Figure 5) [61]. Therefore, modern comprehensive rehabilitation for patients with CKD does not simply aim to add life to years, but to add life to years and years to life, which is a new rehabilitation concept [61].

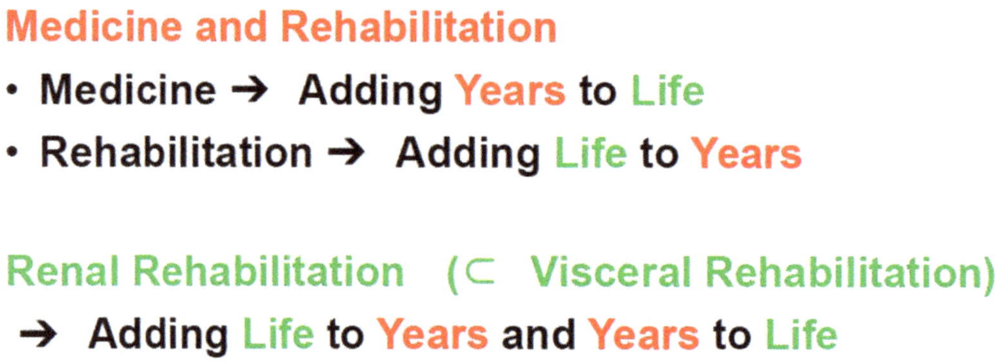

Medicine and Rehabilitation
- Medicine → Adding Years to Life
- Rehabilitation → Adding Life to Years

Renal Rehabilitation (⊂ Visceral Rehabilitation)
→ Adding Life to Years and Years to Life

Figure 5. Renal rehabilitation is a new target in rehabilitation (based on [61]). Medical science basically aims to add years to life by increasing life expectancy. Rehabilitation generally aims to add life to years by helping patients with impairment to achieve and use their full physical, mental, and social potential. However, accumulating evidence suggests that rehabilitation in patients with visceral impairments, such as renal, cardiac, and pulmonary impairments, can not only improve exercise performance and HR-QOL, but can also increase survival (adding life to years and years to life).

11. Conclusions

RR is a coordinated, multifaceted intervention designed to optimize a patient's physical, psychological, and social functioning in addition to stabilizing, slowing, or even reversing the progression of renal deterioration, improving exercise tolerance and preventing the onset and worsening of heart failure, thereby reducing morbidity and mortality. RR is an effective, feasible, and safe secondary prevention strategy in CKD and is a promising model for a new field of rehabilitation.

Future large RCTs should focus more on the effects of rehabilitation and exercise programs, as these topics and exercise types have not been studied as extensively as cardiovascular and pulmonary rehabilitation. Moreover, efforts to increase RR implementation rates are urgently needed.

Funding: This research received no external funding.

Institutional Review Board Statement: Not applicable.

Informed Consent Statement: Not applicable.

Data Availability Statement: Not applicable.

Acknowledgments: I have been conducting basic research, clinical research, and academic activities related to renal rehabilitation, but I was not able to do this alone. I would like to take this opportunity to thank the many seniors, colleagues, graduate students, and colleagues who have been involved with me thus far.

Conflicts of Interest: The author declares no conflicts of interest.

References

1. The Japanese Society for Dialysis Therapy. Available online: https://docs.jsdt.or.jp/overview/index.html (accessed on 23 November 2023). (In Japanese)
2. Kooman, J.P.; Kotanko, P.; Schols, A.M.W.J.; Shiels, P.G.; Stenvinkel, P. Chronic kidney disease and premature ageing. *Nat. Rev. Nephrol.* **2014**, *10*, 732–742. [CrossRef] [PubMed]
3. O'Hare, A.M.; Tawney, K.; Bacchetti, P.; Johansen, K.L. Decreased survival among sedentary patients undergoing dialysis: Results from the dialysis morbidity and mortality study wave 2. *Am. J. Kidney Dis.* **2003**, *41*, 447–454. [CrossRef] [PubMed]
4. Go, A.S.; Chertow, G.M.; Fan, D.; McCulloch, C.E.; Hsu, C.-y. Chronic Kidney Disease and the Risks of Death, Cardiovascular Events, and Hospitalization. *N. Engl. J. Med.* **2004**, *351*, 1296–1305. [CrossRef]
5. Johansen, K.L. Exercise in the End-Stage Renal Disease Population. *J. Am. Soc. Nephrol.* **2007**, *18*, 1845–1854. [CrossRef] [PubMed]
6. Kohzuki, M. Renal rehabilitation: Definition and evidence. In *Renal Rehabilitation*; Kohzuki, M., Ed.; Ishiyaku Publishers, Inc.: Tokyo, Japan, 2012; pp. 10–17. (In Japanese)
7. Kohzuki, M. Renal rehabilitation: Present and future perspectives. In *Hemodialysis*; Suzuki, H., Ed.; Intech: Oakville, ON, Canada, 2013; pp. 743–751.
8. Tentori, F.; Elder, S.J.; Thumma, J.; Pisoni, R.L.; Bommer, J.; Fissell, R.B.; Fukuhara, S.; Jadoul, M.; Keen, M.L.; Saran, R.; et al. Physical exercise among participants in the Dialysis Outcomes and Practice Patterns Study (DOPPS): Correlates and associated outcomes. *Nephrol. Dial. Transplant.* **2010**, *25*, 3050–3062. [CrossRef]
9. Smart, N.; Steele, M. Exercise training in haemodialysis patients: A systematic review and meta-analysis. *Nephrology* **2011**, *16*, 626–632.
10. Sieverdes, J.C.; Sui, X.; Lee, D.C.; Church, T.S.; McClain, A.; Hand, G.A.; Blair, S.N. Physical activity, cardiorespiratory fitness and the incidence of type 2 diabetes in a prospec-tive study of men. *Br. J. Sports Med.* **2010**, *44*, 238–244. [CrossRef]
11. Blair, S.N.; Kohl, H.W., III; Paffenbarger, R.S., Jr.; Clark, D.G.; Cooper, K.H. Physical fitness and all-cause mortality: A prospective study of healthy men and women. *JAMA* **1989**, *262*, 2395–2401.
12. Blair, S.N.; Sallis, R.E.; Hutber, A.; Archer, E. Exercise therapy—The public health message. *Scand. J. Med. Sci. Sports* **2012**, *22*, e24–e28. [CrossRef]
13. Caspersen, C.J.; Powell, K.E.; Christenson, G.M. Physical activity, exercise, and physical fitness: Definitions and distinctions for health-related research. *Public Health Rep.* **1985**, *100*, 126–131.
14. Kohzuki, M. New Ideas on Limitations to VO2max: Five Major Determinants for VO2max. *Pulm. Res. Respir. Med. Open J.* **2018**, *5*, e1–e2. [CrossRef]
15. Caso, G.; Garlick, P.J. Control of muscle protein kinetics by acid-base balance. *Curr. Opin. Clin. Nutr. Metab. Care* **2005**, *8*, 73–76. [CrossRef] [PubMed]
16. Bailey, J.L.; Wang, X.; England, B.K.; Price, S.R.; Ding, X.; Mitch, W.E. The acidosis of chronic renal failure activates muscle proteolysis in rats by augmenting transcription of genes encoding proteins of the ATP-dependent ubiquitin-proteasome pathway. *J. Clin. Investig.* **1996**, *97*, 1447–1453. [CrossRef]
17. Mitch, W.E. Influence of metabolic acidosis on nutrition. *Am. J. Kidney Dis.* **1997**, *29*, XLVI–XLVIII. [CrossRef] [PubMed]
18. Fahal, I.H. Uraemic sarcopenia: Aetiology and implications. *Nephrol. Dial. Transplant.* **2014**, *29*, 1655–1665. [CrossRef]
19. Kolb, E.M.; Kelly, S.A.; Middleton, K.M.; Sermsakdi, L.S.; Chappell, M.A.; Garland, T., Jr. Erythropoietin elevates VO_2, max but not voluntary wheel running in mice. *J. Exp. Biol.* **2010**, *213*, 510–519. [CrossRef]
20. Bach, T.M.; Clement, D.B. Exercise induced acute renal failure in an athlete. *Can. Fam. Physician* **1980**, *26*, 591–595.
21. Jackson, C.R. Exercise-induced renal failure and muscle damage. *Proc. R. Soc. Med.* **1970**, *63*, 566–570.
22. Kohzuki, M.; Kamimoto, M.; Wu, X.M.; Xu, H.L.; Kawamura, T.; Mori, N.; Nagasaka, M.; Kurosawa, H.; Minami, N.; Kanazawa, M.; et al. Renal protective effects of chronic exercise and antihypertensive therapy in hyper-tensive rats with chronic renal failure. *J. Hypertens.* **2001**, *19*, 1877–1882. [CrossRef]
23. Kanazawa, M.; Kawamura, T.; Li, L.; Sasaki, Y.; Matsumoto, K.; Kataoka, O.; Ito, O.; Minami, N.; Sato, T.; Ootaka, T.; et al. Combination of Exercise and Enalapril Enhances Renoprotective and Peripheral Effects in Rats With Renal Ablation. *Am. J. Hypertens.* **2006**, *19*, 80–86. [CrossRef]

24. Tufescu, A.; Kanazawa, M.; Ishida, A.; Lu, H.; Sasaki, Y.; Ootaka, T.; Sato, T.; Kohzuki, M. Combination of exercise and losartan enhances renoprotective and peripheral effects in spontaneously type 2 diabetes mellitus rats with nephropathy. *J. Hypertens.* **2008**, *26*, 312–321. [CrossRef] [PubMed]
25. Ito, D.; Cao, P.; Kakihana, T.; Sato, E.; Suda, C.; Muroya, Y.; Ogawa, Y.; Hu, G.; Ishii, T.; Ito, O.; et al. Chronic Running Exercise Alleviates Early Progression of Nephropathy with Upregulation of Nitric Oxide Synthases and Suppression of Glycation in Zucker Diabetic Rats. *PLoS ONE* **2015**, *10*, e0138037. [CrossRef] [PubMed]
26. Bogataj, S.; Pajek, M.; Pajek, J.; Ponikvar, J.B.; Paravlic, A.H. Exercise-based interventions in hemodialysis patients: A systematic review with a me-ta-analysis of randomized controlled trials. *J. Clin. Med.* **2019**, *9*, 43. [PubMed]
27. Hu, H.; Liu, X.; Chau, P.H.; Choi, E.P.H. Effects of intradialytic exercise on health-related quality of life in patients undergoing mainte-nance haemodialysis: A systematic review and meta-analysis. *Qual. Life Res.* **2022**, *31*, 1915–1932. [CrossRef]
28. Scapini, K.B.; Bohlke, M.; Moraes, O.A.; Rodrigues, C.G.; Inácio, H.F.; Sbruzzi, G.; Leguisamo, C.P.; Sanches, I.C.; Filho, H.T.; Irigoyen, M.C. Combined training is the most effective training modality to improve aerobic capaci-ty and blood pressure control in people requiring haemodialysis for endstage renal disease: Systematic review and network meta-analysis. *J. Physiother.* **2019**, *65*, 4–15. [CrossRef]
29. Sheng, K.; Zhang, P.; Chen, L.; Wu, C.; Chen, J. Intradialytic exercise in hemodialysis patients: A systematic review and meta-analysis. *Am. J. Nephrol.* **2014**, *40*, 478–490. [CrossRef]
30. Song, Y.-Y.; Hu, R.-J.; Diao, Y.-S.; Chen, L.; Jiang, X.-L. Effects of Exercise Training on Restless Legs Syndrome, Depression, Sleep Quality, and Fatigue Among Hemodialysis Patients: A Systematic Review and Meta-analysis. *J. Pain Symptom Manag.* **2018**, *55*, 1184–1195. [CrossRef]
31. Liu, Y.; Luo, X.; Deng, S.; Chen, J.; Zhang, L.; Huang, Y.; Hu, H. Combined aerobic and resistance exercise in maintenance hemodialysis patients: A meta-analysis. *Semin. Dial.* **2023**, *36*, 278–293. [CrossRef]
32. Baria, F.; Kamimura, M.A.; Aoike, D.T.; Ammirati, A.; Rocha, M.L.; de Mello, M.T.; Cuppari, L. Randomized controlled trial to evaluate the impact of aerobic exercise on visceral fat in overweight chronic kidney disease patients. *Nephrol. Dial. Transplant.* **2014**, *29*, 857–864. [CrossRef]
33. Greenwood, S.A.; Koufaki, P.; Mercer, T.H.; MacLaughlin, H.; Rush, R.; Lindup, H.; O'Connor, E.M.; Jones, C.; Hendry, B.; Macdougall, I.; et al. Effect of exercise training on estimated GFR, vascular health, and cardiorespira-tory fitness in patients with CKD: A pilot randomized controlled trial. *Am. J. Kidney Dis.* **2015**, *65*, 425–434. [CrossRef]
34. Chen, I.-R.; Wang, S.-M.; Liang, C.-C.; Kuo, H.-L.; Chang, C.-T.; Liu, J.-H.; Lin, H.-H.; Wang, I.-K.; Yang, Y.-F.; Chou, C.-Y.; et al. Association of Walking with Survival and RRT Among Patients with CKD Stages 3–5. *Clin. J. Am. Soc. Nephrol.* **2014**, *9*, 1183–1189. [CrossRef] [PubMed]
35. Ma, Q.; Gao, Y.; Lu, J.; Liu, X.; Wang, R.; Shi, Y.; Liu, J.; Su, H. The effect of regular aerobic exercise on renal function in patients with CKD: A systematic review and meta-analysis. *Front. Physiol.* **2022**, *13*, 901164. [CrossRef]
36. Swamy, S.; Noor, S.M.; Mathew, R.O. Cardiovascular Disease in Diabetes and Chronic Kidney Disease. *J. Clin. Med.* **2023**, *12*, 6984. [CrossRef] [PubMed]
37. Xanthopoulos, A.; Papamichail, A.; Briasoulis, A.; Loritis, K.; Bourazana, A.; Magouliotis, D.E.; Sarafidis, P.; Stefanidis, I.; Skoularigis, J.; Triposkiadis, F. Heart Failure in Patients with Chronic Kidney Disease. *J. Clin. Med.* **2023**, *12*, 6105. [CrossRef] [PubMed]
38. Sato, T.; Kohzuki, M.; Ono, M.; Muto, M.; Osugi, T.; Kawamura, K.; Naganuma, W.; Sato, M.; Shishito, N. Association between physical activity and change in renal function in patients after acute myocardial infarction. *PLoS ONE* **2019**, *14*, e0212100. [CrossRef]
39. Séronie-Vivien, S.; Delanaye, P.; Piéroni, L.; Mariat, C.; Froissart, M.; Cristol, J.-P. Cystatin C: Current position and future prospects. *Clin. Chem. Lab. Med.* **2008**, *46*, 1664–1686. [CrossRef] [PubMed]
40. Poortmans, J.R.; Gulbis, B.; De Bruyn, E.; Baudry, S.; Carpentier, A. Limitations of serum values to estimate glomerular filtration rate during exercise. *Br. J. Sports Med.* **2012**, *47*, 1166–1170.
41. Robinson-Cohen, C.; Littman, A.J.; Duncan, G.E.; Weiss, N.S.; Sachs, M.C.; Ruzinski, J.; Kundzins, J.; Rock, D.; de Boer, I.H.; Ikizler, T.A.; et al. Physical Activity and Change in Estimated GFR among Persons with CKD. *J. Am. Soc. Nephrol.* **2014**, *25*, 399–406. [CrossRef]
42. Burlacu, A.; Covic, A. Special Issue: "Cardiovascular Complications in Renal Diseases". *J. Clin. Med.* **2023**, *12*, 5307.
43. Bishop, N.C.; Burton, J.O.; Graham-Brown, M.P.M.; Stensel, D.J.; Viana, J.L.; Watson, E.L. Exercise and chronic kidney disease: Potential mechanisms underlying the physiological benefits. *Nat. Rev. Nephrol.* **2023**, *19*, 244–256. [CrossRef]
44. Kirkman, D.L.; Sequeira-Lopez, M.L.S. Call for Papers: Exercise and the kidneys in health and disease. *Am. J. Physiol. Ren. Physiol.* **2023**, *324*, F461–F463.
45. K/DOQI Workshop. K/DOQI clinical practice guidelines dor cardiovascular disease in dialysis patients. *Am J Kidney Dis.* **2005**, *45*, S16–S153. [CrossRef]
46. Delgado, C.; Johansen, K.L. Deficient Counseling on Physical Activity among Nephrologists. *Nephron Clin. Pract.* **2010**, *116*, c330–c336. [CrossRef] [PubMed]
47. Delgado, C.; Johansen, K.L. Barriers to exercise participation among dialysis patients. *Nephrol. Dial. Transplant.* **2012**, *27*, 1152–1157. [CrossRef] [PubMed]

48. Konstantinidou, E.; Koukouvou, G.; Kouidi, E.; Deligiannis, A.; Tourkantonis, A. Exercise training in patients with end-stage renal disease on hemodialysis: Comparison of three rehabilitation programs. *J. Rehabil. Med.* **2002**, *34*, 40–45. [CrossRef] [PubMed]
49. Wilund, K.R.; Painter, P. Formation of an Exercise in CKD Working Group. *Am. J. Kidney Dis.* **2016**, *67*, 812. [CrossRef] [PubMed]
50. Krause, R.; WGRR-European Working Group on Renal Rehabilitation and Exercise Physiology (affiliated to the ERA-EDTA); KfH-Kuratorium für Dialyse und Nieren transplantation e.V.; Nephrological Centre Berlin-Moabit. Nephrologists' view on exercise training in chronic kidney disease (results of the questionnaire at the WCN 2003). *Clin. Nephrol.* **2004**, *61*, S2–S4.
51. Schrag, W.F.; Campbell, M.; Ewert, J.; Hartley, S.; Niemann, J.; Ross, D. Multidisciplinary Team Renal Rehabilitation: Interventions and Outcomes. *Adv. Ren. Replace. Ther.* **1999**, *6*, 282–288. [CrossRef]
52. Japanese Society of Renal Rehabilitation. Available online: https://jsrr.smoosy.atlas.jp/ja/ (accessed on 23 November 2023). (In Japanese).
53. Bennett, P.N.; Kohzuki, M.; Bohm, C.; Roshanravan, B.; Bakker, S.J.; Viana, J.L.; MacRae, J.M.; Wilkinson, T.J.; Wilund, K.R.; Van Craenenbroeck, A.H.; et al. Global Policy Barriers and Enablers to Exercise and Physical Activity in Kidney Care. *J. Ren. Nutr.* **2022**, *32*, 441–449. [CrossRef]
54. Kidney Disease: Improving Global Outcomes (KDIGO) Blood Pressure Work Group. KDIGO clinical practice guideline for the management of blood pressure in chronic kidney disease. *Kidney Int.* **2012**, *2*, 337–414.
55. American College of Sports Medicine. *ACSM's Guidelines for Exercise Testing and Prescription*, 11th ed.; Liguori, G., Feito, Y., Fountaine, C., Roy, B.A., Eds.; Wolters Kluwer: Philadelphia, PA, USA, 2022; pp. 336–341.
56. Japanese Society of Renal Rehabilitation. *Guideline for Renal Rehabilitation*; Nankodo, Inc.: Tokyo, Japan, 2018; pp. 1–87. (In Japanese)
57. Yamagata, K.; Hoshino, J.; Sugiyama, H.; Hanafusa, N.; Shibagaki, Y.; Komatsu, Y.; Konta, T.; Fujii, N.; Kanda, E.; Sofue, T.; et al. Clinical practice guideline for renal rehabilitation: Systematic reviews and recommendations of exercise therapies in patients with kidney diseases. *Ren. Replace. Ther.* **2019**, *5*, 4. [CrossRef]
58. Williams, A.D.; Fassett, R.G.; Coombes, J.S. Exercise in CKD: Why is it important and how should it be delivered? *Am J Kidney Dis.* **2014**, *64*, 329–331. [CrossRef] [PubMed]
59. Zelle, D.M.; Klaassen, G.; van Adrichem, E.; Bakker, S.J.; Corpeleijn, E.; Navis, G. Physical inactivity: A risk factor and target for intervention in renal care. *Nat. Rev. Nephrol.* **2017**, *13*, 152–168. [CrossRef] [PubMed]
60. Kohzuki, M. Paradigm shift in rehabilitation medicine in the era of multimorbidity and multiple disabilities (MMD). *Phys. Med. Rehabil. Int.* **2014**, *1*, 4.
61. Kohzuki, M.; Sakata, Y.; Kawamura, T. A paradigm shift in rehabilitation medicine: From "adding life to years" to "adding life to years and years to life". *Asian J. Hum. Serv.* **2012**, *2*, 1–8.

Disclaimer/Publisher's Note: The statements, opinions and data contained in all publications are solely those of the individual author(s) and contributor(s) and not of MDPI and/or the editor(s). MDPI and/or the editor(s) disclaim responsibility for any injury to people or property resulting from any ideas, methods, instructions or products referred to in the content.

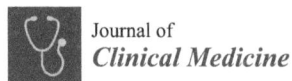

Review

The Effects of Physiotherapy in the Treatment of Cubital Tunnel Syndrome: A Systematic Review

Tomasz Wolny [1,*], César Fernández-de-las Peñas [2], Tomasz Buczek [3], Magdalena Domin [1], Arkadiusz Granek [4] and Paweł Linek [1]

[1] Institute of Physiotherapy and Health Sciences, Musculoskeletal Elastography and Ultrasonography Laboratory, The Jerzy Kukuczka Academy of Physical Education, Mikołowska 72A, 40-065 Katowice, Poland; magdalena.rutka@wp.pl (M.D.); p.linek@awf.katowice.pl (P.L.)
[2] Department of Physical Therapy, Occupational Therapy, Rehabilitation and Physical Medicine, Universidad Rey Juan Carlos, 28922 Madrid, Spain; cesar.fernandez@urjc.es
[3] Physiotherapy Clinic, "FizjoMedical", 44-251 Rybnik, Poland; tomaszbuczek91@gmail.com
[4] Hospital of the Ministry of Interior and Administration, 25-316 Kielce, Poland; arkadiusz.granek@gmail.com
* Correspondence: t.wolny@twreha.com

Abstract: Background: To date, various forms of physiotherapy are used in the treatment of cubital tunnel syndrome (CuTS). The effectiveness of physiotherapy for CuTS is inconclusive. The aim of this systematic review was to evaluate the effects of physiotherapy in the conservative treatment of CuTS. Methods: The six databases were searched from December 2020 to March 2022. The inclusion criteria were randomised controlled trials, case series, and case reports that evaluate the effects of physiotherapy in the treatment of adult participants with diagnosis CuTS. A total of 11 studies met the eligibility criteria, capturing a total of 187 participants. Results: In three types of papers, pain, muscle strength, and limitation of upper limb function were the most frequently assessed characteristics. Physiotherapy was most often based on manual therapy, neurodynamic techniques, and electrical modalities. One clinical trial rated the risk of bias "high" and the other two "some concerns". In case-series designs, five studies rated the risk of bias as "serious" and three as "moderate". Most of the studies showed a significant improvement in the clinical condition, also in the follow-up study. Only one clinical trial showed no therapeutic effect. Conclusion: There is no possibility of recommending the best method of physiotherapy in clinical practice for people with CuTS based on the results of this systematic review. More high-quality studies are required.

Keywords: cubital tunnel syndrome; ulnar neuropathy; physiotherapy modalities; treatment outcomes; review

1. Introduction

Cubital tunnel syndrome (CuTS) is a compressive neuropathy of the ulnar nerve. It is the second most prevalent peripheral neuropathy of the upper extremity after carpal tunnel syndrome [1,2]. The mean annual incidence of CuTS is estimated at 24.7 cases per 100,000 people [3], and its prevalence is 2–6% in the general population [4]. In the early stages of CuTS, sensory symptoms such as paraesthesia and slight hypoesthesia are reported, occurring mostly paroxysmally and related to the position of the elbow. Over time, these symptoms worsen. This is followed by motor disturbances, mostly weakness and atrophy of the intrinsic muscles of the hand [1,5]. The stages of this neuropathy can be divided into three degrees of severity: mild, moderate, and severe [6]. The progressive course of CuTS over time leads to the impairment of hand function, which adversely affects the activities of daily living, and professional life, and deteriorates the overall health-related quality of life. With the significant prevalence of CuTS, this neuropathy is a major medical, economic, and social problem.

CuTS is referred to as compression neuropathy that occurs around the cubital tunnel. The most common sites of potential compression of the ulnar nerve are the arcade of Struthers, the medial intermuscular septum, the medial epicondyle, the cubital tunnel, and the deep flexor–pronator aponeurosis [7]. This neuropathy is usually divided into primary (idiopathic) and secondary (symptomatic) [8]. In idiopathic forms of CuTS, no morphological abnormalities can be found in the tissues surrounding the ulnar nerve [8]. Furthermore, there are several causes of secondary forms of CuTS (anatomical changes after trauma, degenerative changes, systemic diseases such as rheumatoid arthritis, lipomas, ganglion cysts, inflammatory processes, etc.) [8–10]. Other risk factors for CuTS are related to upper extremity motor activity, overhead activity, heavy physical work, obesity, and nicotinism [11]. Therefore, it can be concluded that CuTS is just a synonym for ulnar nerve neuropathy occurring in the elbow area. The difficulty in finding the aetiology of CuTS also affects the choice of the most appropriate treatment modality for this neuropathy.

The treatment of CuTS is divided into surgical and conservative [12]. Palmer and Hughes [10] showed various surgical techniques for ulnar nerve decompression and emphasised that no "gold standard" for surgical treatment has been developed to date. In situ decompression, intramuscular transposition, subcutaneous transposition, submuscular transposition, medial epicondylectomy, and endoscopic techniques are most commonly used [10]. However, surgical treatment is only recommended when muscle strength is weakened, and conservative methods do not bring the expected therapeutic effect [13]. Hence, conservative treatment is used as first-line therapy, usually in the early and mild-to-moderate stages of CuTS [5]. Conservative treatment includes modification of activities of daily living with the avoidance of prolonged elbow joint flexion [10], nonsteroidal anti-inflammatory drugs, steroid injections, and physical therapy approaches [14]. To the best of our knowledge, there is also no standardised procedure for CuTS conservative treatment with well-documented effectiveness. It seems that physiotherapy is one of the most important forms of conservative treatment, which has been proven to be effective in other peripheral neuropathies [15–19]. To date, various forms of physiotherapy have been used in the treatment of CuTS [20–23]. However, the effectiveness of physiotherapy intervention as a conservative treatment of CuTS is inconclusive. Therefore, it was decided to conduct, for the first time, a systematic review of papers evaluating the effectiveness of physiotherapy treatment for CuTS. Such an analysis determines the quality of the research conducted to date and provides directions for future research.

2. Methods

This systematic review adheres to the Preferred Reporting Items for Systematic Reviews and Meta-Analyses (PRISMA) statement [24]. The protocol was registered in the International Prospective Register of Systematic Reviews (PROSPERO) database, registration number CRD 42020219297.

2.1. Data Sources and Searchers

The literature review was conducted between December 2020 and March 2022. Six electronic databases (MEDLINE via PubMed, Cochrane, Embase, Web of Science, Scopus, and PEDro) were searched to identify relevant papers. The search strategy was developed during a panel meeting after an initial article search. It was based on the use of key phrases and/or their abbreviations based on a metadata system (MeSH) and various combinations of these phrases to increase search efficiency. An extensive list of terms to describe the target population based on the PICO acronym was formulated:

P (population)—cubital tunnel syndrome;
I (intervention)—physiotherapy treatment;
C (comparator)—control group, placebo group, and sham therapy;
O (outcomes)—nerve conduction study, discrimination and threshold sensation, functional assessment, and ultrasound imaging measurements (Supplementary Material S1).

All papers were accepted regardless of the year of publication. However, the search was limited to papers available in English. Titles and abstracts of scientific papers retrieved from the databases were analysed for inclusion criteria. The papers that did not show relevance to the subject area studied were excluded. The lists of references in the publications included in the review were also analysed to make sure that other papers that may meet the inclusion criteria were not missed. The resulting papers were combined using the EndNote x9 software (version 19.2.0.13018, Philadelphia, PA, USA).

2.2. Study Selection

The review of the retrieved papers was conducted in two stages. The first step was to review the titles and abstracts of papers identified as potentially relevant to the research questions. In the next step, the full texts of the papers identified during the initial selection were reviewed. In both stages, the review was performed by two independent reviewers (T.W., T.B.), and by a third independent reviewer (P.L.) in contentious cases. The inclusion criteria were all experimental studies such as randomised controlled trials (RTCs) and case reports that evaluate the effects of physiotherapy in the treatment of adult participants (>16 years old) with diagnosis CuTS. Participants not diagnosed as CuTS or exposed to any form of surgical procedure and/or with other neuropathies of the upper limb were excluded from the study. The characteristics of the RTC and CS types of studies were presented separately.

2.3. Data Extraction

Two reviewers independently extracted and documented data from each included study using Excel (Microsoft, Redmond, WA, USA) according to the Centre for Reviews and Dissemination recommendations [25]. We extracted data including the year of publication, study design, sample size, gender, age, target population, description of interventions, outcome measures, and study results. The main study outcomes expressed as means and SDs were also extracted.

2.4. Methodological Quality Assessment

The methodological quality of randomised clinical trials was assessed using the revised Cochrane risk-of-bias tool for randomised trials (RoB 2) [26]. According to the Cochrane guidelines, this tool evaluates possible errors as follows: "low risk", "some concern", or "high risk". Due to the fact that the remaining works that qualified for the review were case studies, their quality was assessed in two stages. In the first stage, the article quality was assessed using The Critical Appraisal Checklist for Case Reports developed by Moola et al. [27]. If five of the eight evaluation criteria are met, the quality is assessed as satisfactory (such a study was included). In the second stage, the quality was assessed using the Risk of Bias in Non-randomised Studies of Interventions (ROBINS-I) assessment tool [28]. This tool evaluates possible errors as follows: "low risk of bias", "moderate risk of bias", "serious risk of bias", "critical risk of bias", or "no information". In both cases, the evaluation was conducted by two independent reviewers (T.W. and T.B.). The Cohen κ statistic was applied to determine the agreement between assessors.

2.5. Data Synthesis and Analysis

The extracted data from all included studies were tabulated, including the study authors and sample characteristics, the measurements of the outcome variables, and key results. All the identified studies were included in a qualitative synthesis and are presented in the tables. Initially, it was intended to synthesise the data quantitatively by conducting a meta-analysis. However, because of high heterogeneity in terms of study design, population examined, and various interventions, we could not perform a meta-analysis.

3. Results

3.1. Study Selection

An initial search of the databases together with a manual search and analysis of the references identified 1719 papers. This number was reduced to 995 after deleting duplicates. Based on exclusion and qualification criteria, 16 papers met the eligibility criteria (Figure 1). Of these papers, five were excluded after further analysis because they neither concerned CuTS patients nor addressed physiotherapy management. One paper discussed ulnar tunnel syndrome, another described the case of a patient who developed CuTS due to venous thrombosis, while another dealt with the ultrasonographic diagnosis of CuTS. One paper focused on the surgical treatment of CuTS caused by anconeus epitrochlearis, and one evaluated the effectiveness of electrostimulation after traumatic ulnar nerve injury. Finally, 11 articles were included in the final review comprising 3 RCT-type studies [13,29,30] (Table 1) and 8 case-series-type studies [20–23,31–34] (Table 2).

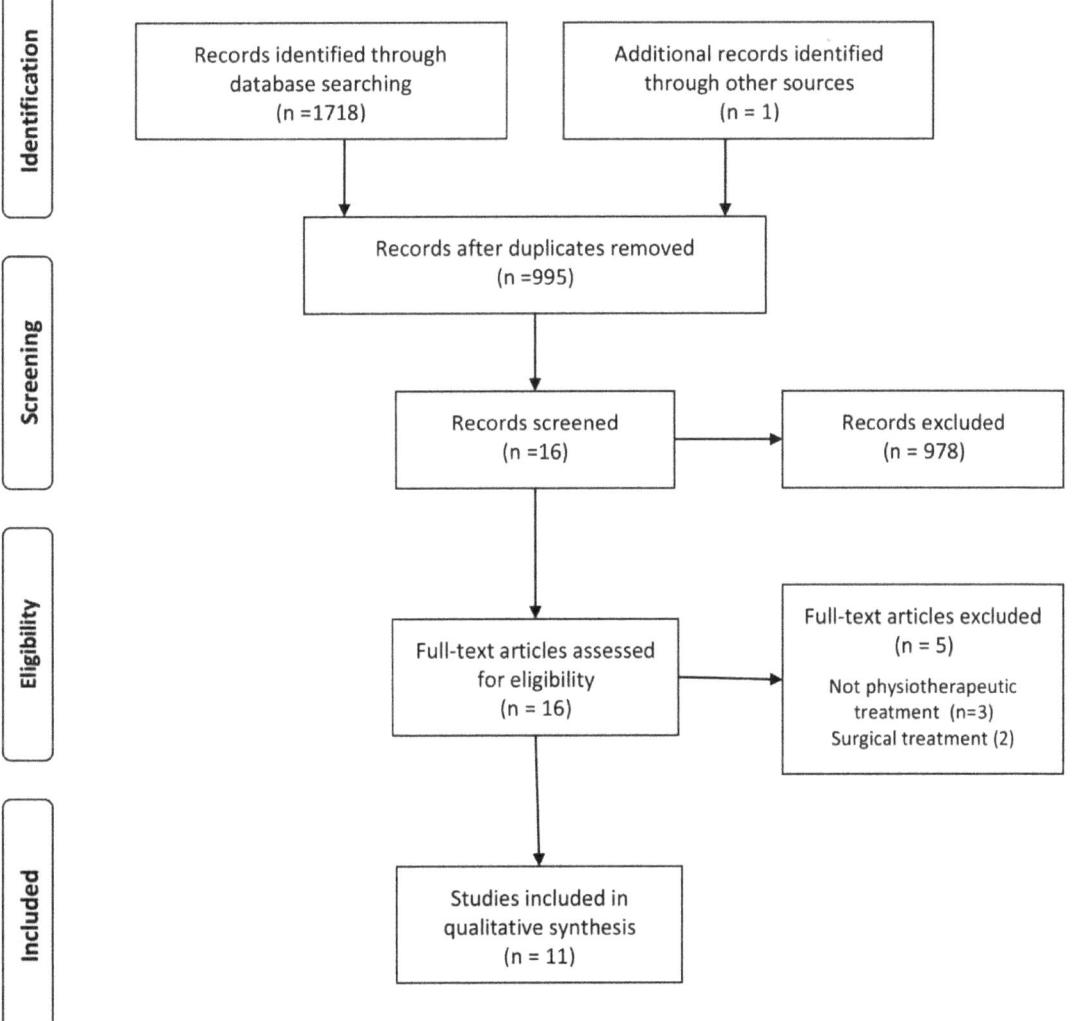

Figure 1. Flowchart.

Table 1. Characteristics of included randomised clinical trials (RTCs).

Study	Participants	Outcome Measures	Control/Comparison	Intervention	Results
Svernlov et al. [13]	n = 70; Sex: 39 female; 31 male; Age: 17–72	Measurement at baseline and 6-month follow-up; Activities scale (COPM); Grip strength (JAMAR dynamometer); Pain (VAS); Neurophysiological examination (NCS, electromyography).	Three groups	Group A—elbow orthosis (3-month treatment); Group B—nerve gliding exercises (3-month treatment); Group C—information (exercise modification).	There was a significant improvement in each group after the applied therapy. There were no between-group differences.
Badur et al. [29]	n = 61; Sex: 32 female; 29 male; Age: 16–79	Measurement at baseline, after treatment, and 1- and 3-month follow-up; Pain (VAS); Upper-extremity disability and symptoms (DASH); Overall health (SF-36 questionnaire); Grip strength (dynamometer).	Two groups	Group 1—continuous shortwave diathermy (10 treatments); Group 2—placebo shortwave diathermy (10 treatments).	There were no changes in the assessed parameters in both groups after the applied therapy.
Ozkan et al. [30]	n = 32; Sex: 16 female; 16 male; Age: mean = 43.5	Measurement at baseline, after treatment, and 1- and 3-month follow-up; Pain (VAS); Grip strength (dynamometer); Sensory threshold (Semmes–Weinstein monofilament test; Neurophysiological examination (NCS); patient satisfaction scale.	Two groups	Group 1—low-level laser therapy (10 treatments); Group 2—ultrasound therapy (10 treatments).	There was a significant improvement in both groups after the applied therapy. There were no between-group.

COPM—Canadian Occupational Performance Measure; VAS—visual analogue scale; NCS—nerve conduction study; DASH—Disabilities of the Arm, Shoulder, and Hand Outcome Measure.

Table 2. Characteristics of included case studies design.

Study	Participants	Outcome Measures	Control/Comparison	Intervention	Results
Kearns and Wang [20]	n = 1; Sex: female; Age: 45	Measured at baseline and 4 weeks post-treatment; Tissue tension (STTT); range of motion (goniometer); symptom provocation (ULTT, elbow flexion test); structural dysfunction (PAM); pain (NPRS).	No	Thrust manipulation (humeroulnar joint 2 treatments, radiocarpal joint 1 treatment).	After 3 treatment sessions, pain and paraesthesia were resolved; all other tests were negative.
Oskay et al. [21]	n = 7; Sex: not specified; Age range: 35–70	Measured at baseline, after treatment, and 12-month follow-up; Symptom provocation (elbow flexion test); palmar gripping and grasping (pinchmeter and grip dynamometer); pain (VAS); loss of sensation (Semmes–Weinstein monofilaments); upper-extremity disability and symptoms (DASH).	No	Cold application; pulsed ultrasound (10 treatments); nerve mobilisation techniques (10 treatments); strengthening exercises; postural adaptations; education; ergonomic modifications.	Pain, Tinel's sign, and Disability of Arm, Shoulder, and Hand Index scores were decreased; grip and pinch strength increased during the observation period.
Shen et al. [22]	n = 7; Sex: not specified; Age: 35–71	Measured at baseline and 4-, 8-, and 12-week follow-up; Severity of paraesthesia/dysaesthesia (VAS); upper-extremity disability and symptoms (DASH).	No	Extracorporeal shock wave therapy (3 treatments).	The VAS and Quick DASH scores demonstrated improvements at all follow-up time points in all treated elbows.
Anandkumar and Manivasagam [23]	n = 3; Sex: 2 male; 1 female; Age: 35,45,50	Measured at baseline, beginning of each treatment session, and at 6-month follow-up; Pain (NPRS); function limitation (PSFS); pain-free grip strength (JAMAR dynamometer); self-reported outcome measure (GROC).	No	Dry needling (4 treatments, twice a week).	All patients achieved complete pain reduction and full recovery of function; the strength of the pain-free grip also improved; all self-reported significant improvement after therapy; the effect lasted 6 months after the therapy.
Illes and Johnson [31]	n = 1; Sex: female; Age: 41	Measured at baseline and after treatment; Severity of numbness (VAS); Symptom provocation (EAST, Tinel sign); Grip strength (Blood pressure cuff).	No	Chiropractic manipulative therapy; myofascial therapy (11 treatments); elastic therapeutic taping (no number specified); home exercises (8 treatments).	After 11 treatment sessions, symptoms resolved completely.

Table 2. Cont.

Study	Participants	Outcome Measures	Control/Comparison	Intervention	Results
Coppieters et al. [32]	$n = 1$ Sex: female Age: 17	Measured at baseline, beginning of each treatment session, and at 6- and 10-month follow-up; Pain (VAS); range of motion (goniometer); clinical tests (neural provocation test, elbow flexion test, Tinel's sign); functional status (NPQ).	No	Neurodynamic mobilisation (5 treatments); Elbow mobilisation (4 treatments); home exercises—active ulnar nerve-sliding (5 treatments); high-velocity distraction/rotation thrust (3 treatments); education (1 instruction).	After the applied therapy, in each of the tests used, the symptoms were eliminated; The effect lasted 10 months after the therapy.
Kwak et al. [33]	$n = 2$ Sex: male Age: 39 and 40	Measured at baseline, after treatment, and at 1, 2, 3, and 6 months post-treatment; Pain (NPRS); NCS; elbow imaging (MRI).	No	PRF (1 treatment).	After 1 treatment session, the pain was completely relieved. At the 1-, 2-, 3-, and 6-month follow-up assessments after the procedure, the previously reported pain had not recurred.
Fernández-de-Las-Peñas al. [34]	$n = 1$ Sex: male Age: 48	Measured at baseline and at 1, 3, 6, and 12 months post-treatment; Upper-extremity disability and symptoms (DASH); neuropathic pain (S-LANSS); self-reported outcome measure (GROC).	No	PENS of the ulnar nerve (3 treatments); self-neural glides as a home program (2–3 weeks).	After three treatment sessions, there was an elimination of pain and symptoms and an improvement in functional status; the effect lasted 12 months after the therapy.

NPRS—Numeric Pain Rating Scale; PSFS—Patient Specific Functional Scale; GROC—global rating of change; VAS—visual analogue scale; NPQ—Northwick-Park Questionnaire; DASH—Disabilities of the Arm, Shoulder, and Hand Outcome Measure; S-LANSS—Leeds Assessment of Neuropathic Symptoms and Signs; PENS—ultrasound-guided percutaneous electrical stimulation; STTT—selective tissue tension test; ULTT—upper-limb tension test; PAM—passive accessory movement; PRF—pulsed radiofrequency; NCS—nerve conduction study; MRI—magnetic resonance imaging.

3.2. Randomised Controlled Trials

3.2.1. Participants

In all RCTs, the subjects were clinically/neurophysiologically diagnosed with CuTS (two studies clinically and neurophysiologically; one study only clinically). A total of 163 subjects aged 16–79 years old were examined and underwent therapy. The RCT involved 87 women and 76 men [13,29,30].

3.2.2. Outcome Measures

All studies evaluated pain (3/3 papers) and muscle strength (3/3 papers) [13,29,30]. Two papers evaluated upper extremity function and nerve conduction [13,30]. In addition, one study assessed sensory threshold [30] and overall health quality [29].

3.2.3. Interventions

Each study used a different therapeutic procedure: orthosis (experimental intervention), neurodynamic techniques (experimental intervention), ergonomic physical activity instruction (control group) [13], continuous shortwave diathermy (experimental intervention) and placebo (control group) [29], and low-level laser therapy (experimental intervention) and ultrasound (experimental intervention) [30].

3.2.4. Risk of Bias

Based on the reviewers' assessment using the ROB 2 tool to evaluate the risk of bias, the overall bias was considered to be "high" in one study [13], while "some concerns" were indicated in the remaining two RCTs [29,30] (Table 3). The most common flaws were the high risk of bias in domain 4 (risk of bias in measurement of the outcome) in one RTC [13] and domain 2 (risk of bias due to deviations from the intended interventions) in all RTC studies [13,29,30].

Table 3. Risk of Bias in randomised clinical trials (RTCs).

Study	Domain 1 Risk of Bias Arising from the Randomisation Process	Domain 2 Risk of Bias Due to Deviations from the Intended Interventions	Domain 3 Missing Outcome Data	Domain 4 Risk of Bias in Measurement of the Outcome	Domain 5 Risk of Bias in Selection of the Reported Result	Overall Risk of Bias
Svernlov et al. [13]	Low	Some concerns	Low	High	Low	High
Badur et al. [29]	Low	Some concerns	Low	Low	Low	Some concerns
Ozkan et al. [30]	Low	Some concerns	Low	Low	Low	Some concerns

3.2.5. Synthesis of the Results

Two RCTs reported significant improvements in the clinical condition of the subjects (pain reduction, improved function, increase in muscle strength, improvement in the sensory threshold, and improvement in nerve conduction), which occurred not only after the therapy but also persisted at 1, 3, and 6 months of follow-up [13,30]. In one study, there were no changes in pain muscle strength, function, and overall health evaluated after therapy in comparison with the control group [29].

3.3. Case Studies

In all case series [21,22] and case reports [20,23,31–34], subjects were clinically and neurophysiologically diagnosed with CuTS (four studies clinically and neurophysiologically; four studies only clinically). In eight case studies, 24 subjects ranging in age from 17 to 71 years were examined and treated. The gender of the subjects was determined in six of the eight papers [20,23,31–34]. Studies by Oskay et al. and Shen et al. [21,22] failed to specify gender. In total, 48 women and 5 men participated in the study, and in 14 cases, the gender was not specified.

3.3.1. Outcome Measures

The most frequently evaluated symptom was pain (six of the eight papers) [20–23,33,34]. Symptom provocation tests (five of the eight papers) [20,21,31,32,34] and functional limitations of the upper extremity (five of the eight papers) were also frequently assessed [21–23,32,34]. Muscle strength was assessed in three of the eight papers [21,23,31]. Range of motion was assessed in two papers [20,32] as was the severity of paraesthesia [20,31]. In two of the eight papers, authors evaluated subjective improvements following therapy [23,33]. Furthermore, one study evaluated nerve conduction [33] and sensory threshold [21].

3.3.2. Interventions

Neurodynamic techniques (3/8 papers) [21,32,34] and chiropractic manipulation (two of the eight papers) [20,31] were the most frequently used in therapy. Other papers used dry needling [23], percutaneous electrical stimulation [34], pulsed radiofrequency [33], combined ultrasound and cold therapy [21], and extracorporeal shock wave therapy [22].

3.3.3. Therapeutic Effect

In all case studies, significant improvements in the clinical status of the subjects (reduction in pain and subjective symptoms, improved function, increase in grip and pinch strength, reduction in symptoms in provocation tests such as Tinel's sign or elbow flexion test) were reported, which occurred not only after therapy [20–23,31–33] but were also maintained in the 6-, 8-, 10- and 12-month follow-up periods [21–23,32–34].

3.3.4. Risk of Bias

The Critical Appraisal Checklist for Case Reports values ranged from 5 to 7 in all case studies, which was considered sufficient [20–23,31–34] (Table 4). In the second stage based on the reviewer's evaluation using the ROBINS-I tool for non-randomised studies of interventions to evaluate the risk of bias, the overall bias was serious in five of the eight papers [20,21,31,32,34] and moderate in three of them [22,23,33] (Table 5). The most common flaws were a serious risk of bias in "bias due to confounding" in five of the eight studies [20,21,31,32,34]; "bias in classification of interventions" in five out of the total eight papers [20,21,31,32,34]; "bias due to deviations from intended interventions" in five of the eight studies [20,21,32,34]; "bias in measurement of outcomes" in another combination of five studies out of the total eight [20,21,31,32,34], and the "overall bias" in five of the eight papers [20,21,31,32,34].

Table 4. Critical appraisal checklist for case studies design.

Critical Appraisal Checklist	Kearns and Wang [20]	Oskay et al. [21]	Shen et al. [22]	Anandkumar and Manivasagam [23]	Illes and Johnson [31]	Coppieters et al. [32]	Kwak et al. [33]	Fernández-de-Las-Peñas et al. [34]
1. Were the patient's demographic characteristics clearly described?	Yes	Unclear	Yes	Yes	Yes	Yes	Yes	Yes
2. Was the patient's history clearly described and presented as a timeline?	Yes	Yes	Yes	Yes	Yes	Yes	Yes	Yes
3. Was the current clinical condition of the patient on presentation clearly described?	Yes	Yes	Yes	Yes	Yes	Yes	Yes	Yes
4. Were diagnostic tests or assessment methods and the results clearly described?	Unclear	Yes	Yes	Unclear	Unclear	Unclear	Yes	Unclear
5. Was the intervention(s) or treatment procedure(s) clearly described?	Yes	Yes	Yes	Yes	Yes	Yes	Yes	Yes
6. Was the post-intervention clinical condition clearly described?	Yes	Yes	Yes	Yes	Yes	Yes	Yes	Yes
7. Were adverse events (harms) or unanticipated events identified and described?	No	Unclear	Unclear	Unclear	No	Unclear	Unclear	No
8. Does the case report provide takeaway lessons?	No	Yes	Yes	Yes	No	No	Yes	Unclear

Table 5. Risk of bias in case studies design.

Study	Bias Due to Confounding	Bias in Selection of Participants in the Study	Bias in Classification of Interventions	Bias Due to Deviations from Intended Interventions	Bias Due to Missing Data	Bias in Measurement of Outcomes	Bias in Selection of the Reported Result	Overall Bias
Kearns and Wang [20]	Serious	Moderate	Serious	Serious	Moderate	Serious	Moderate	Serious
Oskay et al. [21]	Serious	Moderate	Serious	Serious	Moderate	Serious	Moderate	Serious
Shen et al. [22]	Moderate	Low	Moderate	Moderate	Low	Moderate	Moderate	Moderate
Anandkumar and Manivasagam [23]	Moderate	Low	Moderate	Moderate	Low	Moderate	Moderate	Moderate
Illes and Johnson [31]	Serious	Moderate	Serious	Serious	Moderate	Serious	Moderate	Serious
Coppieters et al. [32]	Serious	Moderate	Serious	Serious	Moderate	Serious	Moderate	Serious
Kwak et al. [33]	Moderate	Low	Moderate	Moderate	Low	Moderate	Moderate	Moderate
Fernández-de-Las-Peñas et al. [34]	Serious	Moderate	Serious	Serious	Moderate	Serious	Moderate	Serious

4. Discussion

The aim of the present systematic review was to evaluate the effects of physiotherapy in the conservative treatment of CuTS. Based on the search strategy used, 11 papers were included in the review, consisting of 3 RCTs [13,29,30] 2 case series [21,22], and 6 case reports [20,23,31–34]. In two-thirds (66.6%) of the RCT included, the authors reported beneficial effects immediately after physiotherapy and in the long-term in pain, function, muscle strength, sensory thresholds, and nerve conduction [13,30]. One RCT reported no significant treatment effect on pain scores, muscle strength, function, and health status [29]. In all case studies, the authors emphasised the positive effects of different physiotherapy procedures concerning the reduction in pain symptoms, improved function, increased pinch-grip strength, and a reduction in symptoms in provocation tests (Tinel's sign, elbow flexion test), both immediately after treatment [20–23,31–33] and in the long-term follow-up [21–23,32–34].

Although 91% of the included papers reported beneficial effects of physiotherapy [13,20–23,31–34], the results obtained have to be viewed with caution. This is due to the fact that 73% of current publications were case studies [20–23,31–34] with small numbers of subjects (24 in total), very heterogeneous research methodology and physiotherapy programs, and a high risk of bias. Furthermore, 3 RCTs [13,29,30] examined 163 people, but even in this case, due to methodological differences, it is difficult to draw firm conclusions about the effectiveness of physiotherapy treatment in CuTS, particularly when one RCT did not observe any significant effect [29].

It should be pointed out that the method used for the diagnosis of CuTS was problematic in most of the papers included in the review. Although a nerve conduction study (NCS) was performed in 54% of papers [13,22,29,30,32,33], the result was negative in one paper, despite the symptoms that could indicate CuTS [32]. In the other papers, the diagnosis was based on clinical and orthopaedic examinations [20,21,23,31,34]. As NCS-based diagnosis of peripheral neuropathies is the gold standard [35] in some compression neuropathies (as is the case in CTS), it appears that it should also apply to other peripheral neuropathies. According to the accepted study protocol, it was decided to include the analysis papers in which patients were diagnosed as CuTS despite the absence of a nerve conduction study but only based on history and clinical and orthopaedic examinations. Therefore, the results of some studies and their findings must be viewed with caution. It seems that electrodiagnostic tests are necessary not only to make an accurate diagnosis of CuTS but also to assess the severity of the condition and objectively evaluate improvements after therapy [36]. Although some authors have demonstrated the high sensitivity and specificity of clinical tests in the diagnosis of CuTS [37,38], there is no agreement [39]. It is important to note that, regardless of the differences in the assessment of the various clinical tests, this will be a much more subjective assessment than it is in the case of NCS. Furthermore, NCS provides specific information such as conduction velocity in nerve fibres, latency, and amplitude, information that cannot be obtained from a functional test. However, it should also be noted that some authors indicated that symptoms often precede nerve conduction disturbances [40,41], especially in the early stages of peripheral neuropathy. In these cases, for obvious reasons, the diagnosis must be based only on clinical symptoms and orthopaedic examination, which can also explain the failure to use NCS study in some papers to some extent. It would be unethical to omit clinical cases or delay therapeutic management in patients who have subjective symptoms but do not have a disrupted NCS. On the other hand, the lack of a certain diagnosis does not allow the use of therapy aimed at the cause but only at reducing the patient's symptoms.

Significant differences in the offered therapeutic programs are another major problem in assessing the effectiveness of physiotherapy approaches in CuTS based on the papers included in this review. In fact, it is difficult to find any similarities in the therapeutic programs used. In 64% of the papers, physiotherapy was based just on one form of therapy [13,20,22,23,29,30,33]. However, in each of them, this was a different type of therapy. The remaining 36% of papers [21,31,32,34] used a total of multiple therapeutic measures, not only targeting the elbow region but also the cervical spine and thorax [31,32]. Neurodynamic techniques were used in 36% of the papers [13,21,32,34] but with different methodologies and often as a component of other treatments. In 18% of the papers, neurodynamic techniques were used as a self-therapy program, which may make it even more difficult to control the correctness of their performance and regular use.

A major weakness of all qualified papers is their low methodological quality, which was confirmed by the RoB results. Regardless of study type (case series, case reports, or RCTs), low RoB was not reported in any of the papers included. Therefore, this review indicated a complete lack of high-quality studies evaluating the effectiveness of physiotherapy in the conservative treatment of CuTS. Taking into account the prevalence of CuTS and the strong evidence confirming the effectiveness of physiotherapy in other peripheral neuropathies [15–19], it is difficult to indicate the reason for such low interest in CuTS conservative treatment.

4.1. Limitations

This systematic review has some potential limitations. The number of papers included in the review was small, and only three RCTs were identified. The sample size was small, with only 186 subjects. Some of the papers lacked clinical information about the patients' condition and severity of CuTS, which may have also affected the obtained results. The lack of an NCS study conducted not only to make an accurate diagnosis but also to assess the effects achieved after the therapeutic cycle is another limitation of many of the included papers and, thus, of the review itself. Only papers published in English were included in this review, which may have resulted in the omission of some studies evaluating the effectiveness of physiotherapy in the conservative treatment of CuTS. Further, the papers included in the review were characterised by different therapeutic programs, which made it difficult to assess the therapeutic effects.

4.2. Implications for Future Research

The results of this review allow for several recommendations for future research. First of all, there is a need for more well-designed RCT studies with two or more representative groups of subjects. Due to the prevalence of CuTS, case series and case reports have no substantive justification. It is also important to perform the diagnosis of CuTS based on NCS and ultrasound imaging, while clinical symptoms and other tests should be considered as supplementary information about the study population. The diagnosis of CuTS should be supplemented with the determination of the CuTS stage, which is also important in the assessment of the effectiveness of the offered therapy. Since most of the papers included in the review had a beneficial therapeutic effect, randomised controlled trials should be conducted based on similar therapeutic programs such as manual therapy including neurodynamic techniques, ultrasound therapy, low-level laser therapy, percutaneous electrical stimulation, or dry needling. Future studies should be multi-central and (if possible) blinded or even double-blinded.

5. Conclusions

Although physiotherapy could have the potential to demonstrate a positive effect in the treatment of CuTS, most published studies to date are of questionable methodological quality. Thus, at this stage of knowledge, there is no possibility to recommend the best method, duration, and interval of physiotherapy in the clinical practice of people with CuTS. More high-quality studies are required.

Supplementary Materials: The following supporting information can be downloaded at: https://www.mdpi.com/article/10.3390/jcm11144247/s1, Supplementary Material S1: Search terms and number of items identified in the PubMed database.

Author Contributions: Conceptualisation, T.W.; methodology, T.W., P.L. and M.D.; software, P.L. and A.G.; formal analysis, T.W. and P.L.; investigation, P.L., T.W., C.F.-d.-l.P., M.D. and T.B.; resources, M.D. and T.B.; data curation, M.D. and T.B.; writing—original draft preparation, T.W.; writing—review and editing, P.L., C.F.-d.-l.P., T.B., M.D. and A.G.; visualisation, M.D.; supervision, T.W.; project administration, T.W.; funding acquisition, P.L. and A.G. All authors have read and agreed to the published version of the manuscript.

Funding: This research received no external funding.

Institutional Review Board Statement: Not applicable.

Informed Consent Statement: Not applicable.

Data Availability Statement: Data are available upon request.

Conflicts of Interest: The authors declare no conflict of interest.

References

1. Elhassan, B.; Steinmann, S.P. Entrapment neuropathy of the ulnar nerve. *J. Am. Acad. Orthop. Surg.* **2007**, *15*, 672–681. [CrossRef] [PubMed]
2. Robertson, C.; Saratsiotis, J. A review of compression ulnar neuropathy at the elbow. *J. Manip. Physiol. Ther.* **2005**, *28*, 345. [CrossRef] [PubMed]
3. Mondelli, M.; Giannini, F.; Ballerini, M.; Ginanneschi, F.; Martorelli, M. Incidence of ulnar neuropathy at the elbow in the province of Siena (Italy). *J. Neurol. Sci.* **2005**, *234*, 5–10. [CrossRef] [PubMed]
4. An, T.W.; Evanoff, B.A.; Boyer, M.I.; Osei, D.A. The Prevalence of Cubital Tunnel Syndrome: A Cross-Sectional Study in a U.S. Metropolitan Cohort. *J. Bone Jt. Surg.* **2017**, *99*, 408–416. [CrossRef]
5. Kooner, S.; Cinats, D.; Kwong, C.; Matthewson, G.; Dhaliwal, G. Conservative treatment of cubital tunnel syndrome: A systematic review. *Orthop. Rev.* **2019**, *11*, 7955. [CrossRef]
6. McGowan, J. The results of transposition of the ulnar nerve for traumatic ulnar neuritis. *J. Bone Jt. Surg. Br.* **1950**, *32*, 293–301. [CrossRef]
7. Ochiai, N.; Honmo, J.; Tsunjino, A.; Nisiura, Y. Electrodiagnosis in entrapment neuropathy by the arcade of struthers. *Clin. Orthop. Relat. Res.* **2001**, *378*, 129–135. [CrossRef]
8. Sunderland, S. *Nerves and Nerve Injuries*; Churchill Livingstone: Edinburgh, UK; London, UK; New York, NY, USA, 1978.
9. Assmus, H.; Antoniadis, G.; Bischoff, C.; Hoffmann, R.; Martini, A.-K.; Preissler, K.; Scheglmann, K.; Schwerdtfeger, K.; Wessels, K.D.; Wustner-Hofmann, M. Cubital tunnel syndrome—a review and management guidelines. *Cent. Eur. Neurosurg.* **2011**, *72*, 90–98. [CrossRef]
10. Palmer, B.A.; Hughes, T.B. Cubital tunnel syndrome. *J. Hand Surg. Am.* **2010**, *35*, 153–163. [CrossRef]
11. Bartels, R.H.; Verbeek, A.L. Risk factors for ulnar nerve compression at the elbow: A case control study. *Acta Neurochir.* **2007**, *149*, 669–674. [CrossRef]
12. Cutts, S. Cubital tunnel syndrome. *Postgrad. Med. J.* **2007**, *83*, 28–31. [CrossRef] [PubMed]
13. Svernlov, B.; Larsson, M.; Rehn, K.; Adolfsson, L. Conservative treatment of the cubital tunnel syndrome. *J. Hand Surg.* **2009**, *34B*, 201–207. [CrossRef] [PubMed]
14. Lund, A.T.; Amadio, P.C. Treatment of cubital tunnel syndrome: Perspectives for the therapist. *J. Hand Ther.* **2006**, *19*, 170–178. [CrossRef] [PubMed]
15. Wolny, T.; Saulicz, E.; Linek, P.; Shacklock, M.; Myśliwiec, A. Efficacy of Manual Therapy Including Neurodynamic Techniques for the Treatment of Carpal Tunnel Syndrome: A Randomized Controlled Trial. *J. Manip. Physiol. Ther.* **2017**, *40*, 263–272. [CrossRef]
16. Wolny, T.; Linek, P. Neurodynamic Techniques Versus "Sham" Therapy in the Treatment of Carpal Tunnel Syndrome: A Randomized Placebo-Controlled Trial. *Arch. Phys. Med. Rehabil.* **2018**, *99*, 843–854. [CrossRef]
17. Wolny, T.; Linek, P. Is manual therapy based on neurodynamic techniques effective in the treatment of carpal tunnel syndrome? A randomized controlled trial. *Clin. Rehabil.* **2019**, *33*, 408–417. [CrossRef]
18. Wolny, T.; Linek, P. Long-term patient observation after conservative treatment of carpal tunnel syndrome: A summary of two randomised controlled trials. *PeerJ* **2019**, *7*, e8012. [CrossRef]
19. Fernández-de-las-Peñas, C.; Cleland, J.; Palacios-Ceña, M.; Fuensalida-Novo, S.; Alonso-Blanco, C.; Pareja, J.A.; Alburquerque-Sendín, F. Effectiveness of manual therapy versus surgery in pain processing due to carpal tunnel syndrome: A randomized clinical trial. *Eur. J. Pain* **2017**, *21*, 1266–1276. [CrossRef]
20. Kearns, G.L.; Wang, S. Medical diagnosis of cubital tunnel syndrome ameliorated with thrust manipulation of the elbow and carpals. *J. Man. Manip. Ther.* **2012**, *20*, 90–95. [CrossRef]
21. Oskay, D.; Meriç, A.; Nuray, K.; Firat, T.; Ayhan, C.; Leblebicioğlu, G. Neurodynamic mobilization in the conservative treatment of cubital tunnel syndrome: Long-term follow-up of 7 cases. *J. Manip. Physiol. Ther.* **2010**, *33*, 156–163. [CrossRef]
22. Shen, Y.P.; Wu, Y.Y.; Chu, H.Y.; Li, T.Y.; Chen, L.C.; Wu, Y.T. Extracorporeal shock wave therapy in cubital tunnel syndrome: A pilot study. *Neurol. Asia* **2018**, *23*, 233–238.

23. Anandkumar, S.; Manivasagam, M. Effect of dry needling on cubital tunnel syndrome: Three case reports. *Physiother. Theory Pract.* **2019**, *35*, 363–372. [CrossRef] [PubMed]
24. Moher, D.; Liberati, A.; Tetzlaff, J.; Altman, D.G.; Group, T.P. Preffered Reporting Items for Systematic Reviews and Mata-Analyses: The PRISMA Statement. *PLoS Med.* **2009**, *6*, e1000097. [CrossRef] [PubMed]
25. Centre for Reviews and Dissemination. *Systematic Reviews: CRD's Guidance for Undertaking Reviews in Health Care*; University of York: York, UK, 2008.
26. Risk of Bias Tools—Current Version of RoB 2. Available online: https://www.riskofbias.info/welcome/rob-2-0-tool (accessed on 8 April 2021).
27. Moola, S.; Munn, Z.; Tufanaru, C.; Aromataris, E.; Sears, K.; Sfetc, R.; Currie, M.; Lisy, K.; Qureshi, R.; Mattis, P.; et al. Chapter 7: Systematic reviews of etiology and risk. In *Joanna Briggs Institute Reviewer's Manual 2017*; Joanna Briggs Institute: Adelaide, Australia, 2017.
28. Sterne, J.A.C.; Hernán, M.A.; Reeves, B.C.; Savović, J.; Berkman, N.D.; Viswanathan, M.; Henry, D.; Altman, D.G.; Ansari, M.T.; Boutron, I.; et al. ROBINS-I: A tool for assessing risk of bias in non-randomized studies of interventions. *BMJ* **2016**, *355*, i4919. [CrossRef]
29. Badur, N.B.; Ozkan, F.U.; Aktas, I. Efficacy of shortwave diathermy in ulnar nerve entrapment at the elbow: A double-blind randomized controlled clinical trial. *Clin. Rehabil.* **2020**, *34*, 1048–1055. [CrossRef]
30. Ozkan, F.U.; Saygi, E.K.; Senol, S.; Kapci, S.; Aydeniz, B.; Aktas, I.; Gozke, E. New treatment alternatives in the ulnar neuropathy at the elbow: Ultrasound and low-level laser therapy. *Acta Neurol. Belg.* **2015**, *115*, 355–360. [CrossRef]
31. Illes, J.D.; Johnson, T.L., Jr. Chiropractic management of a patient with ulnar nerve compression symptoms: A case report. *J. Chirop. Med.* **2013**, *12*, 66–73. [CrossRef]
32. Coppieters, M.W.; Bartholomeeusen, K.E.; Stappaerts, K.H. Incorporating nerve-gliding techniques in the conservative treatment of cubital tunnel syndrome. *J. Manip. Physiol. Ther.* **2004**, *27*, 560–568. [CrossRef]
33. Kwak, S.; Daeun, J.; Choo, Y.J.; Chang, M.C. Management of neuropathic pain induced by cubital tunnel syndrome using pulsed radiofrequency: Two case report. *Medicine* **2019**, *98*, e15599. [CrossRef]
34. Fernández-de-Las-Peñas, C.; Arias-Buría, J.L.; El Bachiri, Y.R.; Plaza-Manzano, G.; Cleland, J.A. Ultrasound-guided percutaneous electrical stimulation for a patient with cubital tunnel syndrome: A case report with a one-year follow-up. *Physiother. Theory Pract.* **2020**, *6*, 1–6. [CrossRef]
35. Johnson, E.W. Diagnosis of carpal tunnel syndrome. The gold standard. *Am. J. Phys. Med. Rehabil.* **1993**, *72*, 1. [CrossRef] [PubMed]
36. David, C.; Preston, D.C.; Barbara, E.; Shapiro, B.E. *Electromyography and Neuromuscular Disorders. Clinical-Electrophysiologic Correlations*, 2nd ed.; Elsevier: Philadelphia, PA, USA, 1998.
37. Nee, R.J.; Jull, G.A.; Vicenzino, B.; Coppieters, M.W. The validity of upper-limb neurodynamic tests for detecting peripheral neuropathic pain. *J. Orthop. Sports Phys. Therapy* **2012**, *42*, 413–424. [CrossRef] [PubMed]
38. Novak, C.B.; Lee, G.W.; Mackinnon, S.E.; Lay, L. Provocative testing for cubital tunnel syndrome. *J. Hand Surg.* **1994**, *19*, 817–820. [CrossRef]
39. Gillard, J.; Perez-Cousin, M.; Hachulla, E.; Remy, J.; Hurtevent, J.F.; Vinckier, L. Diagnosis thoracic outlet syndrome: Contribution of provocative test, ultrasonography, electrophysiology, and helical computed tomography in 48 patient. *Jt. Bone Spine* **2001**, *68*, 416–424. [CrossRef]
40. Carlson, H.; Colbert, A.; Frydl, J.; Arnall, E.; Elliot, M.; Carlson, M. Current options for nonsurgical management of carpal tunnel syndrome. *Int. J. Clin. Rheumtol.* **2010**, *5*, 129–142. [CrossRef]
41. Chang, M.H.; Chiang, H.T.; Ger, L.P.; Yang, D.A.; Lo, Y.K. The cause of slowed forearm median conduction velocity in carpal tunnel syndrome. *Clin. Neurophysiol.* **2000**, *111*, 1039–1044. [CrossRef]

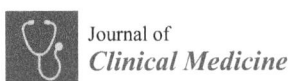

Study Protocol

Study Protocol for a Multicenter, Randomized Controlled Trial to Improve Upper Extremity Hemiparesis in Chronic Stroke Patients by One-to-One Training (NEURO®) with Repetitive Transcranial Magnetic Stimulation

Daigo Sakamoto [1,2], Toyohiro Hamaguchi [2,*], Kai Murata [1], Atsushi Ishikawa [1], Yasuhide Nakayama [3] and Masahiro Abo [3,*]

[1] Department of Rehabilitation Medicine, The Jikei University School of Medicine Hospital, Tokyo 105-8471, Japan
[2] Department of Rehabilitation, Graduate School of Health Science, Saitama Prefectural University, Saitama 343-8540, Japan
[3] Department of Rehabilitation Medicine, The Jikei University School of Medicine, Tokyo 105-8461, Japan
* Correspondence: hamaguchi-toyohiro@spu.ac.jp (T.H.); abo@jikei.ac.jp (M.A.); Tel.: +81-48-973-4125 (T.H.); +81-3-3433-1111 (M.A.)

Abstract: During recovery from upper limb motor paralysis after stroke, it is important to (1) set the exercise difficulty level according to the motor paralysis severity, (2) provide adequate exercises, and (3) motivate the patient to achieve the goal. However, these factors have not been well-formulated. This multicenter, randomized controlled trial study aims to examine the therapeutic effects of these three factors on patients undergoing a novel intervention using repetitive transcranial magnetic stimulation and intensive one-to-one training (NEURO®) and to formulate a corresponding research protocol. The control group will receive conventional NEURO® occupational therapy. In the intervention group, four practice plans will be selected according to the Fugl-Meyer assessment (FMA-UE) scores of the upper extremity. The goal is to predict the post-treatment outcomes based on the pre-treatment FMA-UE scores. Based on the degree of difficulty and amount of practice required, we can formulate a practice plan to promote upper limb motor recovery. This occupational therapy plan will be less influenced by the therapist's skill, facilitating effective rehabilitation. The study findings may be utilized to promote upper limb motor paralysis recovery and provide a basis for proposing activities of daily living adapted to upper limb function.

Keywords: occupational therapy; upper limb function; study protocol; stroke

1. Introduction

Approximately 80% of stroke patients develop motor paralysis [1]. Motor paralysis of the upper extremity limits patients' activities of daily living (ADL) and reduces their quality of life [2,3]. To improve the motor function of the upper extremity in stroke patients, it is necessary to induce neuroplasticity in the patient's brain through continuous rehabilitation [4–6]. Novel intervention using repetitive transcranial magnetic stimulation (rTMS) and intensive one-to-one training (NEURO®) is one such approach.

The role of rTMS in NEURO® is to pre-condition for rehabilitation by regulating movement-related neural activation. The effects of rTMS depend on the location, frequency, and intensity of the stimulation [7,8]. For example, in transcranial magnetic stimulation in NEURO®, the primary motor cortex of the patient's intact cerebral hemisphere is irradiated at 2400 pulses per day [6]. The stimulation intensity is defined as 90% of the resting motor threshold, with the first dorsal interosseous muscle of the non-paralyzed side as the target muscle. rTMS attenuates abnormal muscle tone by decreasing the excitability of cortical and spinal anterior horn cells and modulating interhemispheric inhibition [9–11]. For stroke patients in the acute and convalescent (with stable symptoms 1 or 2 months after onset) phases, methods have been developed to increase neural excitability by applying high-frequency rTMS (>4 Hz) to the affected cerebral hemisphere [12–14]. Methods have also been developed to stimulate the bilateral cerebral hemispheres [15]. Rehabilitation in NEURO® is intended to promote use-dependent plasticity of the brain by repeated motor exercises under the condition that the patient's interhemispheric inhibition is regulated by rTMS. Occupational therapists instruct the patients on NEURO® regarding the (1) functional motor exercises in the proximal and distal parts of the upper limb, (2) movement exercises including reaching and manipulating objects, (3) ADL exercises using the paralyzed side, and (4) ADL instruction and self-exercises to encourage the usage of the paralyzed side in daily life [4–6].

The goal of patients treated with NEURO® is to reacquire ADL using the paralyzed side. In occupational therapy, compensatory movements using the non-paralyzed side, assistive devices, and assistive technology may be applied to supplement the patient's motor function to reacquire the target activities [16–18]. However, in some cases, improving the motor function of the affected side may increase the possibility of patients acquiring the desired ADL. A hemiplegic patient needs at least 20 h of practice during a two-week hospitalization to recover upper limb motor function [19]. The number of stimulated upper limb movements is estimated to be 420 per session [19,20]. Rehabilitation is also more effective when patients are aware of their goals for the recovery of motor function and achievement of ADL [21,22]. Clinical occupational therapists presumably share the treatment goals with patients based on the physician's prediction of recovery after treatment and provide selected exercises in appropriate amounts according to the characteristics of individual patients' motor paralysis. The motor function of patients undergoing NEURO® can be predicted using the Fugl-Meyer assessment of the upper extremity (FMA-UE) score [23]. NEURO® reportedly improves upper limb motor function in patients regardless of the stroke type [24]. The content of rehabilitation provided by the therapist presumably affects the patient's recovery; however, this has not been verified.

Occupational therapists intervene with the aim of helping patients acquire their target movements. They induce neuroplasticity by rTMS after considering the severity of motor paralysis. In previous studies on NEURO®, occupational therapy exercises were determined by the physician and therapist-in-charge with the consent of the patient, and 40 to 60 min of treatment were provided twice a day [4–6]. However, when compared with the well-established stimulation method of rTMS, the difficulty level, amount of practice, and goal settings in NEURO® are not yet formalized and are dependent on the discretion of the physicians and therapists. Motor paralysis and related disability in daily life are highly individualized; while it is difficult for patients to have an idea of the training and recovery needed, this is not a problem for therapists with sufficient clinical experience. The issues faced include: (1) unclear criteria for selecting upper limb motor exercises based on the severity of motor paralysis, (2) unavailability of guidelines for the number of upper limb exercises to be performed by patients, and (3) unclear goal-sharing between patients and therapists regarding the recovery of upper limb motor function and the use of upper limbs in ADL. Therefore, a formalized occupational therapy in NEURO® will uniformize the treatment method and stabilize the functional recovery of patients.

This study aims to evaluate the therapeutic effect of NEURO® on patients by providing a certain amount of selected functional exercises based on the severity of the patients' motor paralysis. We also define a research protocol in this study. It is hypothesized that the occupational therapy intervention used in this study will improve the patients' upper limb motor function compared to the conventional intervention method used for patients who receive NEURO®. We believe that if the treatment plan for NEURO® occupational therapy is established according to the characteristics of the patients' motor paralysis, the patients will be less influenced by the skills and years of experience of the assigned occupational therapist, and the effectiveness of rehabilitation will be more stable than that of conventional occupational therapy. This stability will contribute to the improvement of the patient's goal for ADL.

2. Materials and Methods

2.1. Aims

The purpose of this study is to evaluate the therapeutic effect of NEURO® on patients by providing a certain amount of selected functional exercises based on the severity of the patients' motor paralysis. We also aim to define a research protocol in this study.

2.2. Study Design

We will use a multicenter, randomized controlled trial design to conduct this study.

2.3. Participants and Settings

The study participants are patients with a history of stroke who are admitted to a NEURO®-certified facility and have undergone NEURO®. NEURO® is performed in 14 registered NEURO®-accredited facilities by trained staff who have passed the examination of the Department of Rehabilitation Medicine, The Jikei University School of Medicine [25]. The inclusion criteria for patients, based on the rTMS guidelines, are as follows: (1) hemiplegia after first stroke, (2) age $\geq$ 20 years, (3) 6 months after stroke onset, and (4) no bilateral cerebrovascular disease [26]. Exclusion criteria are as follows: (1) patients with a diagnosis of dementia based on a Mini Mental State Examination score below the cutoff point, (2) patients with physical or psychiatric diseases requiring medical management, (3) patients with seizures within 1 year, (4) patients with intracranial clips or cardiac pacemakers, (5) patients with a history of subarachnoid hemorrhage, and (6) patients with fever ($\geq$37 °C), upper respiratory tract inflammation, malaise, and taste or olfactory symptoms when seen by a rehabilitation physician affiliated with a NEURO® -accredited facility prior to admission.

2.4. Participant Characteristics

Participant characteristics such as age, sex, height, weight, body mass index (BMI), and dominant hand will be investigated. Medical information regarding the type of disease (cerebral infarction, cerebral hemorrhage, etc.), paralyzed side, post-onset period, and the years of clinical practice of the treating therapists will be investigated (Table 1).

Table 1. Demographic data of patients.

		Intervention Group	Control Group	Total
Number of patients		N = XX	N = XX	N = XX
Age		XX	XX	XX
Sex		Female = XX	Female = XX	Female = XX
		Male = XX	Male = XX	Male = XX
Height		XX	XX	XX
Weight		XX	XX	XX
BMI		XX	XX	XX
Affected side		Left = XX,	Left = XX,	Left = XX,
		Right = XX	Right = XX	Right = XX
Dominant hand		Left = XX,	Left = XX,	Left = XX,
		Right = XX	Right = XX	Right = XX
Diagnosis	CI	N = XX	N = XX	N = XX
	ICH	N = XX	N = XX	N = XX
Time from onset		XX	XX	XX
FMA-UE severity				
No (<23)		N = XX	N = XX	N = XX
Poor ($\leq$23–$\leq$31)		N = XX	N = XX	N = XX
Limited ($\leq$32–$\leq$47)		N = XX	N = XX	N = XX
Notable ($\leq$48–$\leq$52)		N = XX	N = XX	N = XX
Full ($\leq$53–$\leq$66)		N = XX	N = XX	N = XX

BMI, body mass index; CI, cerebral infarction; ICH, intracranial hemorrhage; FMA-UE, Fugl-Meyer assessment of the upper extremity.

2.5. Sample Size

The sample size was estimated via a priori analysis using G*Power. We selected goodness-of-fit (F test) and analysis of covariance (ANCOVA) (for fixed effects, main effects, and interactions) for finding the sample fitness and size. The other data were set as $\alpha = 0.05$, $1 - \beta$ (power) = 0.8, numerator df = 1, number of groups = 4, and number of covariates = 4. Based on this calculation, the minimum sample size was estimated to be 128 (64 in each group). Since the subjects were hemiplegic patients, the minimum sample size was defined as 128 subjects (64 subjects in each group).

2.6. Randomization

A random number table, created using Microsoft Excel (Microsoft, Redmond, WA, USA), will be used for the allocation of patients into the intervention and control groups. The random number table is created at each hospital and maintained by the allocation manager at each hospital.

2.7. Sequence Generation

Simple randomization will be used for allocation. Once patients who meet the eligibility criteria are enrolled, they will be assigned using a random number table generated at each hospital.

2.8. Allocation Concealment Mechanism

Allocation will be performed by random assignment using a table of random numbers created at each hospital. The order of patient allocation will not be concealed from the person in charge of allocation. Patients will be assigned in the order in which they are registered according to the random number table (Figure 1).

	STUDY PERIOD			
	Enrollment	Allocation	Post-allocation	
TIMEPOINT	$-t_1$	0	t_1	t_2
ENROLLMENT:				
Eligibility screen	X			
Informed consent	X			
Allocation		X		
INTERVENTIONS:				
Control group			•────────•	
Intervention group			•────────•	
ASSESSMENTS:				
Participant characteristics		X		
FMA-UE, ARAT, JASMID			X	X

Figure 1. Schedule of enrollment, interventions, and assessments. FMA-UE, Fugl-Meyer assessment of the upper extremity; ARAT, Action Research Arm Test; JASMID, Jikei Assessment Scale for Motor Impairment in Daily Living. Investigators will obtain informed consent from patients who meet the eligibility criteria. Patient allocation will be performed by random assignment using a table of random numbers created at each hospital. Participant characteristics and medical information will be investigated. The control and intervention groups will receive treatment for two weeks. Patients will be evaluated on the day of admission and on the day of discharge.

2.9. Blinding

This study will be double-blind. (1) Patients who meet eligibility criteria and are enrolled will be blinded to the treatment received and to the group to which they are assigned. Physicians and occupational therapists will not be blinded to the group assignment. The evaluator is not blinded. (2) The data will be analyzed by an analyst using a dataset that has been processed in such a way that the group assignment is unknown. In order to confirm the success or failure of the patients' blinding, therapists will ask patients which treatment they thought they received after completing NEURO® treatment and then confirm whether it was the treatment actually performed.

2.10. Interventions

2.10.1. rTMS

All patients undergoing NEURO® will be hospitalized for 2 weeks. The rTMS will be directed at the primary motor cortex of the patient's healthy cerebral hemisphere at 2400 pulses a day at a low frequency of 1 Hz, as in the conventional NEURO® protocol (Table 2). The rehabilitation physicians affiliated with NEURO®-accredited facilities who are in charge of the patient will administer rTMS. The stimulation intensity is set at 90% of the resting motor threshold for the first dorsal interosseous muscle of the non-paralyzed side. This is the lowest intensity that activates motor-evoked potentials in a muscle. A figure-8 coil with a 70 mm diameter and a Mag Pro R 30 stimulator (Mag Venture Company, Farum, Denmark) are used for stimulus irradiation. The duration of treatment with NEURO® and the method of rTMS irradiation are not changed between the control and intervention groups.

Table 2. NEURO® study protocol and momentum settings.

First Week	Monday	Tuesday	Wednesday	Thursday	Friday	Saturday	Sunday
Event	Admission						
rTMS (pulse)	2400	2400	2400	2400	2400	2400	-
One-to-one training (time)	-	500	500	500	500	500	-
Second week	Monday	Tuesday	Wednesday	Thursday	Friday	Saturday	Sunday
Event						Discharge	
rTMS (pulse)	2400	2400	2400	2400	2400	2400	
One-to-one training (time)	500	500	500	500	500	-	

rTMS, repetitive transcranial magnetic stimulation. The protocol for admission on Monday is shown. In the columns of one-to-one training, the momentum of joint exercises for the functional exercises set up in this study is shown. Patients will perform the functional exercises of one-to-one training for a total of 1000 times. Patients are exposed to a total of 28,800 rTMS stimuli and 2400 pulses per day, except on Sundays. Patients will be evaluated on the day of admission and on the day of discharge.

2.10.2. Rehabilitation

Rehabilitation, as in the previous NEURO® protocols, will consist of up to six 20 min intervention sessions per day for all patients, except on Sundays and the days of admission and discharge. Rehabilitation in NEURO® is delivered according to prescribed methods by therapists who practice NEURO® at certified medical institutions. Occupational therapy will be provided for a minimum of three sessions per day. The assignment of occupational therapy and physical therapy sessions will be determined by the attending physician with the patient's consent, considering the patient's needs, goals, and physical function. Moreover, all patients will be required to perform 60 min of independent training twice a day [4–6]. The method of assigning occupational and physical therapy sessions will be kept consistent between the control and intervention groups. In this study, the goals of occupational therapy and the content of the exercises provided in the intervention group will be defined.

2.11. Intervention for the Control Group

The control group will receive occupational therapy as per conventional NEURO® [4–6]. Functional exercises, such as proximal and distal upper extremity joint movements, muscle mobilization, movement exercises including reaching and manipulation of objects, and daily living exercises to promote the patient's goals and use in daily life will be performed. The patient will be encouraged to use the paralyzed side of the body for self-training and to manage daily life situations.

2.12. Treatment for the Intervention Group

In the intervention group, (1) the difficulty level of practice will be set according to the severity of motor paralysis, (2) the amount of practice necessary for the recovery of motor paralysis will be set, and (3) the treatment goals of the patient and therapist will be set with regard to the functional practice performed in occupational therapy. Movement practice including reaching and manipulation of objects and daily living practice to promote the patient's goals and use in daily life will be performed using the same intervention methods as in conventional occupational therapy [4–6].

The exercise difficulty level will be selected from four plans, according to the scores of shoulder flexion to 90° during elbow extension in Part A and finger extension in Part C of FMA-UE (Figure 2). In studies investigating the hierarchy of difficulty levels of FMA-UE, the synergic movement difficulty level was lower than the difficulty level in shoulder flexion to 90° during elbow extension [27–29]. The ability or inability to perform shoulder flexion to 90° during elbow extension is considered a criterion to determine whether a patient is able to perform movements other than the synergic movement (Figure 3). Shoulder flexion to 90° during elbow extension and finger extension reportedly play a role in the functional prognosis of motor paralysis [30–32]. In the case of ADL, reaching movements to the target body part or object are planned, followed by skillful finger movements. Therefore, the patient's ability to perform shoulder flexion to 90° during elbow extension is considered an indicator of whether the practice of the proximal or distal part of the upper limb should be prioritized. Each plan is assigned a menu of exercises with reference to studies that have examined the hierarchy of difficulty levels in the sub-items of FMA-UE [27–29]. Each plan includes five exercises for one-to-one practice with the occupational therapist and self-training for the patient (Table 3). We will introduce one of the five functional exercises after a discussion between the patient and therapist and after obtaining the patient's agreement on the exercises that are highly relevant to their daily activities and those that are requested by the patient. Different training menus may be set for one-to-one training and self-training. However, they cannot be changed during the hospitalization period or mid-session. The exercises can be divided into the following three types, depending on the amount of assistance required and load of the exercise: (1) exercises to move the paralyzed limb with resistance (active resistive exercises), (2) exercises to move the paralyzed limb without resistance or assistance (active free exercises), and (3) exercises to move the paralyzed limb with manual guidance from the therapist or with assistance from the patient's non-paralyzed limb (active assistive exercises). The exercises are categorized based on whether the joints are moved by the therapist or external forces (passive exercise) [33,34]. In the present study, exercises including voluntary movements are assigned under four plans. Passive exercises, such as stretching to decrease muscle tension and joint exercises to increase range of motion are not included in these four plans. Passive exercises are to be performed by the therapist while conditioning the patient's body prior to the functional exercises or when relaxing between treatments, as appropriate.

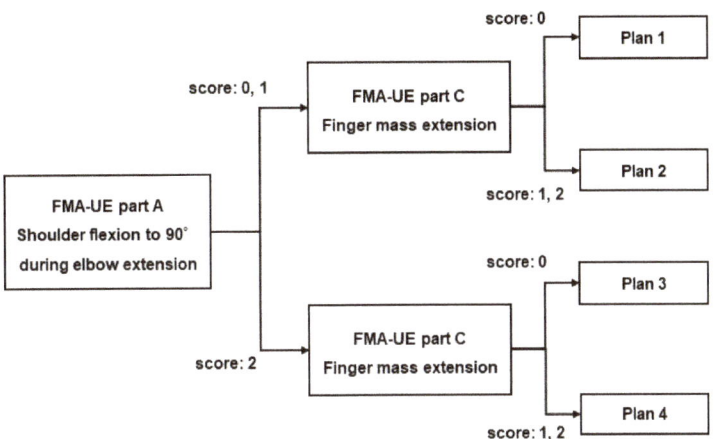

Figure 2. Chart of procedures for determining a functional practice plan. FMA-UE, Fugl-Meyer assessment of the upper extremity. The FMA-UE Part A (shoulder flexion to 90° during elbow extension) and Part C (finger mass extension) scores, evaluated on the day of admission, are used to determine the plan of functional exercises. The functional exercise plans are classified from 1 to 4 according to the scores from the two tests.

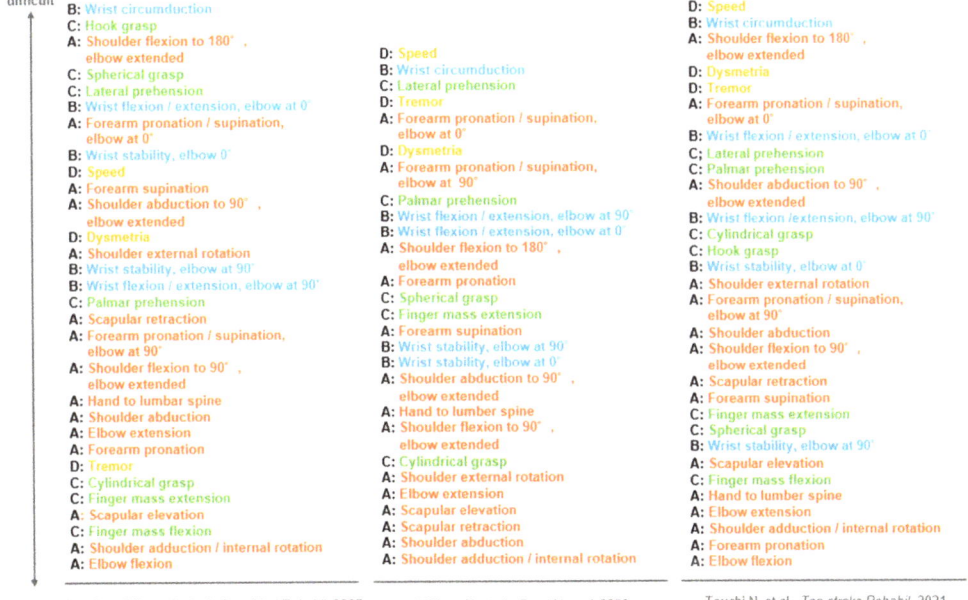

Figure 3. Item difficulty of Fugl-Meyer assessment for upper extremity. The results of three studies examining the difficulty of FMA-UE sub-items are presented. The sub-items with higher difficulty are located toward the top. A, B, C, and D next to the lower-level items indicate the corresponding subsection. As for the participants' characteristics, Woodbury ML et al. reported that the participants were mainly patients with acute mild hemiplegia. Hijikata et al. reported that the participants were mainly patients with moderate-to-severe chronic-stage hemiplegia. Tauchi et al. reported that the participants were mainly patients with mild-to-moderate subacute-stage hemiplegia. This figure has been partly modified from the articles published by Woodbury, M.L., et al., 2007 [27], Hijikata, et al., 2020 [28], and Tauchi, et al., 2021 [29].

Table 3. Training menu for each plan.

	One-to-One Training	Self-Training
Plan 1	Scapular retraction/protraction Shoulder flexion to 0–180°, elbow extended Shoulder flexion to 0–90°, elbow extended Elbow extension	Scapular retraction/protraction Shoulder flexion to 0–180°, elbow extended Shoulder flexion to 0–90°, elbow extended Elbow extension
Plan 2	Shoulder flexion to 0–180°, elbow extended Shoulder flexion to 0–90°, elbow extended Elbow extension Finger extension, elbow extended	Scapular retraction/protraction Shoulder flexion to 0–180°, elbow extendedElbow extension Finger extension
Plan 3	Shoulder flexion to 90–180°, elbow extended Shoulder abduction to 0–180°, elbow extended Wrist flexion/extension, elbow extended Finger extension	Shoulder flexion to 90–180°, elbow extended Forearm supination/pronation Wrist flexion/extension Finger extension
Plan 4	Shoulder abduction to 0–180°, elbow extended Forearm supination/pronation, elbow extended Wrist flexion/extension, elbow extended Finger extension, elbow extended	Shoulder flexion to 90–180°, elbow extended Forearm supination/pronation Wrist flexion/extension Finger extension

Ten exercises are set for each of the four plans, five for one-to-one training and five for self-training. The five exercises in the blank columns are determined by the patient and the therapist based on the patient's consent, the discussion between the patient and the therapist regarding the exercises that are expected to be highly necessary for the patient to acquire the activities of daily living, and the exercises that meet the patient's needs. Different practice menus may be introduced for one-to-one training and self-training, but the determined practice plan and the practice menus introduced in the plan should not be changed during the hospitalization period or in the middle of the session. The posture and the amount of load during the exercises are determined according to Figures 4 and 5, respectively, and the occupational therapist may change them according to the patient's condition and the purpose of the exercises.

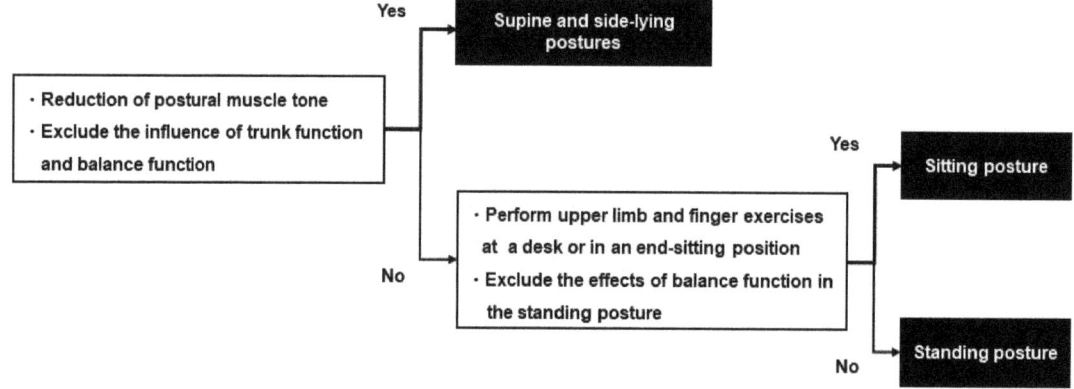

Figure 4. Chart practice posture determination methods. A method for determining the posture of functional exercises is presented. The supine and side-lying postures are chosen when the influence of postural muscle tone reduction, trunk function, and balance function are excluded. The sitting posture is selected when the patient wants to perform upper limb and finger exercises at a desk or in an end-sitting position or when the patient wants to exclude the effects of balance function in the standing posture. The standing posture is selected when the patient's goal is to perform ADL in the standing posture.

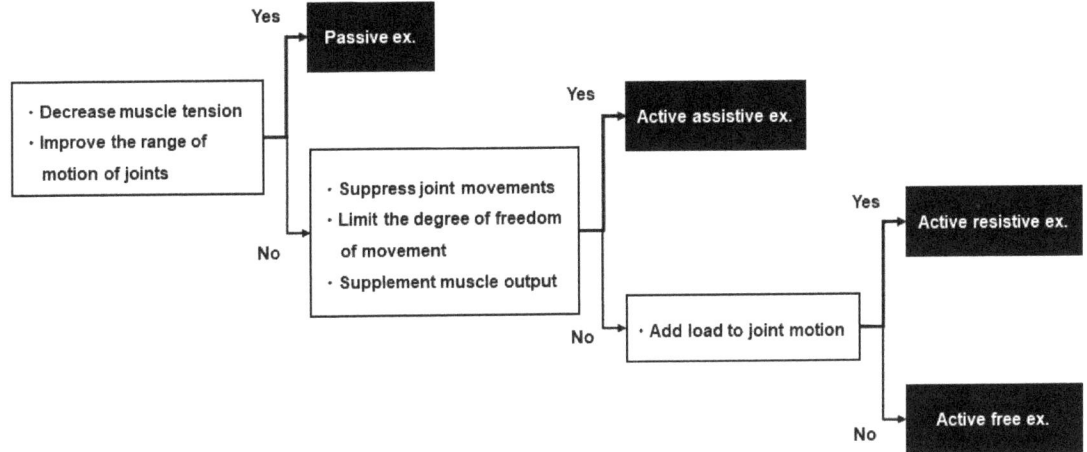

Figure 5. Chart of methods to determine the amount of practice assistance. A method for determining the amount of assistance for performing functional exercises is presented. Passive exercise is selected when the goal is to decrease muscle tension and improve the range of motion of joints. Active assistive exercise is selected when the patient wants to suppress joint movements, limit the degree of freedom of movement, and supplement muscle output. Active resistive exercise is selected to add load to joint motion. Active free exercise is selected to perform upper-extremity movements without adding load to the joint motion.

The patient's posture during practice and the load of the exercise are determined according to the patient's physical function, such as motor paralysis, muscle tone and balance, and the purpose of the exercise to be performed. The occupational therapist is not allowed to change the content of the set joint exercises but is allowed to change the posture and the amount of load during the exercises according to changes in the patient's muscle tone, muscle output, and motor paralysis. Figure 4 shows the method for determining the posture, and Figure 5 shows the method for determining the practice load.

The upper-extremity movements will be performed 100 times each per day for a total of 500 times, from a menu of five exercises. These exercises should be performed on a one-to-one basis between the occupational therapist and the patient. The number of upper-extremity movements in self-training will not be included in the number of five exercises. The patient is expected to perform a total of 500 joint exercises per day, including occupational therapy for functional exercises, except on Sundays, the day of admission, and the day of discharge. For example, when a patient is admitted on Monday and discharged on the following Saturday, they will perform a minimum of 5000 joint movements for functional exercises (Table 2).

We estimate that patients will perform more than 5000 upper-extremity movements during their hospitalization because, in addition to regular training, functional exercises, object handling practices, and ADL training will be scheduled. Peurala et al. reported that during a two-week period of hospitalization in which constraint-induced movement therapy was performed, a practice period of 20–56 h was effective in improving upper limb function [20]. Han et al. simulated the number of reaching movements to increase voluntary use of the paralyzed upper limb and reported that 420 movements per session were the threshold [19]. All patients undergoing NEURO® will receive two hours of therapist-led rehabilitation and two hours of patient-led training per day, except on the day of admission, the day of discharge, and Sundays, during a two-week inpatient treatment period.

The minimum number of functional exercises in the intervention group will be 500 per day. The protocol of the intervention group meets the requirements of the amount and duration of exercises reported in previous studies. This study is planned in 14 NEURO®-certified facilities in Japan: The Jikei University Hospital, The Jikei University Daisan Hospital, Tokyo General Hospital, Nishi-Hiroshima Rehabilitation Hospital, Kimura Hospital, Kyoto Ohara Memorial Hospital, Izumi Memorial Hospital, Hakodate Shintoshi Hospital, Aomori Shintoshi Hospital, Hattanmaru Rehabilitation Hospital, Atsuchi Rehabilitation Hospital, Ainomiyako Neurosurgery Hospital, Shinagawa Rehabilitation Hospital, and International University of Health and Welfare Ichikawa Hospital. A total of 15 professionals with at least five years of experience in NEURO® rehabilitation were selected as therapists. The level of difficulty of functional exercises in the occupational therapy intervention used in this study was discussed with them and decided upon via consensus. In the past, the treatment and evaluation of patients undergoing NEURO® have been performed by occupational therapists who have completed the prescribed training at NEURO®-accredited facilities. The treatment and evaluation procedures for the intervention group will be fully explained to the occupational therapists by at least one expert selected at each site who has discussed this study protocol with the occupational therapists. The expert at each site will supervise the occupational therapists to ensure that they fully understand and implement the study protocol for the intervention group.

The treatment goal is set according to the study by Hamaguchi et al. [23], and the predicted value of recovery of upper limb motor function by NEURO® is calculated using the FMA-UE score obtained on the first day of hospitalization [23]. The physician-in-charge will explain to the patients the predicted score at discharge, the target ADL, and the plan of functional exercises to be performed to achieve the goal. They also promote the patient's understanding of these plans. These procedures are performed by the physician and occupational therapist within two days of admission.

2.13. Outcome Evaluation

The outcomes will be evaluated primarily by FMA-UE. FMA-UE is a comprehensive battery of tests that examines motor function, balance, range of motion of the joints, and degree of joint pain in stroke patients [35]. The motor function items of the upper limb are scored on a 66-point scale using a 3-point ordinal scale. Joint and isolated movements are evaluated in accordance with the recovery stage of motor paralysis. The total score of FMA-UE is classified into no (<23), poor (≤ 23–≤ 31), limited (≤ 32–≤ 47), notable (≤ 48–≤ 52), and full (≤ 53–≤ 66) capacities using the severity reported by Hoonhorst et al. [36].

The secondary assessment is an Action Research Arm Test (ARAT). ARAT is an upper extremity functional assessment tool based on the upper extremity test [37,38]. It consists of four sub-items and includes tasks of grasping and carrying objects, manipulation, and reaching to one's own body. It is scored on a 57-point scale using a 4-point ordinal scale. As a second secondary evaluation, the Wolf Motor Function Test (WMFT) will be used. The WMFT consists of six tasks involving upper-extremity movements and nine tasks of object manipulation [39]. In the WMFT, the performance time of each task is measured, and the quality of movement is scored using a 6-level ordinal scale. In addition, the Jikei Assessment Scale for Motor Impairment in Daily Living (JASMID) will be used to examine the use of the affected upper limb in daily life [40]. JASMID is a patient-reported outcome that was developed based on Motor Activity Log and adapted to the Japanese lifestyle [41,42] and has been used in a previous NEURO® study [23]. JASMID consists of 20 questions related to upper limb movement and evaluates the frequency of use and quality of movement of the upper limb on the affected side on a 5-point ordinal scale. The FMA-UE and ARAT will be used to measure the therapeutic effects of mild motor paralysis, which may be underestimated due to the ceiling effect. For patients with mild symptoms, the WMFT and JASMID will be used to evaluate the treatment effect using the task performance time, frequency of use of the upper extremity on the affected side, and quality of movement [43,44]. Since sleep duration influences the promotion of neuroplasticity in the brain, we investigate patients' sleep duration and sleep quality using a questionnaire [45]. Patients are asked to respond to the sleep quality questions using a 3-point scale (1: did not sleep well, 2: unsure, 3: slept well).

2.14. Statistical Analysis

A multivariate ANCOVA will be conducted to test the hypothesis that the occupational therapy intervention in this study will improve motor function in chronic stroke patients undergoing NEURO® when compared with conventional occupational therapy interventions. The dependent variable will be the date or period of assessment, and the independent variables will be the change in scores of the primary assessment (FMA-UE) and the secondary assessments (ARAT and JASMID). The covariates are age, sex, BMI, and time since onset. JAMOVI version 2.2.1 (JAMOVI Project, Sydney, Australia) will be used for statistical analysis.

The primary analysis will be conducted when the intervention and control group samples reach a total of 64 cases each in all settings. The secondary analysis will be conducted when the number of patients in each group exceeds 60% of all participating centers (Figure 6).

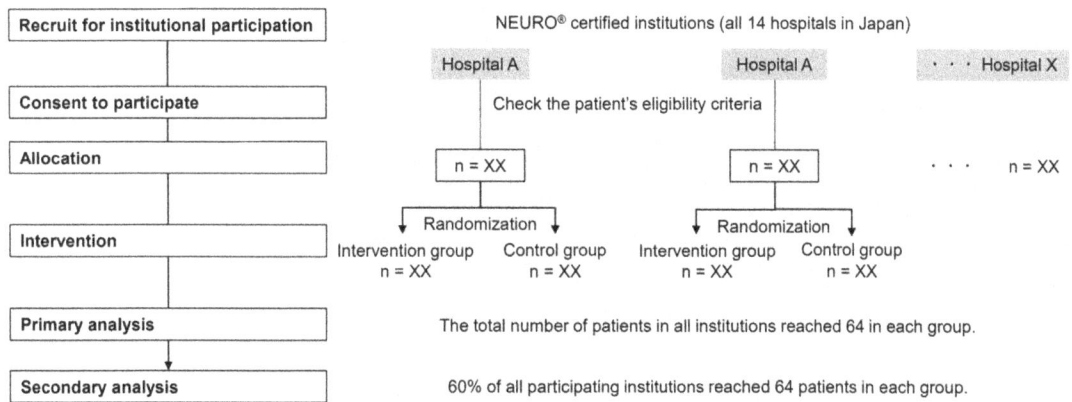

Figure 6. Research procedure. The study setting includes 14 NEURO®-accredited facilities in Japan that have agreed to participate in the study. Once patients who meet the study eligibility criteria are enrolled, they will be assigned to the intervention and control groups using a random number table generated for each facility.

2.15. Ethical Considerations and Declarations

All patients will provide written consent to participate in this study. This study was approved by the Jikei University School of Medicine Ethics Committee (approval number 32-33810423). The study has been registered in the Clinical Trials Registry of the University hospital Medical Information Network (UMIN) Center (UMIN Test ID: UMIN000047489).

Doctors and occupational therapists will wear masks, wash their hands and sterilize with alcohol when providing treatment.

2.16. Status and Timeline of the Study

This study was approved by the ethics committee and registered as a clinical trial. This study will begin in December 2022 and end in August 2024.

3. Discussion

We predict that the occupational therapy interventions in this study will improve patients' motor function compared to conventional occupational therapy interventions. The occupational therapy intervention in this study specifies (1) the level of practice difficulty, (2) the amount of practice, and (3) the method of goal setting. (1) The difficulty levels of the exercise menus in the four plans are set according to the item-specific difficulty levels of FMA-UE. Functional exercises are selected in accordance with the severity of the patient's motor paralysis [27–29]. (2) The amount of practice is specified with reference to studies that have verified the threshold of the number of joint movements required for the recovery of motor paralysis [19]. Patients will be provided with an adequate amount of practice according to the selected practice plan. (3) Goal setting is based on the FMA-UE scores at the initial evaluation to predict recovery; the treatment goals and the selected practice plan will be explained to the patients [23]. One of the five functional exercises will be introduced based on the patient's preference. The patient's understanding of the set goals and the performance of active practice are reportedly important for the recovery of motor paralysis [21,22]. Therefore, the occupational therapy intervention in this study can promote the use-dependent plasticity of patients' brains more effectively than conventional occupational therapy interventions and is expected to improve patients' motor functions.

If the occupational therapy intervention used in this study improves the patients' upper limb motor function when compared to that of the conventional occupational therapy intervention, the level of practice difficulty and the amount of practice used in this study can act as a guideline to formulate a new practice method to improve the upper limb function of patients. Occupational therapists can provide a sufficient amount of joint movement exercises according to the severity of the patient's upper limb motor paralysis to encourage use-dependent plasticity in the patient. Standardization of occupational therapy treatment content and equalization of treatment allow efficient and effective rehabilitation of patients. Improvement in motor function contributes to the improvement of the patient's ADL (Figure 7). The results obtained after the implementation of this protocol will assure that the ADL and certain results of occupational therapy can be attained by patients with upper motor paralysis, in any facility.

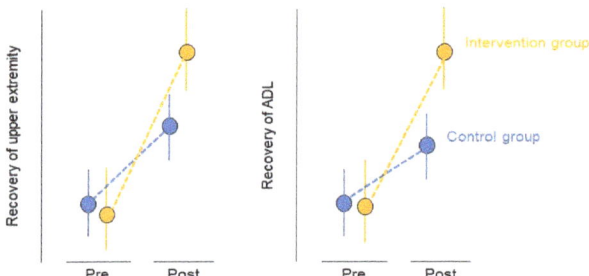

Figure 7. Expected results. ADL, activities of daily living. In the administered occupational therapy, the intervention group is defined by (1) setting the difficulty level of functional exercises, (2) providing an adequate amount of exercise, and (3) the method of goal setting. Therefore, the use-dependent plasticity can be promoted more effectively in the interventional group than in the conventional occupational therapy group, and the patients' motor functions are expected to improve. Improvement of motor function is expected to contribute to the improvement of patients' ADL.

This study has a few limitations. Since this study will be conducted at a facility in Japan, it is unclear whether similar results will be obtained in other countries. We speculate that there is a limitation to the generalization of this study's results. In countries other than Japan, the medical systems are different, and it is difficult to implement the same treatment methods since insurance for hospitalization of patients with chronic stroke and the roles of doctors and therapists vary. There are also cultural differences in the ADL required by patients. Multinational studies are needed to clarify this point. In addition, the patient's nutritional status may affect the recovery of motor paralysis. In this study, it will not be possible to obtain data on the nutritional status of patients prior to inpatient treatment.

Author Contributions: Conceptualization: D.S., T.H. and M.A.; methodology: D.S., T.H. and K.M.; software: T.H.; validation: A.I. and Y.N.; formal analysis: T.H.; investigation: D.S., K.M. and A.I.; resources: Y.N. and M.A.; data curation: K.M. and T.H.; writing—original draft preparation: D.S.; writing—review and editing: T.H. and M.A.; visualization: K.M.; supervision: Y.N. and M.A.; project administration: M.A. All authors have read and agreed to the published version of the manuscript.

Funding: This research received no external funding.

Institutional Review Board Statement: This study was approved by the Jikei University School of Medicine Ethics Committee (approval number 32-33810423).

Informed Consent Statement: All patients will provide written consent to participate in this study.

Acknowledgments: We would like to thank all occupational therapists from the Department of Rehabilitation at The Jikei University Hospital, The Jikei University Daisan Hospital, Hakodate Shintoshi Hospital, Aomori Shintoshi Hospital, Tokyo General Hospital, Izumi Memorial Hospital, Kyoto Ohara Memorial Hospital, Nishi-Hiroshima Rehabilitation Hospital, and Hattanmaru Rehabilitation Hospital for their cooperation and advice in this study.

Conflicts of Interest: The authors declare no conflict of interest.

References

1. Langhorne, P.; Bernhardt, J.; Kwakkel, G. Stroke rehabilitation. *Lancet* **2011**, *377*, 1693–1702. [CrossRef]
2. Palstam, A.; Sjödin, A.; Sunnerhagen, K.S. Participation and autonomy five years after stroke: A longitudinal observational study. *PLoS ONE* **2019**, *14*, e0219513. [CrossRef]
3. van Mierlo, M.L.; van Heugten, C.M.; Post, M.W.; Hajós, T.R.; Kappelle, L.J.; Visser-Meily, J.M. Quality of life during the first two years post stroke: The Restore4Stroke cohort study. *Cerebrovasc. Dis.* **2016**, *41*, 19–26. [CrossRef] [PubMed]
4. Kakuda, W.; Abo, M.; Kobayashi, K.; Momosaki, R.; Yokoi, A.; Fukuda, A.; Ishikawa, A.; Ito, H.; Tominaga, A. Low-frequency repetitive transcranial magnetic stimulation and intensive occupational therapy for poststroke patients with upper limb hemiparesis: Preliminary study of a 15-day protocol. *Int. J. Rehabil. Res.* **2010**, *33*, 339–345. [CrossRef] [PubMed]
5. Kakuda, W.; Abo, M.; Shimizu, M.; Sasanuma, J.; Okamoto, T.; Yokoi, A.; Taguchi, K.; Mitani, S.; Harashima, H.; Urushidani, N.; et al. A multi-center study on low-frequency rTMS combined with intensive occupational therapy for upper limb hemiparesis in post-stroke patients. *J. Neuroeng. Rehabil.* **2012**, *9*, 4. [CrossRef]
6. Abo, M.; Kakuda, W.; Momosaki, R.; Harashima, H.; Kojima, M.; Watanabe, S.; Sato, T.; Yokoi, A.; Umemori, T.; Sasanuma, J. Randomized, multicenter, comparative study of NEURO versus CIMT in poststroke patients with upper limb hemiparesis: The NEURO-VERIFY study. *Int. J. Stroke* **2014**, *9*, 607–612. [CrossRef] [PubMed]
7. Hoogendam, J.M.; Ramakers, G.M.; Di Lazzaro, V. Physiology of repetitive transcranial magnetic stimulation of the human brain. *Brain Stimul.* **2010**, *3*, 95–118. [CrossRef] [PubMed]
8. Goldsworthy, M.R.; Hordacre, B.; Rothwell, J.C.; Ridding, M.C. Effects of rTMS on the brain: Is there value in variability? *Cortex* **2021**, *139*, 43–59. [CrossRef]
9. Sasaki, N.; Abo, M.; Hara, T.; Yamada, N.; Niimi, M.; Kakuda, W. High-frequency rTMS on leg motor area in the early phase of stroke. *Acta Neurol. Belg.* **2017**, *117*, 189–194. [CrossRef]
10. Ueda, R.; Yamada, N.; Abo, M.; Ruwan, P.W.; Senoo, A. MRI evaluation of motor function recovery by rTMS and intensive occupational therapy and changes in the activity of motor cortex. *Int. J. Neurosci.* **2020**, *130*, 309–317. [CrossRef] [PubMed]
11. Wang, Q.; Zhang, D.; Zhao, Y.Y.; Hai, H.; Ma, Y.W. Effects of high-frequency repetitive transcranial magnetic stimulation over the contralesional motor cortex on motor recovery in severe hemiplegic stroke: A randomized clinical trial. *Brain Stimul.* **2020**, *13*, 979–986. [CrossRef] [PubMed]
12. Watanabe, K.; Kudo, Y.; Sugawara, E.; Nakamizo, T.; Amari, K.; Takahashi, K.; Tanaka, O.; Endo, M.; Hayakawa, Y.; Johkura, K. Comparative study of ipsilesional and contralesional repetitive transcranial magnetic stimulations for acute infarction. *J. Neurol. Sci.* **2018**, *384*, 10–14. [CrossRef]
13. Du, J.; Yang, F.; Hu, J.; Hu, J.; Xu, Q.; Cong, N.; Zhang, Q.; Liu, L.; Mantini, D.; Zhang, Z.; et al. Effects of high- and low-frequency repetitive transcranial magnetic stimulation on motor recovery in early stroke patients: Evidence from a randomized controlled trial with clinical, neurophysiological and functional imaging assessments. *NeuroImage Clin.* **2019**, *21*, 101620. [CrossRef] [PubMed]
14. Vabalaite, B.; Petruseviciene, L.; Savickas, R.; Kubilius, R.; Ignatavicius, P.; Lendraitiene, E. Effects of high-frequency (HF) repetitive transcranial magnetic stimulation (rTMS) on upper extremity motor function in stroke patients: A systematic review. *Medicina* **2021**, *57*, 1215. [CrossRef]
15. Sasaki, N.; Kakuda, W.; Abo, M. Bilateral high- and low-frequency rTMS in acute stroke patients with hemiparesis: A comparative study with unilateral high-frequency rTMS. *Brain Inj.* **2014**, *28*, 1682–1686. [CrossRef] [PubMed]
16. Legg, L.A.; Lewis, S.R.; Schofield-Robinson, O.J.; Drummond, A.; Langhorne, P. Occupational therapy for adults with problems in activities of daily living after stroke. *Cochrane Database Syst. Rev.* **2017**, *7*, CD003585. [CrossRef] [PubMed]
17. Nam, J.H.; Kim, H. How assistive devices affect activities of daily living and cognitive functions of people with brain injury: A meta-analysis. *Disabil. Rehabil. Assist. Technol.* **2018**, *13*, 305–311. [CrossRef] [PubMed]
18. Fudickar, S.; Kiselev, J.; Frenken, T.; Wegel, S.; Dimitrowska, S.; Steinhagen-Thiessen, E.; Hein, A. Validation of the ambient TUG chair with light barriers and force sensors in a clinical trial. *Assist. Technol.* **2020**, *32*, 1–8. [CrossRef]
19. Han, C.E.; Arbib, M.A.; Schweighofer, N. Stroke rehabilitation reaches a threshold. *PLoS Comput. Biol.* **2008**, *4*, e1000133. [CrossRef] [PubMed]

20. Peurala, S.H.; Kantanen, M.P.; Sjögren, T.; Paltamaa, J.; Karhula, M.; Heinonen, A. Effectiveness of constraint-induced movement therapy on activity and participation after stroke: A systematic review and meta-analysis of randomized controlled trials. *Clin. Rehabil.* **2012**, *26*, 209–223. [CrossRef]
21. Rice, D.B.; McIntyre, A.; Mirkowski, M.; Janzen, S.; Viana, R.; Britt, E.; Teasell, R. Patient-centered goal setting in a hospital-based outpatient stroke rehabilitation Center. *PM R.* **2017**, *9*, 856–865. [CrossRef] [PubMed]
22. Stewart, J.C.; Lewthwaite, R.; Rocktashel, J.; Winstein, C.J. Self-efficacy and reach performance in individuals with mild motor impairment due to stroke. *Neurorehabil. Neural Repair.* **2019**, *33*, 319–328. [CrossRef]
23. Hamaguchi, T.; Yamada, N.; Hada, T.; Abo, M. Prediction of motor recovery in the upper extremity for repetitive transcranial magnetic stimulation and occupational therapy goal setting in patients with chronic stroke: A retrospective analysis of prospectively collected data. *Front. Neurol.* **2020**, *11*, 581186. [CrossRef] [PubMed]
24. Tatsuno, H.; Hamaguchi, T.; Sasanuma, J.; Kakita, K.; Okamoto, T.; Shimizu, M.; Nakaya, N.; Abo, M. Does a combination treatment of repetitive transcranial magnetic stimulation and occupational therapy improve upper limb muscle paralysis equally in patients with chronic stroke caused by cerebral hemorrhage and infarction?: A retrospective cohort study. *Medicine* **2021**, *100*, e26339. [CrossRef] [PubMed]
25. Introducing NEURO®. Available online: https://www.j-sts.jp/about_neuro.html (accessed on 12 January 2022).
26. Rossi, S.; Hallett, M.; Rossini, P.M.; Pascual-Leone, A.; Safety of TMS Consensus Group. Safety, ethical considerations, and application guidelines for the use of transcranial magnetic stimulation in clinical practice and research. *Clin. Neurophysiol.* **2009**, *120*, 2008–2039. [CrossRef] [PubMed]
27. Woodbury, M.L.; Velozo, C.A.; Richards, L.G.; Duncan, P.W.; Studenski, S.; Lai, S.M. Dimensionality and construct validity of the Fugl-Meyer Assessment of the upper extremity. *Arch. Phys. Med. Rehabil.* **2007**, *88*, 715–723. [CrossRef] [PubMed]
28. Hijikata, N.; Kawakami, M.; Ishii, R.; Tsuzuki, K.; Nakamura, T.; Okuyama, K.; Liu, M. Item difficulty of Fugl-Meyer assessment for upper extremity in persons with chronic stroke with moderate-to-severe upper limb impairment. *Front. Neurol.* **2020**, *11*, 577855. [CrossRef] [PubMed]
29. Tauchi, Y.; Kyougoku, M.; Takahashi, K.; Okita, Y.; Takebayashi, T. Dimensionality and item-difficulty hierarchy of the Fugl-Meyer assessment of the upper extremity among Japanese patients who have experienced stroke. *Top. Stroke Rehabil.* **2021**, *29*, 579–587. [CrossRef] [PubMed]
30. Massie, C.L.; Fritz, S.; Malcolm, M.P. Elbow extension predicts motor impairment and performance after stroke. *Rehabil. Res. Pract.* **2011**, *2011*, 381978. [CrossRef] [PubMed]
31. McPherson, J.G.; Chen, A.; Ellis, M.D.; Yao, J.; Heckman, C.J.; Dewald, J.P.A. Progressive recruitment of contralesional corticoreticulospinal pathways drives motor impairment post stroke. *J. Physiol.* **2018**, *596*, 1211–1225. [CrossRef]
32. Lotze, M.; Ladda, A.M.; Stephan, K.M. Cerebral plasticity as the basis for upper limb recovery following brain damage. *Neurosci. Biobehav. Rev.* **2019**, *99*, 49–58. [CrossRef] [PubMed]
33. Brunnstrom, S. Motor testing procedures in hemiplegia: Based on sequential recovery stages. *Phys. Ther.* **1966**, *46*, 357–375. [CrossRef] [PubMed]
34. Doering, T.J.; Resch, K.L.; Steuernagel, B.; Brix, J.; Schneider, B.; Fischer, G.C. Passive and active exercises increase cerebral blood flow velocity in young, healthy individuals. *Am. J. Phys. Med. Rehabil.* **1998**, *77*, 490–493. [CrossRef] [PubMed]
35. Fugl-Meyer, A.R.; Jääskö, L.; Leyman, I.; Olsson, S.; Steglind, S. The post-stroke hemiplegic patient. 1. A method for evaluation of physical performance. *Scand. J. Rehabil. Med.* **1975**, *7*, 13–31. [PubMed]
36. Hoonhorst, M.H.; Nijland, R.H.; van den Berg, J.S.; Emmelot, C.H.; Kollen, B.J.; Kwakkel, G. How do Fugl-Meyer arm motor scores relate to dexterity according to the action research arm test at 6 months poststroke? *Arch. Phys. Med. Rehabil.* **2015**, *96*, 1845–1849. [CrossRef] [PubMed]
37. Carroll, D. A quantitative test of upper extremity function. *J. Chronic Dis.* **1965**, *18*, 479–491. [CrossRef]
38. Lyle, R.C. A performance test for assessment of upper limb function in physical rehabilitation treatment and research. *Int. J. Rehabil. Res.* **1981**, *4*, 483–492. [CrossRef] [PubMed]
39. Wolf, S.L.; Catlin, P.A.; Ellis, M.; Archer, A.L.; Morgan, B.; Piacentino, A. Assessing Wolf motor function test as outcome measure for research in patients after stroke. *Stroke* **2001**, *32*, 1635–1639. [CrossRef] [PubMed]
40. Ishikawa, A.; Kakuda, W.; Taguchi, K.; Uruma, G.; Abo, M. The reliability and validity of a new subjective assessment scale for poststroke upper limb hemiparesis, the Jikei assessment scale for motor impairment in daily living. *Tokyo Jikei Med. J.* **2010**, *125*, 159–167.
41. van der Lee, J.H.; Beckerman, H.; Knol, D.L.; de Vet, H.C.; Bouter, L.M. Clinimetric properties of the motor activity log for the assessment of arm use in hemiparetic patients. *Stroke* **2004**, *35*, 1410–1414. [CrossRef] [PubMed]
42. Uswatte, G.; Taub, E.; Morris, D.; Vignolo, M.; McCulloch, K. Reliability and validity of the upper-extremity Motor Activity Log-14 for measuring real-world arm use. *Stroke* **2005**, *36*, 2493–2496. [CrossRef] [PubMed]
43. Lin, J.H.; Hsu, M.J.; Sheu, C.F.; Wu, T.S.; Lin, R.T.; Chen, C.H.; Hsieh, C.L. Psychometric comparisons of 4 measures for assessing upper-extremity function in people with stroke. *Phys. Ther.* **2009**, *89*, 840–850. [CrossRef] [PubMed]
44. Gladstone, D.J.; Danells, C.J.; Black, S.E. The fugl-Meyer assessment of motor recovery after stroke: A critical review of its measurement properties. *Neurorehabil. Neural Repair* **2002**, *16*, 232–240. [CrossRef] [PubMed]
45. Pickersgill, J.W.; Turco, C.V.; Ramdeo, K.; Rehsi, R.S.; Foglia, S.D.; Nelson, A.J. The combined influences of exercise, diet and sleep on neuroplasticity. *Front. Psychol.* **2022**, *13*, 831819. [CrossRef] [PubMed]

MDPI
St. Alban-Anlage 66
4052 Basel
Switzerland
www.mdpi.com

Journal of Clinical Medicine Editorial Office
E-mail: jcm@mdpi.com
www.mdpi.com/journal/jcm

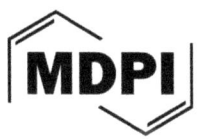

Disclaimer/Publisher's Note: The statements, opinions and data contained in all publications are solely those of the individual author(s) and contributor(s) and not of MDPI and/or the editor(s). MDPI and/or the editor(s) disclaim responsibility for any injury to people or property resulting from any ideas, methods, instructions or products referred to in the content.

www.ingramcontent.com/pod-product-compliance
Lightning Source LLC
LaVergne TN
LVHW070620100526
838202LV00012B/693